The Contact Lens Manual
A practical fitting guide

2nd edition

Andrew Gasson FCOptom, DCLP, FAAO
Contact Lens Practitioner, London, UK

and

Judith Morris MSc, FCOptom, FAAO, FIACLE
Director, Institute of Optometry, London, UK

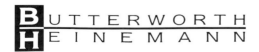

OXFORD   BOSTON   JOHANNESBURG   MELBOURNE   NEW DELHI   SINGAPORE

Butterworth-Heinemann
Linacre House, Jordan Hill, Oxford OX2 8DP
225 Wildwood Avenue, Woburn, MA 01801-2041
A division of Reed Educational and Professional Publishing Ltd

 A member of the Reed Elsevier plc group

First published 1992
Reprinted 1992, 1993, 1994
Second edition 1998

British Library Cataloguing in Publication Data
A catalogue record for this book is available from the British Library

Library of Congress Cataloguing in Publication Data
A catalogue record for this book is available from the Library of Congress

ISBN 0 7506 3187 2

Composition by Scribe Design, Gillingham, Kent, UK
Printed and bound in Great Britain by
Biddles Ltd, Guildford and King's Lynn

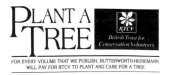

Contents

Foreword

The practice of contact lenses is without doubt one of the most rapidly changing fields of primary eye care. Recent developments in polymeric material formulation and moulding technology have heralded the introduction of contact lens types and modalities that would have been thought of as virtually impossible a decade ago.

Numerous advances in the contact lens field have taken place since the first edition of this book was published in 1992. These include the production of daily disposable contact lenses, the development of novel biocompatible lens materials, the use of grading scales to assist in recording the severity of ocular complications of lens wear, the application of modern accelerated orthokeratology (albeit controversial), the introduction of slit lamp-interfaced computer-assisted digital image capture and the demise of the re-usable glass lens vial in favour of the disposable blister pack, to name a few.

In view of these changes, the authors and their publishers – Butterworth-Heinemann – are to be congratulated for undertaking a thorough and timely update of *The Contact Lens Manual*. The subject material has been expanded, and in some cases contracted, to reflect a truly modern approach to contact lens practice, while at the same time preserving the essential character of this work as a 'manual' in the true sense.

My dictionary defines 'manual' as 'a book of instructions or information' ... and that is exactly what this text is all about. It is a ready reference of practical, useful information of immediate clinical relevance. Notwithstanding this fundamental approach, the book does offer a comprehensive coverage of all aspects of contact lens practice, including specialist topics such as bifocal lenses, lenses for presbyopia, and therapeutic and post-refractive surgery fitting. Unlike other contact lens textbooks, practitioners will not find it necessary to have to plough through pages of heavy theory to find the clinical information they need. Not that there is anything wrong with heavy theory – it is just that this book gets straight to the heart of the matter. Key references are given for those who require additional information about specific topics.

Judith Morris and Andrew Gasson are two of the most outstanding contact lens practitioners in the UK. Their approach and thinking derives from their extensive personal clinical experience, and their continual attendance at, and contributions to, major national and international contact lens conferences and continuing education events. It is difficult to imagine who would be better placed to write such an authoritative chair-side manual of contact lens practice. The authors have been ably assisted by Tony Hough, an accomplished lens designer, industrial consultant and electronic publishing expert, who has produced the enclosed CD-ROM which contains useful lens fitting and design programs.

All in all, *The Contact Lens Manual* is the perfect chair-side reference to accompany contact lens practitioners as we launch into the 21st century.

Nathan Efron, PhD, DSc
Professor of Clinical Optometry
UMIST, Manchester, UK

Preface to the second edition

Since the publication of *The Contact Lens Manual* in 1992, the authors have been encouraged at its generous reception by both student and experienced practitioners alike. The field of contact lenses continues to develop at a rapid rate and this second edition is intended to bring *The Manual* up to date with new clinical and fitting procedures whilst maintaining the essentially practical approach of the original format.

There are new chapters on Record Keeping and Ortho-keratology whilst several sections such as those on disposable lenses, materials classification, tears assessment and instrumentation have been enlarged. A Glossary of contact lens related terms is included for the first time. Recently introduced lens forms and care products have been included whilst obsolete products have been eliminated. Emphasis on the now rarely fitted PMMA has been reduced and the authors continue to take a very cautious approach to the subject of extended wear. Aftercare – always inextricably linked to fitting – will in the future assume an even more important role in contact lens practice. The relevant sections have therefore been enlarged with new diagrams and include details on severe ocular infections as well as indicating the sort of written advice which should be provided to all contact lens wearers.

Terminology in *The Manual* continues to be based on British and International Standards with descriptive terms such as Hard Gas-Permeable (HGP) and Contact Lens Induced Papillary Conjunctivitis (CLIPC) brought in line with current usage.

The main wholly new feature of this edition is the inclusion of a CD-ROM. This gives the opportunity to explore the effect of changing lens parameters on simulated fluorescein patterns for several designs of lens. It also includes a toric lens calculator and several colour photographs to illustrate commonly encountered aftercare problems. The production of the CD-ROM is entirely due to the arcane computing skills and boundless enthusiasm of Tony Hough without whom it would not have been possible. Acknowledgement is also due Keith Edwards for undertaking the slide scanning, to Ken Pullum for updating the chapter on Scleral Lenses, as well as to all of the contact lens companies that provided up to date information on their lenses and products. With special thanks to No. 7 for their sponsorship of the CD-ROM and to Howard Gee for all his advice on contact lens materials.

Preface to the first edition

The Manual is designed as an essentially practical guide to all aspects of contact lens fitting. It follows the authors' own approach to patient management, initial assessment and lens selection as well as giving detailed fitting procedures for both basic and complex lenses. Significant space is allocated to after-care as this is considered an inextricably linked continuation of fitting, whereas theoretical aspects have been kept deliberately concise, supplemented by detailed references and suggestions for further reading.

The introductory chapters and basic fitting are directed mainly at the student or practitioner without recent experience. *The Manual*, however, also covers advanced fitting techniques for the more experienced and the specialist sections on therapeutic lenses and the management of children requiring contact lenses should be of interest both to hospital fitters and to those who encounter the occasional medical case.

Terminology is based on the relatively new British and International Standards. The most common lens types are referred to as either 'hard' or 'soft'. The term 'hard' has been used throughout to indicate specifically modern materials which have been described elsewhere as 'gas-permeable'. PMMA is now considered a little-fitted sub-group.

Inevitably, it is impossible to include details of every lens or solution currently available and the authors have been forced to select representative examples. Mention of a particular product is not intended as an endorsement and any omission, however obvious, should not be construed as an implied criticism.

Finally, the authors would like to acknowledge all of the contact lens companies which have kindly made available detailed information concerning their products; the ACLM for the use of their materials classification system; Allergan-Hydron, Bausch and Lomb and Igel International for their permission to reproduce tables and illustrations; Tony Hough of Microturn for his assistance in producing the tear lens thickness diagrams; Ken Pullum for providing the basis of the section on scleral lenses and for his diagrams; and to the publishers for their constant help and encouragement.

APG
JAM

How to use this book

Please note that for accuracy some of the composite illustrations have been reproduced from the CD-ROM. These illustrations have been generated using mathematical values and are thus not as neat as the figures drawn by our artist, however they are very accurate!

Every time that the CD-ROM icon appears in the text, it indicates that there is an illustration available for viewing on the CD-ROM. Some of these are in full colour.

There are instructions on how to use the CD-ROM at the back of this book. Please contact Butterworth-Heinemann by fax on +(0) 1865 314426 if you experience any difficulties.

Chapter 1

Background

1.1 Applied anatomy

1.1.1 The cornea

Corneal tissue is transparent and avascular, consisting of three layers and two membranes. It protects the interior ocular structures and contributes 70% of the refractive power of the eye. It has the following average dimensions:

Radius of front surface 7.86 mm

Horizontal diameter   11.8 mm

Centre thickness   0.52 mm

Peripheral thickness   1.00 mm

EPITHELIUM

Provides a layer of protective cells. It is enhanced by microvilli, which are prominent irregularities increasing the surface area and providing a roughened surface to assist the adherence of the precorneal tear film.

Very minor corneal insult is covered in about 3 hours by neighbouring cells. Larger areas of damage are covered by the migration of cells from all layers of the surrounding epithelium. Lesions close to the limbus show conjunctival cells taking part in the cell migration.

Practical advice

Newly regenerated epithelium is very susceptible to damage. Lens wear should be suspended for a few days following any significant degree of corneal trauma such as overwear or severe abrasion.

BOWMAN'S MEMBRANE

The relatively tough anterior limiting layer of the cornea. It consists of a very fine non-orientated fibrillar meshwork. If Bowman's membrane is damaged, fibrous scar tissue is laid down, resulting in a permanent opacity.

STROMA

An avascular, regular structure which ensures both the mechanical strength and optical transparency of the cornea. Approximately 78% water, it represents about 90% of the corneal thickness.

DESCEMET'S MEMBRANE

The posterior limiting layer of the cornea. It is the basement layer of the endothelium and is elastic in nature.

ENDOTHELIUM

A single layer of cells in direct contact with the aqueous humour. Its pump mechanism maintains the cornea's fluid balance, which is in turn responsible for transparency. No mitosis occurs, but enlargement and spreading of existing cells take place. Irregularity in the size of endothelial cells is termed *polymegathism*.

CORNEAL SENSITIVITY

Innervation is by 70–80 sensory nerves entering the epithelium and usually losing their myelin sheaths within 0.5 mm of the limbus. The sensitivity of the cornea is greatest centrally and in the horizontal meridian. It reduces towards the vertical and is least at the periphery. Conjunctival sensitivity increases from a minimum at the limbus towards a maximum at the fornix and lid margins.

Sensitivity reduces with age and with contact lens wear. The first indication of reduced oxygen is a drop in corneal sensitivity, although clinically this may not be evident until there is a significant and measurable decrease. Sensitivity varies in women during the menstrual cycle and there is also a diurnal variation, being greatest in the evening.

1.1.2 The conjunctiva

A mucous membrane, continuous with the corneal epithelium. It is divided into a bulbar portion which covers the anterior sclera and a palpebral portion which lines the tarsal plate of the eyelids. The conjunctival glands or goblet cells secrete the mucoproteins found in the tears.

1.1.3 The eyelids

The orbicularis oculi muscle makes up almost one-third of the eyelid thickness. Behind lies the tarsal plate which consists of dense fibrous tissue. The openings to the sebaceous meibomian glands lie in a single row along the lid margin. There are about 25 in the upper lid and 20 in the lower, and they are best observed by eversion.

Practical advice

- Several contact lens problems relate to the eyelids so that lid eversion and thorough examination are essential prior to fitting.
- Meibomian gland dysfunction and blockage can contribute to dry-eye symptoms.
- Infection of meibomian glands causes styes or cysts.
- The average blink rate is about once every 5 seconds.

1.1.4 The tear film

FUNCTIONS

- Maintains a smooth optical surface over the cornea.
- Keeps the surface of the cornea moist.
- Acts as a lubricant for eyes and lids on blinking.
- Provides bacteriocidal action to protect corneal epithelium.
- Removes foreign bodies.

COMPOSITION

- An outermost oily, lipid layer secreted by the meibomian glands. Helps prevent evaporation.

- A central aqueous phase produced by the lacrimal gland and accessory glands of Krause and Wolfring.
- A mucoid layer, covering the epithelium, secreted by the conjunctival goblet cells.

The tear film is approximately 0.7 µm in thickness and about 90% of its volume is contained in the tear prism along the lid margin. The preocular tear film is adversely affected by the presence of a contact lens (*see* Section 6.3.3).

1.2 Applied physiology

A contact lens effectively occludes the cornea from its normal environment of oxygen, tears and ocular secretions. The effect depends upon lens thickness, size, method of fitting and material.
In this context, the following definitions are used:

- Anoxia occurs where no oxygen is present.
- Hypoxia occurs where there is reduced oxygen supply to the ocular tissues.
- Hypercapnia is the accumulation of CO_2.

CORNEAL METABOLISM

Constant metabolic activity in the cornea maintains transparency, temperature, cell reproduction and the transport of tissue materials. The main nutrients needed for these functions are glucose, amino acids and oxygen. Glucose and amino acids are provided by the aqueous humour, whereas oxygen is mainly derived from the tears.

Each layer of the cornea consumes oxygen at a particular rate. Oxygen enters the cornea from both surfaces so that there is minimum tension in the stroma. *Oxygen tension* is the driving force that moves oxygen into the cornea. At sea level, it is 155 mmHg for the open eye. Oxygen is supplied to the closed eye by the palpebral conjunctiva, where the tension is about 55 mmHg.[1]

Corneal swelling as a result of anoxia can be explained by biochemical theory.[1] In simple terms, there is not enough oxygen available to convert the glucose by means of glycolysis into sufficient energy and allow the waste product, lactic acid, to diffuse quickly out of the tissue. Less energy is therefore available for cellular activity, more lactic acid is produced and this builds up in the stroma. Sufficient osmotic pressure is created to allow water to be drawn into the stroma faster than the endothelial pump can remove it, and so corneal swelling occurs.

CORNEAL TEMPERATURE

The normal corneal temperature of 33–36°C may alter during contact lens wear. The effect becomes more significant under closed eye conditions. The change in temperature may be only 3°C, but the rate of metabolic activity is so dependent on ambient temperature that the fine balance between available oxygen and corneal demands under the closed lid may be stressed by such a small temperature change.

STROMAL ACIDOSIS

A drop in stromal pH induces a state of acidosis in contact lens wearers as a result of corneal hypoxia and hypercapnia. It appears that hypercapnia accounts for about 30% of the total pH drop which can occur even without a change in corneal thickness.[2] Chronic acidosis may explain some of the alterations seen in both corneal structure and function following contact lens wear.

TEAR OSMOLARITY

Corneal thickness is also affected by the osmolarity of the tears. In the normal, open eye, the salt content of the tear film is about 10% greater than that of freshly produced tears due to evaporation. When the eye is closed during sleep, it is bathed by fresh isotonic tears. The cornea responds to the less concentrated solution by drawing water into the stroma faster than it can be pumped out by the endothelium. Hence, on wakening, the cornea is found to have increased in thickness by about 5%.[3] Deswelling occurs rapidly during the first 2 hours the eyes are open.

TISSUE FRAGILITY

Reduced oxygen supply to the corneal epithelium, for example with extended wear, causes a decrease in the level of metabolic activity, including the rate of cell mitosis. The thickness of the epithelium reduces as cell production rate and wastage reach a new equilibrium. Such thinning has been observed in long-term extended wear patients. In addition, cell life increases and those at the anterior surface of the epithelium may not retain normal functional resistance. As a result of these changes, the overall resistance of the epithelium is lowered and the risk of infection increased.

CORNEAL SENSITIVITY

One of the first, important effects of hypoxia, of which the patient is unaware, is a drop in corneal sensitivity.[4]

CLOSED EYELID CONDITIONS DURING SLEEP

The following changes are induced:

- Increase in temperature.
- Hypotonic shift in tear osmolarity as a result of increased evaporation.
- Slight acidic shift in tear pH as a result of retardation of carbon dioxide efflux from the cornea.
- Corneal oxygenation reduced from 155 mmHg (open eye) to 55 mmHg (closed eye).

1.3 Physical properties of materials

1.3.1 Oxygen permeability, oxygen transmissibility and equivalent oxygen percentage

OXYGEN PERMEABILITY

The oxygen permeability of a material is generally referred to as the Dk. The units of 10^{-11} cm^2/s ml O$_2$/ml $\times$ mmHg (sometimes referred to as Fatt units) are often omitted for convenience. In this nomenclature, D is the diffusion coefficient – a measure of how fast dissolved molecules of oxygen move within the material – and k is a constant representing the solubility coefficient or the number of oxygen molecules dissolved in the material.

The Dk value is a physical property of a contact lens material and describes its intrinsic ability to transport oxygen. It is defined as 'the rate of oxygen flow under specified conditions through unit area of contact lens material of unit thickness when subjected to unit pressure differences.'[5] It is not a function of the shape or thickness of the material sample, but varies with temperature. The higher the temperature, the greater the Dk.[6]

OXYGEN TRANSMISSIBILITY

Oxygen transmissibility is referred to as Dk/t, with units of 10^{-9} cm/s ml O_2/ml $\times$ mmHg. Here, t is the thickness of the lens or sample of material, and D and k are as defined above.

The Dk/t for a particular lens under specified conditions defines the ability of the lens to allow oxygen to move from anterior to posterior surface. The value of t is generally an average lens thickness for powers between ±3.00 dioptres (D). Outside of this range it is necessary to apply a nomogram.[7] Oxygen transmissibility is not a physical property of a contact lens material, but is a specific characteristic related to the sample thickness.

Surface effects

High Dk materials do not always give the oxygen performance on the eye that would be expected from laboratory results. The corneal swelling is equivalent to that of a lens with a Dk only 55% of the measured value.[8] This barrier effect is due to an intermediate water layer used in measurement. There is also an edge effect due to oxygen flow around the sample periphery.[9]

Boundary effects

The boundary effect (or boundary layer effect) is important for hard gas-permeable materials as there is resistance to oxygen permeation at the boundary between the tears and polymer surface when measurement is made under water/water conditions. For a clean lens, the boundary effect is constant whether the lens is thick or very thin. The effect therefore has a relatively greater influence on a thin lens. This means that a particular Dk/t value with a lens, for example, of thickness 0.35 mm will not be significantly improved compared with a thin 0.10 mm lens. For thin lenses, the boundary effect becomes more important in determining the dissolved oxygen permeability as the Dk of the material increases. There are virtually no boundary effect implications for polymethyl methacrylate (PMMA) and low Dk materials.

EQUIVALENT OXYGEN PERCENTAGE

The equivalent oxygen percentage (EOP) refers to the level of oxygen at the surface of the cornea under a contact lens. For the uncovered cornea exposed to the atmosphere, the amount of oxygen available is 20.9%. With the eye closed the cornea receives

8%, whereas to avoid oedema the EOP should be over 10%[11] (*Dk/t* = 24.1), and for no overnight swelling it needs to be as high as 18% (*Dk/t* = 87). An EOP profile (Figure 1.1) for a lens of known material and thickness shows whether it can provide enough oxygen to avoid corneal oedema.

Practical advice

Consistently reliable comparisons of various materials can be made only by the same person using the same instrument under identical conditions. Care is therefore required in comparing *Dk* measurements from different sources.[10]

1.3.2 Water content and water uptake

The water content is the amount of fluid taken up by a lens material as a percentage of the whole under specified conditions:

Water content (%) =

$$\frac{\text{Wt of fully hydrated lens} - \text{Wt of fully dehydrated lens}}{\text{Wt of fully hydrated lens}} \times 100$$

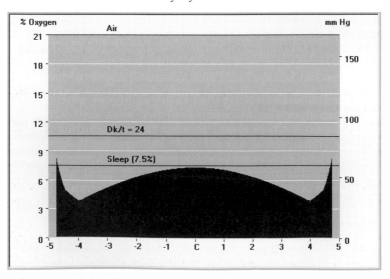

Figure 1.1 Equivalent oxygen percentage profile

Water uptake (%) =

$$\text{Wt of fully hydrated lens} - \text{Wt of fully dehydrated lens} \over \text{Wt of fully dehydrated lens} \times 100$$

Water is lost by evaporation when a hydrogel lens is worn on the eye. This is in part caused by a rise in temperature and is accompanied by a tightening of the fit (*see* Section 17.3).

1.3.3 Wettability

Wettability is the ability of a drop of liquid to adhere to a solid surface. The lower the cohesive forces within a liquid, the greater the attraction between the fluid and surface. Thus, superior wettability enhances the spread of liquid over a surface.

Contact angle is a measure of the hydrophilicity of a surface. The contact angle may be measured in a variety of ways:

- Sessile drop method: measures the tangent to a drop of liquid placed on a sample surface (Figure 1.2).

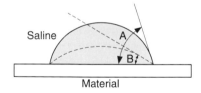

Figure 1.2 Sessile drop method (A, advancing angle; B, receding angle)

- Captive bubble method: measures the tangent to an air bubble formed on the surface of an immersed sample.
- Wilhelmy balance method. A sample is immersed or withdrawn vertically from a liquid.[12]
- Direct meniscus method.[12]

Both the advancing and receding angles are measured. These are formed when liquid is added to or removed from the controlled liquid drop used for measurement (Figure 1.2).

The lower the contact angle, the more wettable the surface (Figure 1.3). Typical values are given in Table 1.1, which demonstrates the great inconsistency between different methods. Comparisons can therefore only be made when the same method has been employed.

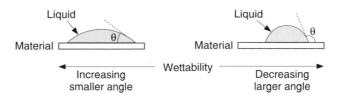

Figure 1.3 Surface wettability

Table 1.1 Wetting angles

Material	Captive bubble*	Captive bubble†	Sessile†	Wilhelmy†		Direct‡	
				Adv.	Rec.	Adv.	Rec.
PMMA	–	59.3	67.3	76.2	34.0	20	11
CAB	20	–	–	–	–	–	–
Boston II	21.5	36.5	82.7	74.0	27.4	46	14
Paraperm O$_2$	23.1	44.4	83.3	77.4	30.6	–	–
Polycon II	15	–	–	–	–	–	–
	receding –	–	–	–	–	–	–
Boston Equalens	30	–	–	–	–	–	–
Fluoromethacrylate (Quantum)	24	–	–	–	–	–	–

*From manufacturers' details.
†After Sarver et al.[13]
‡After Madigan, Holden and Fonn[14]

PMMA, polymethyl methacrylate; CAB, cellulose acetate butyrate.

1.4 Methods of manufacture

The current trend is for soft lenses to be made cheaper and more reproducible by means of mass production, since the raw materials are relatively inexpensive. With hard lenses, however, the emphasis is on careful, stress-free manufacture, because the raw materials are costly and the laboratory is concerned to avoid waste.

REGULATION

One of the most important influences on contact lens manufacture during the 1990s has been *CE marking*. Under the European Medical Device Directive (MDD), contact lenses are treated as medical devices and care products are treated as their accessories. Devices conforming to the directive should show the European standard CE marking, and from June 1998 it is illegal to buy or sell a contact lens which does not have affixed the CE mark from a 'Notified Body'. To be on the approved list, manufacturers are generally required to have implemented a formal quality control system such as ISO 9002.

1.4.1 Hard lens manufacture

• Conventional lathes to cut the back and front lens surfaces from buttons.

• Computer numerically controlled (CNC) lathes. Four types are available with different types of automation, so that both spherical and aspheric surfaces can be cut.[15]

POLISHING

The time and speed of polishing, together with the wetness and composition of the polish, are all very important. Frictional heating and over-polishing of the lens surface cause poor lens wettability.

1.4.2 Soft lens manufacture

• Lathing as with hard lenses, using buttons cut from rods. The finished lens is then hydrated.

• Spin casting, in which polymerization of the monomer and solvent takes place in open, spinning moulds (*see* Section 17.6).

• Cast moulding, which uses closed, disposable moulds with two components. Polymerization is by means of heat. The two methods are dry moulding, where the lens is moulded in the dry state and the edges finished by buffing; and wet moulding, in which the material is already hydrated (e.g. for disposable lenses).

• Liquid edge moulding, in which lenses are cast in polypropylene moulds in the dry state. The contact lens edge is formed by accurate control of pressure on the mould and the volume of polymer employed, leaving the edge intact when the excess polymer (termed *flash*) has been squeezed out.[16] There is no need to polish the edge with this process.

• Lightstream Technology which eliminates the need for solvents and extraction of toxic residues e.g. with CIBA Vision's PVA based nelfilcon A. Rigid quartz moulds are used but the front curve and base curve moulds never actually touch. A mechanical system holds them microns apart. A circular mask blocks the UV lightstream at the edge of the mould, preventing light interaction with the liquid material at the lens edge. This liquid is washed away whilst the photo-lithographic process forms the edge.

1.4.3 Toric lens manufacture

Soft lenses

- For conventional (non-disposable) torics, the method of choice is lathing using CNC lenticular back surface lathes and purposeful crimps to form the toric back surface under pressure. For the front surface, manual lenticular lathes with prism ballast capability are needed. The finished lens is polished before hydration.

- Disposable torics, which have a rather simpler design, are moulded.

- Recent developments are lathe waveform generators capable of generating complex, non-symmetrical geometries on surfaces that can be rotated off-axis.

Hard gas-permeable lenses

- Conventional lathes in conjunction with crimping devices can be used to manufacture toric peripheries, back surface torics, bi-torics and front surface torics.[17] The lens is lathed in the conventional manner, with a radius halfway between the required steeper and flatter meridians. It is then lathed a second time while held under a specified tension within the crimping device. The peripheral curves are then cut and the lens polished.

- Toric lathes that can generate a specified toric back surface.

References

1. Fatt, I. and Weissman, B.A. (1992) *Physiology of the Eye. An Introduction to the Vegetative Functions.* 2nd edn. Butterworth-Heinemann, Boston
2. Rivera, R.K. and Polse, K.A. (1996) Effects of hypoxia and hypercapnia on contact lens- induced corneal acidosis. *Optometry and Vision Science* **73** (3), 178–183
3. Mandell, R. and Fatt, I. (1965) Thinning of the human cornea on awakening. *Nature*, **208**, 292

4. Millodot, M. and O'Leary, D.J. (1980) Effect of oxygen deprivation on corneal sensitivity. *Acta Ophthalmologica*, **58**, 434

5. Fatt, I. and St Helen, R. (1971) Oxygen tension under an oxygen permeable contact lens. *American Journal of Optometry*, **48**, 545

6. Morris, J.A. (1985) An overview of the hard gas permeable oxygen race. *Optometry Today* (March), 168–172

7. Brennan, N.A. (1984) Average thickness of a hydrogel lens for gas transmissiblity calculations. *American Journal of Optometry* **61**, 627

8. Brennan, N., Efron, N. and Holden, B.A. (1986) Further developments in the RGP *Dk* controversy. *International Eyecare*, **2**, 508–509

9. Fatt, I. (1986) Now do we need 'effective permeability'? *Contax* (July), 6–23

10. Holden, B.A., Newton-Howes, J., Winterton, L., Fatt, I., Hamano H. and La Hood, D. *et al.* (1990) The *Dk* project: An interlaboratory comparison of *Dk/L* measurements. *Optometry and Vision Science*, **67**, 476–481

11. Holden, B.A. and Mertz, G.W. (1984) Critical oxygen levels to avoid corneal oedema for daily and extended wear contact lenses. *Investigative Ophthalmology and Visual Science*, **25**, 1161–1167

12. Pearson, R.M. (1987) Rigid gas permeable wettability and maintenance. *Contax* (Sept), 8–16

13. Sarver, M., Bowman, L., Bauman, E., Dimartino, R and Umeda, W. (1984) Wettability of some gas permeable hard contact lenses. *International Contact Lens Clinic*, **11**, 479–490

14. Madigan, M., Holden, B.A. and Fonn, D. (1986) A new method for wetting angle measurement. *International Eyecare*, **2**, 45–48

15. Hough, A. (1997) Rigid lens manufacture in the 1990s. *Optician*, **214** (5612), 24–28

16. Hough, A. (1997) Soft lens manufacture in the 1990s: managing unit costs to compete effectively. *Optician*, **213** (5599), 35–41

17. Meyler, J. and Ruston, D. (1995) Toric RGP contact lenses made easy. *Optician*, **209** (5504), 30–35

Chapter 2

Instrumentation

2.1 Slit lamp

The slit lamp provides the best method of observing ocular tissue in section under high magnification.

2.1.1 Instrument controls and focus

Instrument controls allow for variation in height, lateral movement and focusing. The illumination and observation systems are focused at a common point unless they are uncoupled to allow independent movement.

The optical system contains an *objective*, typically with ×3 to ×3.5 magnification, and an *eyepiece* with variable or interchangeable power. The normal range of total magnification gives ×6, ×10, ×16, ×25 and ×40.

Focus is achieved by rotating the slit beam about its fulcrum[1] (Figure 2.1).

- If the illuminated area moves with the direction of the arm, the projected slit is in front of the focus position.

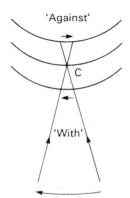

Figure 2.1 Focusing the slit beam (C, focus point)

- If the illuminated area moves against the direction of the arm, the projected slit is beyond the focus position.
- If the illuminated area remains stationary as the arm moves, the slit is exactly in focus.

2.1.2 Methods of illumination

DIRECT METHODS

The slit beam and microscope are focused at the same point to give:

- Diffuse illumination.
- Direct focal illumination.
- Indirect illumination.
- Specular reflection.
- Sclerotic scatter.

INDIRECT METHODS

The beam and microscope are uncoupled so that they are no longer focused at the same point to give:

- Indirect proper illumination.
- Sclerotic scatter.
- Retroillumination.

2.1.3 Recommended slit lamp routine

- The instrument height is set for a halfway point in its travel range. The eyepieces are adjusted for the observer's prescription and pupillary distance (PD).
- A drop of fluorescein is instilled into each eye.
- The patient is made comfortable in relation to the height of the headrest and the instrument table.
- The patient closes the eyes and a slit beam is focused onto the eyelids. The beam is moved to the outer canthus without moving the instrument out of its range of focus, and the patient asked to open the eyes.
- Diffuse illumination is used for a general look at the ocular tissues under low magnification.

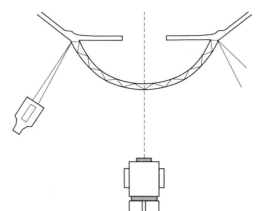

Figure 2.2 Sclerotic scatter

- In a darkened room, the cornea is examined with sclerotic scatter using either the microscope or the unaided eye for signs of opacities or oedema (Figure 2.2).

- Starting at the temporal limbus, the corneal tissue is scanned using direct focal illumination and a parallelepiped at least 2 mm wide. The slit beam is set between 40° and 60° to the temporal side of the centrally placed microscope. Magnification should be about ×20. From the corneal apex to the nasal limbus, the illumination system can be swung to the nasal side of the microscope (Figure 2.3).

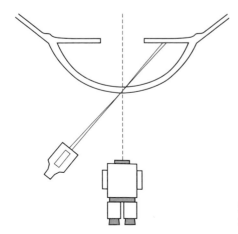

Figure 2.3 Direct focal illumination

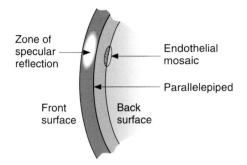

Zone of
specular
reflection

Endothelial
mosaic

Parallelepiped

Front
surface

Back
surface

Figure 2.4 Specular reflection
showing the endothelium

- The beam is reduced to an optic section and the cornea examined in the same manner, localizing any abnormality discovered with the wide beam.

- The patient looks up and down, to take in the superior and inferior limbal areas.

- The direct slit beam is oscillated as the cornea is traversed. Any abnormality changes the scattering of light in the tissues and aids identification. The whole field of view contained by the beam and its surrounds is continuously observed with a combination of direct and indirect illumination.

- As the direct beam is moved across the cornea, specular reflection of the tear film occurs. Examination of this bright area, looking for any debris or oiliness, gives a qualitative assessment of the tear film. Changing focus to the rear of the beam section brings an area of endothelium into view (Figure 2.4).

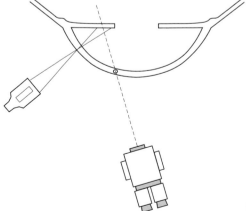

Figure 2.5 Retro-illumination

A general idea of endothelial regularity is obtained, rather than specific cell details. Each zone appears double, as the reflected light using this method enters only one eyepiece at a time.

N.B. The endothelium looks like a patch of beaten gold to the side of the much brighter specular zone.

- The slit lamp is uncoupled to examine the cornea by means of retroillumination. Direct, marginal and indirect retroillumination ascertain whether any abnormality is more or less dense than the surrounding tissue. This is revealed by the way the light converges or diverges around the abnormality, and aids in its identification (Figure 2.5).[2]

- Both the cornea and conjunctiva are then examined for evidence of epithelial staining using a broad scanning beam and the cobalt blue filter. A yellow filter (Kodak Wratten 12) in the observation system gives enhanced contrast and assists identification. Other stains used are rose bengal and, less commonly, alcian blue.

Practical advice

Correct use of the slit lamp requires the co-ordinated use of both hands – one to control the joystick and the other the slit beam.

2.2 Keratometers and autokeratometers

Keratometers measure the curvature of the central cornea over an area of approximately 3–6 mm to determine:

- The radii of curvature.
- The directions of the principal meridians.
- The degree of corneal astigmatism.
- The presence of any corneal distortion.

2.2.1 Types of keratometer

There are two types of instrument, depending on the system of doubling employed to measure the separation of the mire images. Doubling helps in taking the reading, since rapid eye movements would otherwise make the measurement extremely difficult.

Practical advice

The same cornea measured with more than one instrument can result in a variety of readings because different keratometers employ:

- Different mire separations, so that the area of cornea used for reflection varies.
- Different refractive indices for calibration, so that the same radius could give a variety of surface powers.

VARIABLE DOUBLING

The mires have a fixed separation. The separation of the mire images is found by varying the doubling power. The Bausch & Lomb keratometer has two variable doubling devices and two sets of fixed mires (Figure 2.6). Both principal meridians can therefore be measured simultaneously, and it is called a *one position* instrument.

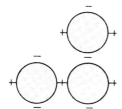

Figure 2.6 Bausch & Lomb mires

FIXED DOUBLING

The doubling is fixed for a particular separation of the mire images. It is only by altering the separation of the mires themselves that a reading can be taken. These keratometers are called *two position* instruments and are based on the Javal–Shiötz design (Figure 2.7).

 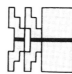

Figure 2.7 Javal–Schiötz mires

2.2.2 Focusing the eyepiece

Most keratometers have a graticule incorporated in the eyepiece. This should be focused prior to taking a reading to prevent accommodation giving an inaccurate result.

2.2.3 Taking a measurement

The patient should be comfortably seated, with the forehead positioned firmly against the headrest. Fixation should be accurate, with the other eye occluded. To help line up the optical system and locate the patient's cornea use:

- The sights attached to the instrument.
- The light from a pen torch directed through the eyepiece, looking for the corneal reflection.

The instrument is positioned initially at a greater distance from the cornea than necessary and slowly moved forward until the mire images come into view and are sharply focused. There should be four images, two of each mire either side of the centre. The middle pair are brought together until lined up in the correct position to take a reading (Figure 2.7).

Similar images need to be superimposed (Figure 2.8), whereas dissimilar mires are required to touch (Figure 2.7). In each case, the instrument is rotated to orientate with the first principal meridian. The measurement is recorded and the second principal meridian found by rotating the instrument through 90°.

Practical advice

- The principal meridians are not at 90° with an irregular cornea.
- Instruments usually show the corneal radius in both millimetres and dioptres.
- The power and radius scales have their maximum and minimum values at opposite ends.
- The axis of the meridian is usually obtained from an external protractor scale.
- Keratometry readings are expressed as *along* a particular meridian.
- Patients fitted in the USA generally have their keratometry and lenses specified in dioptres.

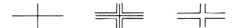

Figure 2.8 Superimposed images – Zeiss (Oberkochen) mires

2.2.4 Extending the range

Radii steeper than the range of the instrument (e.g. keratoconus) can be obtained by placing a +1.25 D trial lens in front of the keratometer objective. At the flatter end, the range can be similarly extended with a –1.00 D lens. Prior calibration is necessary using steel balls of known radius.[3]

Practical advice

- For keratoconus, the Javal-Schiötz instrument is particularly useful, because the range at the steep end extends as far as 5.50 mm.
- Keratometers with circular mires (e.g. Rausch and Lomb) give a qualitative assessment of corneal distortion.

2.2.5 Topographical keratometer

The keratometer can also be used to explore the paracentral and peripheral areas of the cornea by means of a graduated fixation attachment.[4]

2.2.6 Autokeratometers

Autokeratometers determine the radii and principal meridians along the visual axis.[5] They can also measure peripheral radii at predetermined positions away from the corneal apex (e.g. at 23° and 30° with the Nikon NRK 8000). Some instruments use computerized image processing to determine the flattest and steepest corneal radii with corresponding meridians and powers.

Autokeratometers achieve the measurement by calculating the distance between the reflected images from light-emitting diodes. The mires are usually circular and designed to reveal any corneal distortion. They also include distance indicators which enable the reading to take place. Despite the speed of measurement, steady fixation by the patient is essential. This is often assisted by a light-emitting diode, but the practitioner should carefully observe the eye during measurement as well as ensuring that the patient maintains a wide palpebral aperture.

Hand-held models (e.g. Nidek KM-500, Alcon Renaissance) allow single-handed operation and offer benefits in dealing with infants and young children.[6] They can also be employed in the operating theatre and where disabilities make conventional instruments impossible to use. The practitioner must be at the same height as the patient, although some models have a levelling device that automatically corrects the measured axis even if the instrument is held up to 15° off axis.

2.3 Corneal topographers

VIDEOKERATOSCOPY

Videokeratoscopy (e.g. Eyesys, Tomey, Humphries) gives a more detailed assessment of overall corneal topography by means of modern computer analysis. These instruments are now coming into more general use and are mainly based on back-lit Placido disk mires, high-resolution CCD video cameras and a computer for data analysis.[7] The results are presented as a topographic contour map of the cornea with colour used to indicate the curvature and power distribution for the area under analysis. The Eyesys, for example, uses 35 colours covering the range from 52 D to 35 D. The colour scale runs from red at the steep end to blue at the flat end. Typical topographical maps are designated:

- Colour, to depict corneal curvature.
- Dioptric, where each colour represents a range of dioptric (curvature) values.
- Absolute, where each colour always corresponds to a fixed 0.50 D range.
- Keratometric.
- Profile.
- Isometric.

It is also possible to overlay or combine the basic plots with grids, angular scales, simulated keratometric readings, Placido rings, corneal image and pupil position.

In contact lens practice, videokeratoscopy is particularly useful for assessing corneal eccentricity (*e*-value, *see* Section 8.4), surface irregularity and irregular astigmatism. Subtractive plots are used to monitor corneal change with orthokeratology (*see* Chapter 14) or when ceasing PMMA wear. Some instruments include a programme for designing the optimum contact lens based on the corneal map (*see* Section 8.5), together with simulated fluorescein patterns. Misalignment of the visual axis during measurement can give misleading results.

Extreme asymmetry or distortion is frequently seen with:

- Irregular astigmatism, distinguished from regular astigmatism in the corneal map by the lack of a symmetrical 'bow tie' pattern. Residual astigmatism, however, is not necessarily revealed by videokeratoscopy.

- Keratoconus.

- Penetrating keratoplasty.

- Contact lens-induced corneal warpage.

- Refractive surgery.

- Trauma.

Light cone systems rather than ring projection are also available (e.g. TMS-1). They permit a closer focusing distance and lower light intensity. A solid-state laser focuses at the corneal apex rather than the periphery used in other instruments.

A more recent version of corneal topographer is based on slit lamp technology using diffusely reflected light from the corneal surfaces, iris and lens (e.g. Orbscan). The images are acquired by video camera. The slit beam scans with over 7000 independently and directly measured data points. Ray trace triangulation determines elevations of the anterior and posterior corneal surface, giving limbus to limbus data. The corneal mapping produced gives a full analysis of the cornea under view, including a variety of refractive power maps; central (optical axis identification) and peripheral measurement data for contact lens fitting; full corneal pachometry (e.g. Pacscan module); and three-dimensional virtual reality models.

PHOTO-ELECTRIC KERATOSCOPE

In the past, the original photo-electric keratoscope (PEK) produced a photographic record of corneal topography and explored the paracentral and peripheral areas of the cornea. The information was used to provide a computer-designed contact lens (e.g. the Wesley–Jessen system).

2.4 Image capture

Video and digital photography are the two methods currently employed to capture images related to contact lens practice. The slit lamp, for optimal recording, should have continuous zoom optics and variable illumination.

Video images are captured using a CCD (charge coupled device) camera attached to the slit lamp, possibly via a beam splitter, and connection to a video recorder or computer. Cameras are either *one-chip* or *three-chip*, with the latter giving considerably better optical resolution.

Digital photography permits true digital imaging where the result is captured through pixels. The images are easy to store, can be copied without degradation and can be manipulated by means of computer technology. High-quality screen and colour resolution, however, requires large computer storage capacity, so CD-ROM technology is often used to deal with this problem.[8]

2.4.1 Advantages of image capture over conventional photography:

- Images are captured in real time, ensuring that the desired picture is recorded.
- Where necessary, results can be demonstrated immediately to the patient.
- Digital images can be transmitted to other locations via a modem.
- There is no degradation of digital images over time.
- Computer technology is now cost-effective

2.5 Other instruments

BURTON LAMP

The Burton lamp uses ultraviolet light at a safe wavelength of about 400 nm. The lamp is also referred to as a *blue light* or *black light* and is used in conjunction with fluorescein (*see* Section 10.2.1).

Most Burton lamps are combined with a low-power magnifier, large enough to permit binocular viewing. Many models combine white light tubes and some incorporate a yellow filter to intensify the fluorescence.

PLACIDO DISC

The Placido disc is a flat, circular disc with alternate black and white concentric rings. The width and separation of the rings increase towards the periphery and are designed so that the reflections appear the same width when reflected from an average cornea. It gives a qualitative assessment of the regularity of the cornea itself. The eye is viewed through a convex lens in the centre of the disc.

KLEIN KERATOSCOPE

The Klein keratoscope is an internally illuminated version of the Placido disc.

References

1. Morris, J. and Hirji, N. (1992) The slit lamp biomicroscope in optometric practice. *Optometry Today*, 2nd edn, Fleet
2. Phelps Brown, N. (1989) Mini pathology of the eye. *Optician*, **197** (5200), 22–29
3. Sampson, W.G. and Soper, J.W. (1970) Keratometry In *Corneal Contact Lenses*, 2nd edn T J Girard (ed.), Mosby, St. Louis
4. Wilms, K H and Rabbetts, R.B. (1977) Practical concepts of corneal topometry. *Optician*, **174** (4502), 7–13
5. Kon, Y.P. (1992) The keratometer and corneal measurement – part II: auto-keratometers and peripheral keratometry. *Contact Lens Journal*, **20** (8), 11–12
6. Edwards, M.H. and Cho, P. (1996) A new, hand-held keratometer: comparison of the Nidek KM-500 auto keratometer with the B & L keratometer and the Topcon RK-3000A keratometer. *Journal of the British Contact Lens Association*, **19** (2), 45–48
7. Maeda, N. and Klyce, S.D. (1994) Videokeratography in contact lens practice. *International Contact Lens Clinic*, **21** (9&10), 163–169
8. Cox, I. (1995) Digital imaging in contact lens practice. *International Contact Lens Clinic*, **22** (3&4), 62–66

Chapter 3

Record keeping

The information in this chapter represents the authors' interpretation of the obligations laid on practitioners by existing regulations; it is not intended as a substitute for legal advice.

Since the NHS Act 1948, optometrists (opticians) have had a common law Duty of Care that 'records should be adequate'. Against the background of increasingly litigious patients and the possibly serious consequences from the misuse of contact lenses or solutions, it is essential for practitioners to maintain comprehensive written notes. Complete and proper records, as a matter of legal precedent, are now the first line of defence in most complaints of a clinical nature.

3.1 Legal implications

Practitioners, for their own protection, must take a full history of both ophthalmic and general medical factors. Negative findings should also be noted and a second opinion sought in case of doubt.

INFORMED CONSENT

The doctrine of informed consent, which is pertinent to the preliminary discussion with all potential contact lens wearers, acknowledges that:

- 'The patient has a right to know and understand the risks as well as the benefits before agreeing to undergo a procedure as well as knowing if examinations revealed any abnormal findings.'
- Patients should also have an opportunity to ask questions and discontinue at any stage of fitting or treatment. Many practitioners prefer to avoid discussing possible negative consequences, but there could be serious legal problems if a patient claims lack of informed consent.

- In the UK, the Department of Health (DoH) has issued a leaflet called *Contact Lenses and You* which practitioners may use for their patients. It summarizes firstly the questions that patients should be asked by the practitioner at the preliminary visit and, secondly, the topics about which they should receive information when contact lenses are dispensed. The final page consists of a form to be signed by patients to acknowledge that they have been given full information and instructions on the type of lens selected, the care of those lenses, and advice should problems arise. The DoH recommends providing an out-of-hours telephone number in case of serious emergency.
- To avoid any misunderstandings, it is important to tell patients the possible adverse consequences of not following directions – i.e. non-compliance. The practitioner should never guarantee success, and at the dispensing visit, patients should be given adequate instructions reinforced by written information. An acknowledgement or consent form may be used if appropriate, particularly in the case of a new or experimental technique.

RECORD KEEPING

When obtaining details of history, signs and symptoms, *open questions* should be used. This means that patients are given the opportunity to explain symptoms or describe their compliance with the instructions. The technique of open questions at aftercare examinations may prove less confrontational and give much more information than a simple 'yes' or 'no' answer. In addition, the use of *closed questions* often allows patients to provide the answer that they feel is expected by the practitioner.

Example:

When asking about the use of solutions at night:

Closed question: Do you use the surfactant cleaner each night?

Open question: What do you do each night?

The open question is much more likely to obtain the truth; the closed question may not.

Record all patients' comments that reveal non-compliance, followed by advice and warnings given. It is both useful and necessary to describe fully the fit and surface condition of the lenses. It is important to record corneal and other changes by means of grading (*see* Section 3.3) and a drawing, but also note negative findings. Thus, 'no staining' indicates that fluorescein has been used during the examination. Do not forget to note down the final advice given to the patient for resolving any problem as well as a suggested date for the next appointment.

In general terms, it is not a legal defence to say:

'I always do that...'
'I didn't write it down because it was normal.'
'I remember telling the patient that...'
'We always tell patients that...'

Legal action could occur several years after an alleged event, and memory alone, unsupported by the written evidence of the record card, will potentially leave the practitioner in a perilous position. Records should be kept for at least 10 years and professional indemnity insurance maintained for a minimum of 5 years after retirement.

If something is incorrectly recorded, cross it out but do not erase it. Never add to a record at a later date, intending to show that it was written at the time of the visit. Untruthful records will always automatically condemn, whatever the true circumstances of the case.

TELEPHONE CONVERSATIONS

Always make a careful record of telephone conversations, particularly in respect of problems. The notes should be dated on the patient's card with details of advice given. The practitioner bears ultimate responsibility for advice given by unqualified staff and their comments should be similarly recorded.

COMPLAINTS

Details of any complaint and the response given must be carefully documented and dated. The details should include what was said by both the practitioner and the patient during the conversation.

PATIENT ACCESS TO RECORDS

The 1990 Access to Health Records Act allows patients access to a copy of their records on written request. It is now important, therefore, not to write any derogatory or other comments that are not intended to be read by patients. They are also entitled to know the meaning of any coded abbreviations. The practitioner is able to charge a fee for the copy of the records.

There is also a duty to keep records in a secure place and to maintain patient confidentiality. If a request for the records is made when patients transfer to another practice, a copy or summary should be sent. The records are the property of the practitioner and the original should remain in the practice for reference and in case of future litigation.

SPECIFICATION AND REPLICATION

The General Optical Council have ruled that opticians have a duty to provide patients with details of their contact lens specification, stating 'An optician who fits a person with a contact lens shall on completing the fitting give to him a written statement of the particulars necessary to enable the lens to be replicated'. The practitioner must make a decision based on clinical judgement when the fitting is complete. Up to this point, followed by an adequate period of time for checking, no contact lens prescription can be said to exist. The specification should be dated and is current for up to 1 year.

If a patient asks for the prescription to obtain contact lenses elsewhere and, in the practitioner's opinion, the fitting has not been completed, this fact should be clearly indicated on the written specification.

If replacement lenses are requested and it is over 1 year since the last examination, the patient should be advised of the need for continuing aftercare before lenses are ordered. In the event of refusal, it is advisable for this to be noted on the patient's record.

The prescription should enable the lens to be replicated accurately. Conversely, a practitioner should decline to order lenses from another practitioner's prescription if it is unclear, incomplete, ambiguous or no longer current. Any modification to the prescription incurs a liability for the practitioner issuing the lenses.

Care should be exercised in repolishing or cleaning lenses fitted elsewhere. Without a full history, including visual acuities, the practitioner will be left in an invidious position if subsequently a complaint is made by the patient about either ocular problems or lens performance.

RESPONSIBILITY

Implicit in the acceptance of a patient are responsibilities towards that patient. The examination should not be limited only to those aspects that concern contact lenses but must also include standard techniques to determine the patient's ocular health, consistent with the common law Duty of Care. In the event, for example, of a retinal problem which should have been apparent at the time of examination, the practitioner would be considered negligent if the problem had not been detected.

The College of Optometrists and the Association of British Dispensing Opticians each has its own set of guidelines relating to contact lens practice. These are intended to guide practitioners and fitters in their responsibilities for all aspects of contact lens practice. Such guidelines could well be used as the peer view in any legal case, and are currently used in this manner by the General Optical Council for complaint procedures. By virtue of their training, optometrists and medical practitioners have a greater duty of care in general than dispensing opticians.

COMMITTEE ON THE SAFETY OF MEDICINES

In dealing with contact lens patients, any adverse reaction with a known cause should be reported using a Yellow Card provided by the Committee on the Safety of Medicines. The scheme, however, relates only to adverse reactions to contact lenses, medicaments or preparations that optometrists have themselves provided. The value of these reports enables the statistical monitoring of adverse reactions to materials and solutions.

PRODUCT LIABILITY

Practitioners incur product liability for all products dispensed, including their accuracy and sterility. All materials must be safe, properly tested, and comply with any licensing regulations from the Committee on the Safety of Medicines, European directives and the Food and Drugs Administration (FDA) in the USA.

General advice

- The golden rule for patient records is *write it down*.
- If it wasn't recorded in writing, it wasn't seen, done or said.
- Always maintain comprehensive cover for professional indemnity.
- Do not treat conditions outside the scope of the practice or professional responsibility.

MEDICAL DEVICE DIRECTIVE

The Medical Device Directive requires manufacturers of contact lenses and contact lens care products to issue information with all devices or packaging so that they may be used safely. Contact lenses are purchased and prescribed by eye-care practitioners but then issued to patients. The information provided by the manufacturer must therefore take into account the backgrounds of both groups.

- The glass vial, blister pack or mailer should include information on the lens material and lens parameters, including BVP.
- Soft contact lenses must indicate sterility and method used, batch code, and intended use of lenses (e.g. daily wear, extended wear or single use).
- Custom-made lenses should be labelled as such.
- Lens details should also include the manufacturer's expiry date and CE marking.
- The manufacturer's name and adddress together with the recommended use of the lens should be included with the packaging.

Manufacturers' leaflets should contain warnings in respect of: bacterial contamination; ocular side effects; circumstances under which contact lens wear should cease (e.g. red eye or pain); not using tap water; washing hands before use; and that tamperproof seals should be unbroken.

Written instructions from the practitioner should include: correct procedures for hand washing; how to insert and remove contact lenses; how to clean and maintain lenses; wearing schedules; arrangements for aftercare; signs and symptoms of adverse effects and how to deal with them; and advice when participating in water sports (*see* Section 27.4).

Despite the potential risks, plano tinted contact lenses with the function only of changing the eye colour are not considered to be medical devices. They may currently be issued by non-professional suppliers

3.2 Record cards

The use of a standard designed record card helps ensure that all procedures are completed and documented. The card is also used as a prompt during the consultation to avoid missing out routine procedures and questions. The use of diagrams aids description and is an ideal method of monitoring any changes. Photographs or image capture, however, are superior (*see* Section 2.4).

The visits that require full documentation are: Initial, Fitting, Dispensing and Aftercare plus adequate space to record order information and subsequent changes to the lens specification.

3.3 Clinical grading

A simple definition of clinical grading is 'putting numbers instead of words'. An important aspect of record keeping is to record findings in a reproducible way that can be easily understood by professional colleagues and provide a comparison between patient visits. Various scales are currently in use, while some practitioners have devised their own systems.[1] Successful grading needs to be simple, consistent and derived from an understanding of the clinical judgement necessary to discriminate between findings.[2]

Scales are either numeric, usually from 0 to 4, or based on identifying symbols. Definitions are helped by photographic or line illustration.

PUBLISHED GRADING SCALES

There are two main published scales currently in use:

The CCLRU Grading Scale

Devised by the Cornea and Contact Lens Research Unit (CCLRU) in Australia and produced by Vistakon. The grading scales are photographically illustrated and include: corneal staining, depth and extent; conjunctival staining; bulbar and limbal redness; lid redness and roughness; and endothelial polymegathism. The CCLRU scheme uses five grades:

0 = normal
1 = very slight
2 = slight
3 = moderate
4 = severe

The Efron Grading Scale for Contact Lens Complications

Devised by Professor Efron of University of Manchester Institute of Science and Technology (UMIST) and produced by Hydron.[3]

The scale is illustrated with drawings by Tarrant on the basis that the desired level of change can be precisely represented whilst all other factors are kept constant. Eight complications are included, two from each of the conjunctiva, corneal epithelium, stroma and endothelium. The UMIST scheme also uses five grades from 0 to 4:

0 = normal
1 = trace
2 = mild
3 = moderate
4 = severe

The Institute of Optometry Grading Scale

Instead of numbers it is possible to introduce + and − signs to be used with a scheme of consistent abbreviations. In this way, several other features can be graded. Such a system has been devised for use at the Institute of Optometry and includes the following items:

Fitting:	Hard and soft lenses
Lens surface spoilation:	Deposits, drying, greasiness and scratches
Tears:	Debris, grease, tear prism and break up
Cornea and conjunctiva:	Staining, oedema, vessels, abnormalities and endothelium
Lids:	Hyperaemia, follicles, papillae, cobblestone and roughness

The combination of scalar grades and measurements in millimetres enables the quantification of most problems. Corneal changes are in addition illustrated with scale diagrams. The location, depth and extent can all be recorded with careful drawing.

Fitting

Hard lenses

Central pattern:	Apical clearance	= Al+, Al++, Al+++
	Alignment	= Al
	Apical touch	= Al−, Al− −, Al− − −
Peripheral pattern:	No edge clearance	= Ec− −
	Minimum edge clearance	= Ec−
	Optimal edge clearance	= Ec
	Excessive edge clearance	= Ec+

Soft lenses

Centration:

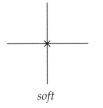

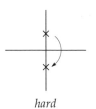

soft   *hard*

Movement: None   = Mov– –
                 Only on upwards gaze   = Mov–
                 Optimal   = Mov
                 Mobile   = Mov+
                 Excessively mobile   = Mov++

Surface spoilation

Deposits: None   = 0
                 1 or 2 small deposits   = +
                 Moderate deposits   = ++
                 Heavy deposits   = +++

Drying: None   = 0
                 Small area   = +
                 Moderate area   = ++
                 Complete dryness   = +++

Greasiness: None   = 0
                 Light greasiness   = +
                 Moderate greasiness   = ++
                 Heavy greasiness   = +++

Scratches: None   = 0
                 Light   = +
                 Moderate   = ++
                 Deep   = +++

Tears

Debris: None   = 0
                 Minimal   = +
                 Moderate   = ++
                 Severe   = +++

Greasiness: None   = 0
                 Minimal   = +
                 Moderate   = ++
                 Severe   = +++

Tear prism:	Minimal	= +
	Moderate, ≤ 0.50 mm	= ++
	Full, > 0.50 mm	= +++

Cornea and conjunctiva

Staining:	No stain	= 0
	Superficial	= +
	Moderate	= ++
	Dense	= +++

(extent and depth by drawing and comment)

Oedema:	Possible	= −
	None	= 0
	Definite	= +
	Unacceptable	= ++

Vessels:

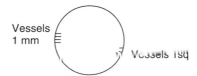

Abnormalities:

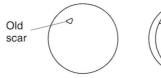

Endothelium:	Regular	= 0
		= +
		= ++
	Irregular	= +++

Lids

Hyperaemia	Absent	= H0
	Minimal	= H+
	Moderate	= H++
	Severe	= H+++

Papillae:	Absent	= P0
	Micro, < 0.3 mm	= P+
	Macro, 0.3–1.0 mm	= P++
	Giant, > 1.0 mm	= P+++

Cobblestone   = C

Follicles   = F

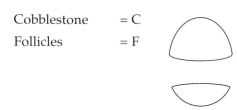

3.4 Computerization of patient records

DATA PROTECTION ACT

Practitioners are increasingly using computers for both practice management and storage of patients' clinical records. It is essential to comply with the provisions of the Data Protection Act in respect of registration and the duty to maintain confidentiality of patient information. Safeguards are therefore necessary to prevent unauthorized access to the records.

The registered entry for a practice must contain particulars of the data held and declare the intended purposes of those data. These are numerically classified into some 200 options and the appropriate category numbers must be declared. On average, there are six options that relate purely to patients. There is a fixed charge for initial registration.

There are eight data protection principles that data users must observe:

1. Data should be obtained and processed fairly and lawfully.
2. Data may be held only for registered uses.
3. Data may not be disclosed contrary to their registered purposes.
4. Only the minimum amount of information required should be kept for each patient.
5. Data must be accurate and, where necessary, kept up-to-date.
6. Data should be held for no longer than required and regularly deleted where necessary.
7. Proper security is essential. All reasonable steps should be taken to ensure that there is no accidental loss of data or improper access.
8. Individuals are entitled to know what personal data may be held on them, and are entitled to a copy of those data. If appropriate, inaccurate data may need to be corrected or erased.

With certain provisos, computer-generated records are admissible as evidence in a court of law. The system must be tamper-proof and needs to incorporate an audit trail that dates, times and records every change to the files as well as identifying the author.

Compared with written notes, there is a greater risk of accidental loss to computer records, so full back-ups must be taken regularly and stored securely. Patient records should be kept for at least 10 years, so any upgrading of the computer system must allow transference of data. To avoid mistakes, the practitioner must maintain supervision over the input of data, although this is frequently delegated to unqualified personnel.

References

1. Lloyd, M. (1992) Lies, statistics, and clinical significance. *Journal of the British Contact Lens Association*, **15** (2), 67–70
2. Hurst, M.A., Mitchell, S.E. and Douthwaite, W.A. (1994) Contact lens opacity grading system (CLOGS). *Journal of the British Contact Lens Association*, **17** (1), 19–24
3. Efron, N. (1997) Clinical application of grading scales for contact lens complications. *Optician*, **213** (5604), 26–35

Further reading

Rosenwasser, H.M. (1991) *Malpractice and Contact Lenses. A guide to limiting liability in contact lens practice.* Butterworth-Heinemann, Oxford

General Optical Council (Contact Lens Qualification etc: Rules), Order of Council 1988

College of Optometrists Guidelines, 1997

Association of Optometrists Members' Handbook. 'Computerised records', current issue

Chapter 4

Consulting room procedures and equipment

4.1 Hygienic procedures to avoid cross-infection

Hygienic procedures within the consulting room are extremely important to avoid any risk of cross-infection between patients as well as between patient and practitioner.[1] Standard practice should include the following:

HAND WASHING BETWEEN PATIENTS

- For routine washing, use an antiseptic hand cleaner such as 4% chlorhexidine gluconate (e.g. Hibiscrub).
- After known contact with a source of infection, use an antibacterial hand cleaner such as 5% chlorhexidine in 70% isopropyl alcohol (e.g. Hibisol).

DISINFECTION OF TRIAL LENSES

- All trial lenses, hard and soft, must be routinely disinfected after use (*see* Section 4.3).

DISINFECTION OF INSTRUMENTATION

- Surfaces of ophthalmic instruments that come into direct contact with the patient, such as chin rests, forehead supports and trial frames should be routinely disinfected (e.g. with wipes containing 70% isopropyl alcohol). Worktops should be similarly treated.

TEMPORARY LENS CONTAINERS

- Containers for temporary storage of patients' lenses during examination should be clean and sterile. With the advent of disposable lenses, the plastic containers in which they are supplied can be kept by the practitioner for single use with future patients. Glass vials can be autoclaved for repeated use.

4.2 Solutions and drugs

Water

Sterile water may be used for rinsing hard lenses, and prior to their insertion with a suitable wetting solution. It should not be used with soft lenses because of the likelihood of hypotonic adhesion to the cornea (*see* Section 17.8).

Tap water should not be used with soft lenses because of the risk of contamination by micro-organisms, particularly *Pseudomonas* and *Acanthamoeba*[2] (*see* Section 29.1.1). For the same reason, it should not be used for rinsing lens cases, although the use of boiled water followed by air drying is acceptable.

Saline (0.9% sodium chloride BP)

Normal saline is extensively used in contact lens practice for a variety of applications:

- Ocular irrigation.
- Rinsing lenses prior to insertion.
- Rinsing and cleaning lenses after fitting.
- Heat disinfection of soft lenses and subsequent storage.
- Wet cells of instruments for soft lens verification.
- Wetting fluorescein strips.
- Rewetting soft lenses.

Practical advice

- For soft lenses, use unpreserved saline.
- For hard lenses, use either preserved or unpreserved. Avoid aerosols for insertion because of air bubbles trapped under the lens.

Proprietary solutions

A range of proprietary wetting, soaking and cleaning solutions is required for both hard and soft lenses (*see* Chapter 26).

STAINING AGENTS

Fluorescein sodium BP

Used in 1% or 2% solution or, more usually, as impregnated paper strips which can be stored indefinitely if kept dry. Cross-infection is avoided by using a different strip for each patient and, in some cases, for each eye.

Fluorescein is the main method of checking hard lens fitting. It makes the tear pattern visible either by means of ultraviolet fluorescence with a Burton lamp or with the cobalt filter of the slit lamp. Fluorescein is almost entirely washed out of the eye within an hour, but a saline rinse is recommended before soft lens re-insertion to avoid any risk of discolouration. It is an important diagnostic aid because it stains damaged living corneal tissue green and the conjunctiva yellow. Contrast with the slit lamp can be enhanced by a combination of filters. A Wratten yellow (6 or 12) is used for observation in conjunction with either the standard cobalt filter or a Wratten 47A blue placed in front of the light source.

Fluorescein is also used to assess dry eyes by evaluating the break-up time and prism height of the tears (*see* Section 5.6).

High molecular weight fluorescein (e.g. Fluoresoft and Fluorexon)

The molecular weight is sufficiently great to prevent immediate penetration into most soft lens materials, although care is still required with high water content lenses as there may be some uptake and discolouration. (NB. Do not subsequently disinfect with hydrogen peroxide since oxidation may well bind molecules of dye to the lens). The degree of fluorescence is less than with standard fluorescein so that a yellow filter is recommended for observation. High molecular weight fluorescein can be used to:

- Assess corneal integrity.
- Evaluate the fitting of soft lenses, or hard/soft combination lenses (*see* Section 32.2).
- Assess break-up time (BUT) and tear prism immediately prior to soft lenses fitting.

- Assess BUT and tear prism with soft lenses in situ.
- Locate axis markings of toric soft lenses.

Rose bengal 1%

Devitalized epithelial cells of the cornea and conjunctiva are stained bright red, indicating abnormal ocular conditions or skin disease. Rose bengal also stains mucus. It can cause mild discomfort if instilled directly into the eye, and takes several hours to absorb. A better technique is to use a cotton wool bud or impregnated paper strip.

Alcian blue

Stains mucus blue. Not generally used in contact lens practice as traces remain in the eye for too long, and rose bengal can be used for the same purpose.

TOPICAL ANAESTHETICS

Benoxinate 0.4%; amethocaine 0.5% and 1.0%

Primarily employed with scleral lenses prior to taking eye impressions. Occasionally used with hard lenses when fitting very sensitive eyes (e.g. keratoconus), where lid spasm prevents lens removal, and for special techniques such as orthokeratology (see Chapter 14). Anaesthetics tend to retard healing of the corneal epithelium, and in cases of trauma and overwear are used only in the presence of extreme pain.

ANTIMICROBIAL AGENTS

Chloramphenicol BP 0.5%

A prescription-only broad-spectrum antibiotic normally used in emergency as a prophylactic, ophthalmic anti-infective.

Brolene (0.1% propamidine isethionate)

Antibiotic with some efficacy against *Acanthamoeba*.[3] Available over the counter.

OTHER DRUGS

Sodium cromoglycate 2% (e.g. Opticrom, Broleze, Vividrin)

An anti-allergic, antihistaminic, over-the-counter preparation to reduce inflammation and mucus secretion. Used generally for a period of 28 days in the treatment of CLIPC to stop irritation, mucus production and growth of papillae. Generally effective in reducing symptoms but not always the size of papillae. Technically a hay fever remedy and not strictly available for optometric treatment. Gives better results in reducing papillae with atopic patients.

Adrenalin 1%

A conjunctival decongestant, often used after taking eye impressions.

Sodium bicarbonate 2%

Use to fill sealed scleral lenses on insertion and for ocular irrigation.

4.3 Trial lens disinfection

All trial lenses, hard and soft, must be thoroughly cleaned before use and properly disinfected after being worn.

Hard gas-permeable and PMMA lenses

After removal from the eye, hard lenses should be carefully cleaned and stored in a proprietary soaking solution. Low-powered PMMA lenses can be stored dry but require careful cleaning and rewetting before insertion.

Practical advice

Avoid very viscous solutions for storage. A lens left for any length of time can be extremely difficult to remove from the vial.

Soft lenses

It is essential that soft lenses are disinfected before use with another patient. A 'quarantine' area can be set aside for this purpose, and several disinfection methods are possible:

- Heat. Autoclaving in 0.9% saline in sealed vials is the safest method, but high temperature can adversely affect the life span of some high water content lenses. An alternative heat method is to use a microwave with the Micro Clens system (*see* Section 26.4.2).

- Preserved solutions are the most convenient method but may be unreliable against *Acanthamoeba*, fungi and yeasts. A minimum of 4–6 hours is required before lenses can be reused, and some patients are sensitive to the preservatives.

- Most two-step hydrogen peroxide systems are more efficient and require less time. The procedures, however, are complicated for routine trial lens storage.

- Chlorine tablets represent a convenient method in practice but demonstrate limited efficacy against fungi and *Acanthamoeba*. Some patients experience stinging with high water content lenses stored in vials too small to permit the correct concentration.

4.4 Other procedures

4.4.1 Professional cleaning and rejuvenation

GAS-PERMEABLE HARD AND PMMA LENSES

A modification unit is used to repolish hard lenses, recondition the lens surface and make other adjustments (see Section 29.6). There is also a Boston professional cleaner for laboratory or practitioner use.

SOFT LENSES

Magnetic stirrers incorporating a hotplate efficiently clean most soft lenses using oxidizing chemicals such as sodium perborate (see Section 26.4.5). Professional cleaning is now less often required with the advent of disposable lenses and frequent replacement schemes.

Ultrasonic devices are claimed to have a cleaning and disinfecting action with both soft and hard lenses, but have not achieved routine use. The same applies to methods employing ultraviolet irradiation.

4.4.2 Lens verification

The instruments for hard and soft lens verification are covered respectively in Sections 12.3 and 20.3.

Practical advice

- Use a projection magnifier in the consulting room both for lens checking and for demonstrating lens condition to the patient.
- Regularly clean and disinfect wet cells filled with saline since they are a potential source of contamination. Hydrogen peroxide is generally the best method, but for any particular instrument seek the manufacturer's advice to ensure that there is no risk of damage.

4.4.3 Ancillary items

The following ancillary items are frequently required during fitting:

- Soft-ended tweezers, a lens lift or a glass rod for removing soft lenses from their vials.
- A glass rod or muscle hook is also useful for removing a dislodged lens from the upper fornix.
- Suction holders for use with hard lenses.
- Clean lens mailers or disposable lens trays for temporary storage when lenses are removed from the eye during examination.
- Glass vials or lens cases for storage when lenses are retained for professional cleaning.
- A crimping device for resealing pharmaceutical lens vials.
- Small self-adhesive labels for identifying lenses temporarily stored in unmarked bottles.
- Miscellaneous items including facial rule, grease pencil, pupil gauge and pen torch.

4.5 Insertion and removal by the practitioner

Practical advice

- Ensure that the patient is as relaxed as possible.
- Avoid the patient actually seeing the lens approach.
- Ensure that both eyes remain open because of Bell's phenomenon.
- Keep the eyes still and slightly depressed by using a fixation target below eye level.
- The head and neck should lean firmly against a carefully positioned headrest.
- Stand to the side of the patient.
- Establish whether the lids are tight or loose, as this may influence the choice of method.
- With hard lenses, have a suction holder readily available for speedy removal in case of a bad reaction.

4.5.1 Hard gas-permeable and PMMA lenses

INSERTION

- The patient looks with both eyes either at a fixation target just below the horizontal or down at the floor.
- The upper lid is retracted.
- The lens is placed onto the cornea from above using either the forefinger or a suction holder.

With very tight-lidded patients and where fixation cannot be controlled:

- The patient looks to the extreme nasal position.
- The lens is placed onto the temporal sclera and slid gently across to the cornea.

Once the lens is in position, the patient is advised not to look up, but to half-close the eyes, looking down to minimize lid sensation.

REMOVAL

- The head is leaned firmly back into the headrest.

- The patient fixates straight ahead.
- The lens is ejected with pressure applied either at the top and bottom lid margins or at the outer canthus.
- Alternatively, the lens is removed from the cornea with a moistened suction holder.

4.5.2 Soft lenses

INSERTION

Soft lenses may be inserted either onto the temporal sclera and slid across or in the same way as hard lenses and placed directly onto the cornea.

Practical advice

- If placed on the cornea with an air bubble, lenses are unstable at the moment of insertion and can be expelled by an involuntary blink.
- Most lenses (except some ultrathin) self-centre onto the cornea.
- Place ultrathin lenses directly onto the cornea.
- In difficult cases, allow the lens to dry on the finger for 15–30 seconds to prevent it from turning inside out and to make it easier for the tear film to attract it onto the cornea.
- Partially fold lenses to cope with very small palpebral apertures.
- With high plus or aphakic lenses, because of the effect of gravity, it may be easier to insert the lenses over a flat mirror with the patient's head in a horizontal position.
- With difficult, tight-lidded patients, it is sometimes much easier to insert the left lens first, since the angle of approach is better for a right-handed practitioner.

Once the lens is correctly centred, the patient should notice only slight lid sensation. Any significant discomfort is probably due to a foreign body, either carried in with the lens or already present in the tear film and subsequently trapped. The lens should be removed, rinsed and reinserted. Mild discomfort, which patients may describe as stinging, is frequently cured by sliding the lens onto the temporal sclera with a circular motion and allowing it to recentre. Other, slightly more efficient, techniques are: (1) to slide the lens in the opposite direction to the discomfort; and (2) to displace the lens first temporally and then nasally to give complete excursion over the cornea.[4]

REMOVAL

Removal is effected by pinching from the eye after moving the lens onto the temporal or inferior sclera, or by applying lid pressure in a way similar to that for hard lenses.

Practical advice

- Hard lens 'scissors methods', using the lids, can be tried with soft lenses but do not always prove effective because of their softness and size, particularly if ultrathin.
- Because of osmotic imbalance, a lens may sometimes appear to stick to the cornea. The eye should be irrigated with 0.9% normal saline, and after a short while the lens may be drawn gently onto the sclera and removed.

References

1. Sheridan, M. (1987) Aids virus in tears. *Optician*, **193** (5083), 15
2. Buckley, R.J. (1991) Acanthamoeba in perspective. Guest Editorial. *Journal of the British Contact Lens Association*, **14**, 5–7
3. Ficker, L. (1988) Acanthamoeba keratitis – the quest for a better prognosis. *Eye*, **2** (Suppl), pp. s37–s45
4. McMonnies, C.W. (1997) The critical initial comfort of soft contact lenses. *Clinical and Experimental Optometry*, **80**, 53–58

Further reading

College of Optometrists Guidelines – *Cross-Infection Control in Optometric Practice*

Chapter 5

Preliminary considerations and examination

5.1 Discussion with the patient

It is important to discuss the various aspects of contact lenses at the first examination and assess potential suitability in relation to patient expectations, spectacle refraction, 'K' readings and slit lamp examination. The discussion, reinforced by introductory patient leaflets, should cover many other related aspects of lens wear and fitting:

- General health, including allergies, hay fever and systemic drugs.
- Ocular health, previous infections or surgery.
- Vision, nature of Rx, amblyopia.
- Previous contact lens history, success or failure.
- Reasons for contact lens wear.
- Types of lens currently available.
- Preconceived ideas and misconceptions.
- Outline of fitting procedures.
- What is required of the patient in terms of aftercare examinations, hygiene and proper use of solutions.
- Fees for both initial fitting and future aftercare.

5.2 Indications and contraindications

5.2.1 Advantages and disadvantages of contact lenses compared with spectacles

ADVANTAGES

- Wider field of view.

- Better for refractive anisometropia.
- Retinal image size almost normal with refractive ametropia (e.g. with aphakia, high minus).
- No unwanted prismatic effects with eye movements.
- Less convergence required by hyperopes for near vision.
- Avoid surface reflections.
- Minimal oblique or other aberrations.
- Cosmetically superior.
- More practical for sports.
- Avoid weather problems (rain, snow, fogging up).
- Provide good acuity for irregular corneas (keratoconus, trauma, and subsequent to refractive surgery).
- Therapeutic uses.
- Vocational uses.

DISADVANTAGES

- Time required for fitting and adaptation.
- Handling skills required by patient.
- Hygienic procedures and lens disinfection necessary.
- Wearing time may be limited.
- Range of useful tints limited.
- For binocular problems, only limited vertical prism possible.
- Greater convergence required by myopes for near vision.
- Lenses can be lost or broken.
- Problems with foreign bodies.
- Peripheral flare (especially at night).
- Deteriorate with use and age.
- Retinal image size disparity in axial anisometropia.
- Maintenance costs.
- Greater overall expense.

5.2.2 Indications and contraindications

INDICATIONS

There are many patients for whom contact lenses are not merely a matter of cosmetic choice, but the best means of providing a satisfactory visual correction.

Visual

- Anisometropia.
- High myopia.
- Aphakia.
- Irregular corneas, scarring, keratoconus, grafts.

Occupational

- Theatre, film and other stage performers.
- Armed forces.
- Professional sports.

Cosmetic

- To avoid spectacles.
- Change eye colour.
- Prosthetic lenses or shells.

Medical

- Therapeutic.
- Bandage.

Psychological

- Where the patient cannot accept wearing spectacles.

Other

- Sports.
- Physical inability to wear spectacles (e.g. allergy to frame materials, nasal problems).

CONTRAINDICATIONS

There are a great many factors that may be considered as contraindications. Few of them are absolute, but all must be carefully assessed prior to fitting.

Visual

- Low refractive errors (e.g. +1.00/−0.75, −0.25/−0.50).
- Correction required only for near vision.
- Acuity with lenses may be worse than with spectacles.
- Prism required horizontally or > 3 vertically.

Occupational

- Where legal constraints apply.

Cosmetic

- Where spectacles are better with a large-angle squint.
- Where spectacles hide facial disfigurement.
- Where a patient has previously been reconciled to a long-standing scarred eye.

Medical

- Active infection or pathology.
- Recurrent corneal erosions.
- Severe sinus or catarrhal problems.
- Allergies.
- Vernal catarrh.
- Diabetes (fragile epithelium).
- Anatomical (e.g. misshapen lid).

Psychological

- Cannot accept the idea of a lens on the eye.
- Cannot tolerate any level of discomfort.
- Unable to cope with insertion and removal.
- Total perfectionist.

Sensitivity

- Cornea too sensitive.
- Lids or lid margins too sensitive.

Dryness

- Poor volume or quality of tears.
- Poor blinking.
- Dry environment.
- Drug-induced (e.g. antihistamine).
- Work-induced (e.g. VDUs).

Environment

- Dust.
- Fumes.
- Dryness (central heating, air conditioning, aeroplanes).
- Altitude (low EOP).

5.3 Advantages and disadvantages of lens types

5.3.1 Soft lenses

ADVANTAGES

- Good initial comfort.
- Ease of adaptation.
- Natural facial expression and head posture.
- Long wearing times.
- Low incidence of oedema.
- Rare occurrence of overwear syndrome.
- Absence of spectacle blur.
- Maintenance of corneal sensitivity.
- Good for intermittent wear.
- Low incidence of photophobia and lacrimation.
- Low incidence of flare, even with large pupils.
- Few problems with foreign bodies.
- Low risk of loss.
- Good for sports.

DISADVANTAGES

- Astigmatism not corrected with spherical lenses.

- Variable vision.
- Near vision problems.
- Lens dehydration.
- Liable to damage.
- Deposits and lens ageing with conventional types.
- Disinfection and hygiene essential.
- Solutions allergies.
- Lens cleaning more difficult.
- Lens contamination.
- Limited life span.
- No modifications possible.
- Difficult to check.
- Corneal vascularization.
- Contact lens-induced papillary conjunctivitis (CLIPC).
- Expensive to maintain.

5.3.2 Hard gas-permeable lenses

ADVANTAGES

- Excellent visual acuity
- Correct corneal astigmatism.
- Variety of complex designs available.
- Ease of maintenance.
- Few solutions allergies.
- Few deposits.
- High oxygen permeabilities (*Dks*).
- Do not cover the entire cornea.
- Tear pump on blinking.
- Good long-term ocular response.
- Easy to check.
- Modifications possible.
- Lenses available in a range of tints.

DISADVANTAGES

- Initial discomfort.
- Precise fitting required.

- Foreign bodies.
- Risk of loss.
- Flare.
- 3 and 9 o'clock staining.
- Lens adhesion.
- Breakage and scratching.
- Greasing with some patients.
- Instability of some materials.

5.3.3 Polymethyl methacrylate (PMMA) lenses

PMMA lenses, despite their historical importance, are now rarely used as a first choice. They may be regarded as a little-fitted sub-group within the general category of hard lenses.

ADVANTAGES

- Inertness of material.
- Stability of material.
- Reproducibility
- Surface wettability.
- Quality of vision.
- Myopia control.
- Ease of manufacture.
- Ease of modification.
- Range of tints.
- Inexpensive.

DISADVANTAGES

- Slow adaptation.
- High incidence of oedema.
- Corneal distortion.
- Spectacle blur.
- Risk of overwear syndrome.
- Endothelial polymegathism.
- Severely reduced corneal sensitivity.

5.4 Visual considerations

CORNEAL AND RESIDUAL ASTIGMATISM

Two basic assumptions are made when assessing the potential success of patients with astigmatism:

1. Total ocular astigmatism = corneal astigmatism + lenticular astigmatism.
2. Most corneal astigmatism is transferred through a soft lens to its anterior surface.

Patients may therefore be divided into four groups at their initial examination by reference to spectacle correction and 'K' readings.

Spherical cornea with spherical refraction

Rx:	−3.00 DS	
'K':	7.85 mm along 180°	(43.00 D)
	7.85 mm along 90°	(43.00 D)

This is the ideal optical case for contact lens fitting. Vision should be equally good with either hard or soft lenses.

Spherical cornea with astigmatic refraction

Rx:	−2.00/−1.75 × 90	
'K':	7.85 mm along 180°	(43.00 D)
	7.90 mm along 90°	(42.75 D)

The astigmatism is almost entirely lenticular, so that the visual result is the same with either a hard or a soft lens. In either case, a front surface toric lens is required to correct the 1.50 D of residual astigmatism.

Toric cornea with astigmatic refraction

Rx:	−2.00/−1.75 × 180	
'K':	7.80 mm along 180°	(43.25 D)
	7.50 mm along 90°	(45.00 D)

All of the astigmatism is corneal. A spherical hard lens, which neutralizes 90% of corneal astigmatism, or a toric soft lens should therefore be fitted.

Toric cornea with spherical refraction

Rx: −3.00 D
'K':   7.80 mm along 180°   (43.25 D)
          7.50 mm along 90°   (45.00 D)

There is 1.75 D of with-the-rule corneal astigmatism together with an equivalent degree of against-the-rule lenticular astigmatism, giving a resultant spherical refraction. A hard lens form would neutralize the corneal but not the lenticular astigmatism. It would therefore leave a residual cylinder of −1.75 × 90. A soft lens should be used *because* it transfers all of the corneal astigmatism through to its front surface without optically neutralizing it.

General advice

Where there is an equal choice between fitting either a toric hard or toric soft, because of the much greater comfort it is generally better to fit a soft lens.

NEAR VISION

Near vision can often cause problems despite good distance acuity. There are several reasons,[1] the main ones being:

- Altered accommodation/convergence ratio.
- Low myopes who previously did not wear spectacles.
- Early presbyopes requiring greater accommodation with lenses compared with spectacles. Conversely, hypermetropes are usually delighted with improved near vision.

INTERMEDIATE VISION

Intermediate visual tasks such as VDU operation or painting can also cause problems. Particular difficulties occur with reading music, especially in dim illumination.

CONTRAST SENSITIVITY AND 'QUALITY OF VISION'

Contact lenses of all types do not always give the absolute stability of vision achieved with spectacles.[2] Variations may be due to either the lens or environmental factors. The 'quality of vision' is very much a subjective interpretation and does not necessarily correlate with Snellen acuity. This can be confirmed by marked differences in contrast sensitivity readings while visual acuity remains the same.[3]

MONOCULAR PATIENTS

Particular care is necessary when fitting essentially monocular patients. They are much more disturbed by factors such as lens mobility, flare, or unstable vision with toric and bifocal lenses.

Practical advice

- Stability of vision is often as important as acuity.
- Snellen acuity is not always a reliable guide to a patient's potential success. In some circumstances a good 6/9 may be more acceptable than a poor 6/6.
- Assess distance, near and intermediate vision separately in relation to work and visual requirements.
- Take particular care with monocular patients.

5.5 External eye examination

External examination prior to fitting is essential to allow the practitioner to:

- Confirm the normality of ocular tissues.
- Discover any condition that would preclude contact lens wear.
- Record for the future any other abnormality.
- Refer for medical treatment any active disease unrelated to contact lens considerations.

Most parts of the examination are carried out using the slit lamp (*see* Section 2.1.3), looking for any evidence of the following conditions.

CORNEA AND LIMBUS

- Vascularization or neovascularization.
- Staining.
- Desiccation.
- Infiltrates or other signs of previous infection.
- Scarring or opacification.
- Other signs of injury.
- Central thinning.
- Peripheral thinning (dellen).
- Pterygium.

BULBAR CONJUNCTIVA

- Injection.
- Desiccation.
- Pinguecula.
- Other irregularity.

LIDS

- Position and size of palpebral aperture.
- Lid tension.
- Irregularity of lid margins.
- Styes and cysts.
- Blepharitis.
- General condition of skin.
- Vesicles on lid margins.
- Patency of meibomian glands.
- Vernal conjunctivitis.
- Contact lens-induced papillary conjunctivitis (CLIPC).
- Concretions.
- Make-up on palpebral conjunctiva.

BLINKING

- Frequency.
- Completeness.

Practical advice

- Lid eversion to examine the tarsal plate and papillary conjunctiva is an essential preliminary.
- Most patients find it rather unpleasant.
- Eversion also gives clues to sensitivity and to how patients will react to having their eyes manipulated.
- Where eversion proves very difficult, it is often possible to examine sufficient of the papillary conjunctiva by instructing the patient to hold the head as far back as possible and look down. The upper lid is gently pulled away from the globe and the light from a pen torch directed towards the upper fornix.

5.6 Assessment of tears

Assessment of tears is an important part of the preliminary examination in order to:

- Predict potential success.
- Eliminate likely failures.
- Discover marginally dry eyes which would be adversely affected by a contact lens.
- Decide on the most appropriate lens type.

There are several ways of assessing the tears. Each has its own limitations depending upon factors such as temperature, humidity and whether the method is invasive or non-invasive.[4]

5.6.1 Assessment of the tear volume

TEAR PRISM OBSERVATION

The upper and lower tear prisms hold 90% of the tears, so that the height and width give a reasonable assessment of tear volume. Reduce the height of the slit lamp beam and adjust it to the horizontal position. The width value can then be used as a measurement guide for the height of the tear prism.

- Slit lamp observation either with or without fluorescein gives an overall view of the entire prism.
- The approximate height of the prism in a normal tear film is 0.2–0.4 mm at the centre and 0.1–0.2 mm at the periphery.[5]

- Reduced height suggests reduced tear volume.
- Increased height could indicate poor drainage because of obstructed puncta or an excessive aqueous layer giving a watery tear film.
- The regularity of the prism along the length of the lid margins indicates the potential of the film to wet the eye consistently. This reduces with age.
- Frothing of the tears within the prism indicates lipid contamination, probably due to meibomian gland dysfunction.

Practical advice

- Measurement of the prism is largely an estimate based on experience.
- To gain this experience, routinely observe all patients to get used to the norm. Initially, aim to recognize an obviously defective prism of half normal height and subsequently refine observation to three-quarters of normal. The value in millimetres is less important than the departure from normal.
- Insertion of fluorescein destabilizes the tear film and can increase the height of the prism.

SCHIRMER TEST

This is a quantitative test of tear production which uses strips of Whatman no. 1 filter paper with notched ends 5 mm wide (Figure 5.1).

The notched end is folded twice to give better balance on the lower lid and placed against the bulbar conjunctiva near the outer

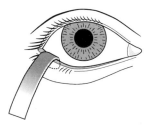

Figure 5.1 Schirmer tear production test

canthus. The eye looks up and in, to avoid contact with the cornea. The lower lid is released to retain the folded part in place. The remainder of the strip projects at right-angles from the lid.

The result is recorded either as the length of paper moistened in 5 minutes (normal = 15 mm) or the time taken to wet a length of 10 mm (normal = 3 minutes).

Practical advice

- The invasive nature of the strip causes reflex tearing.
- The results do not necessarily represent the patient's norm, but do indicate the presence or absence of reflex lacrimation.
- The result is quantitative and can be recorded for future comparison.

PHENOL RED THREAD

The test consists of a cotton, two-ply thread impregnated with phenol red phenolsulphonphthaloin). The thread is pH-sensitive and changes from yellow to red as it is wetted by the tears.[6] The normal result gives 10–20 mm moistened in 15 seconds.

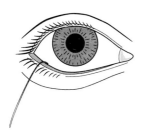

Figure 5.2 Phenol red thread

5.6.2 Tear film stability

INVASIVE TEAR BREAK-UP TIME

The tear break-up time (BUT) is the time in seconds for the breakup of the precorneal tear film in a non-blinking eye. It is a convenient and simple test to perform, but its invasive nature requires careful interpretation of the results.

A drop of fluorescein is instilled into the eye. The slit lamp with blue light is used to observe the patient after a few blinks have mixed the fluorescein completely into the tear film. The patient stares while a wide blue beam is focused onto the cornea. The time is recorded for the first break in the tear film, shown as a dark blue patch against the otherwise green background of fluorescein.

A normal result gives a BUT of 15 seconds or greater.

Practical advice

- If 15 seconds elapse with no break in the tear film, ask the patient to relax since the tear film is well within normal limits and the test can become uncomfortable after about 20 seconds.
- The position of the first break is often significant, especially if it corresponds to an area of staining or occurs at the lower limbus, since it suggests potential problems of desiccation.
- A supplementary test, possibly of even greater value, is to observe the relaxed patient blinking normally to determine whether the tear film breaks up between blinks or remains unbroken until the next blink.
- The use of fluorescein destabilizes the tear film and can give erroneous results.
- The temperature and humidity of the consulting room can affect the result.
- Only a large variation in results (5–10 seconds) is significant.

NON-INVASIVE TEAR BREAK-UP TIME

Non-invasive break-up time (NIBUT) methods measure the stability of the tear film without a staining agent. Most only show tear thinning rather than a true break in the tear film.

- One position keratometer with circular mires (e.g. Bausch & Lomb). The time is recorded when distortion is first seen in any part of the mire pattern. The three mires cover only a very limited amount of the central 3.00 mm of corneal surface, making this a rather inaccurate method.
- Hir-Cal grid. An extension of the above technique using a circular grid set within the Bausch & Lomb keratometer.[7] Observation is still made only of the central corneal cap so that the first signs of break-up may be missed if they occur in the periphery.

- Loveridge grid. A modification of the Klein keratoscope (*see* Section 2.5) with a fine grid pattern and +22.00 D observation lens. A convenient hand-held method with inbuilt stopwatch.[8]
- Tearscope. Uses a cold cathode ring light source[9] (*see* Section 5.6.3). Observation of the reflected light will show a true NIBUT, the norm being about 40 seconds.

5.6.3 Tear film analysis

SLIT LAMP TECHNIQUES

- Specular reflection. Observes the bright zone of specular reflection with the slit lamp (*see* Section 2.1.3). Allows debris in the tears to show up as dark spots which move on blinking.
- Narrow-field specular reflection. The first Purkinje image, seen with reduced slit lamp illumination, appears either plain or enhanced with coloured fringes. It gives a relative estimate of tear film thickness and can indicate contamination of the lipid layer. Coloured fringes alone are difficult to assess, but when found together with irregularity of the tear prism, they strongly suggest a poor teal film.

KEELER TEARSCOPE-PLUS

The original Tearscope was devised to make use of specular observation of the tear film over the entire cornea. The Tearscope-Plus has been redesigned with a range of inserts for more extensive tear film and ocular surface imaging.[10] These include:

- Concentric rings for Placido disc type observation.
- A coarse grid for hand-held observation.
- A fine grid insert for tear film observation and NIBUT using the slit lamp.
- Blue and yellow filters for fluorescein observation (*see* Section 2.1.3).
- Dark field observation of contact lenses. Made possible by limiting the effect of retro-illumination within the observation system.

The illumination source of the Tearscope-Plus is a double concentric, cold cathode light. The design positions the light away from the corneal surface eliminating heat transfer and avoiding tear evaporation.

Other observations can be made for the pre-ocular tear film (POTF):

- Lipid layer contamination and classification.
- Lipid layer spread during blinking.
- Tear prism classification for regularity.
- Tear prism continuity in the corneal and conjunctival area.
- Measurement of NIBUT with or without a grid.
- Meibomian gland manipulation and observation of lipid secretion spreading over the tear surface.

Only the lipid layer is visible by specular reflection. As it thickens, a pattern of flowing lipids appears. An amorphous pattern (i.e. devoid of detail) is seen with increased thickness. The ideal picture appears without coloured patterns. These are produced by interference and relate to abnormal clumps and irregularity in the thickness of the lipid layer. If the aqueous layer is observed, it will be seen as a dark grey surface where the lipid layer has broken (Table 5.1).[11]

Table 5.1 Description of the appearance and the approximate thickness of the lipid layer patterns (with abbreviations) observed by specular reflection with the Tearscope

Lipid layer pattern	Code	Appearance	Estimated thickness (nm)
Absent	Abs	No lipid layer visible	<10
Open meshwork marmoreal	M(o)	Indistinct, grey, marble-like pattern, frequently visible only by the postblink movement	10–20
Closed meshwork marmoreal	M(c)	Well defined, grey, marble-like pattern with a tight meshwork	20–40
Flow	F	Constantly changing, wave-like pattern	30–90
Amorphous	A	Blue-whitish appearance with no discernible features	80–90
Normal coloured fringes	CF(n)	Appearance of coloured interference fringes	>100
Abnormal coloured fringes	CF(ab)	Discrete areas of highly variable coloured fringes. These change rapidly in colour over a small area	Variable

Similar observations can be made on contact lenses for the pre-lens tear film (PLTF):

- Lipid layer when present.
- Coloured interference fringes of the aqueous layer.
- NIBUT.
- Surface contamination.

For soft lens wearers, the most common use of the Tearscope-Plus is the early detection of dry-eyed patients. This in turn can be used to suggest the optimum frequency of replacement for disposable lenses. With dry eyes, the lipid layer may be absent and the thin aqueous layer will display coloured fringes with surface contamination and a reduced NIBUT.

With hard gas-permeable lenses the lipid layer rapidly disappears. The aqueous layer consequently thins, showing a coloured fringe distribution over the lens surface. The NIBUT recorded when the tear film is seen breaking is typically about 5 seconds.

The non-invasive drying-up time (NIDUT) is recorded when the coloured fringes have all disappeared, on average at about 20 seconds. At this point, the surface is devoid of tears.

STAINING AGENTS (see Section 4.2)

Fluorescein

Fluorescein staining in the horizontal or inferior sectors of the cornea is an indication of tear film dehydration. Staining of the conjunctiva will also be seen at the nasal and temporal positions and in the region of any elevated tissue.

Under normal conditions, fluorescein blends immediately with the tear film. If there is poor mixing, the tear prism and any conjunctival staining may both present a dull orange hue. This effect is often unilateral, and with time the colour changes to the more usual bright fluorescein green.

Rose bengal

Rose bengal can be used to assess the severity of any staining and help decide on the future management of the patient. Any significant uptake of the dye prior to fitting suggests that it is unwise to proceed with contact lenses.

PATIENT QUESTIONNAIRE ON DRY EYES

Screening with the aid of a questionnaire prior to contact lens fitting can give valuable information in assessing a marginally dry-eyed patient. Questionnaires have been published by McMonnies[12] and, in a modified version, by Biocompatibles Ltd. The topics covered are:

- Symptoms experienced and extent of problems.
- Atmospheric conditions that make the eyes sensitive.
- Effects of alcohol.
- Medication taken (e.g. hormone-replacement therapy, antihistamines, tranquillizers).
- Presence of systemic conditions with dry eye side effects.
- Reports of dryness in other parts of the body.
- Sleep-induced problems.

5.7 Patient suitability for lens types

The majority of patients are now fitted with either hard or soft lenses. PMMA, scleral or other lens forms are needed only occasionally. It is often immediately obvious from the preliminary examination and discussion which type is likely to be more suitable. Many patients can be successful with either hard or soft lenses, but it is quite often necessary actually to use trial lenses of each type in order to evaluate lens performance on the eye.

5.7.1 Hard gas-permeable lenses

Hard gas-permeable lenses are the likely first choice in the following cases:

NEW PATIENTS

- Soft trial lenses give unsatisfactory vision.
- Significant corneal astigmatism is present (> 1.00 D).
- Corneal irregularity is present.
- Dry eyes have been diagnosed.
- An extremely high Dk is required.
- VDUs are used full-time.
- Dry geographic or working environment.
- There is a history of hay fever, vernal conjunctivitis or giant papillary conjunctivitis prior to fitting.

- The appearance of the limbal vessels prior to fitting suggests that vascularization is a likely consequence with soft lenses.
- Patients are unlikely to comply with soft lens disinfection.
- Handling difficulties are likely with soft lenses (e.g. low myopes with ultra-thin lenses; very small palpebral apertures).
- Lenses are likely to require future power modification.

REFITS OR PREVIOUS FAILURES

Where soft lenses have failed because of:

- Poor vision.
- Poor comfort.
- Dry eyes.
- Poor centration or fitting.
- Poor handling or repeated breakage.
- Corneal vascularization.
- CLIPC
- Repeated infections.
- Unacceptably short life span with conventional lenses.
- Frequent deposits.
- Solutions allergies.
- Materials allergy.

5.7.2 Soft lenses

Soft lenses are the likely first choice in the following cases:

NEW PATIENTS

- Hard trial lenses give unsatisfactory comfort because the lids or cornea are obviously too sensitive.
- Hard trial lenses give poor centration.
- The *Rx* is spherical and hypermetropic.
- The *Rx* is spherical with astigmatic 'K' readings (*see* Section 5.4).
- The pupils are very large or decentred.
- Rapid adaptation is required.

- An irregular wearing schedule is expected.
- Where there is poor or incomplete blinking prior to fitting.
- Older patients.
- There are awkward anatomical features likely to give poor hard lens positioning (e.g. low lower lid; proptosed eyes; decentred corneal apex).
- Dusty geographic or working environment.
- Patients need the security of a lens which it is almost impossible to dislodge from the eye (e.g. professional sports use).

REFITS OR PREVIOUS FAILURES

Where hard lenses have failed because of:

- Poor comfort.
- Poor vision.
- Flare and reflections.
- Poor centration.
- Oedema.
- Poor blinking.
- 3 and 9 o'clock staining or vascularization.
- Other persistent corneal staining.
- Persistent conjunctival injection.
- Poor handling or repeated loss.

References

1. Stone, J. (1967) Near vision difficulties in non-presbyopic corneal lens wearers. *Contact Lens Journal*, **1**, 14–16
2. Guillon, M., Lydon, D.P.M. and Wilson, C. (1983) Variations in contrast sensitivity function with spectacles and contact lenses. *Journal of the British Contact Lens Association*, **6**, 120–124
3. Applegate. R.A. and Massof, R.W. (1975) Changes in the contrast sensitivity function induced by contact lens wear. *American Journal of Optometry*, **52**, 840–846
4. Craig, J. and Blades, K. (1997) Preocular tear film assessment. *Optician*, Part I **213** (5588), 15–21, Part II **213** (5596), 20–27
5. Osbourne, G., Zantos, S., Robboy, M., Medici, L. and Petrzala, ?. (1989) Evaluation of tear meniscus heights on marginal dry eye soft lens wearers. *Investigative Ophthalmology and Visual Science*, **30** (Suppl), 501
6. Hamano, H. and Kaufman, H.E. (1987) *The Physiology of the Cornea and Contact Lens Applications.* Churchill Livingstone, New York
7. Hirji, N., Patel, S. and Callender, M. (1989) Human tear film pre-rupture

phase time (TP-RPT) – A non-invasive technique for evaluating the pre-corneal tear film using a novel keratometer mire. *Ophthalmic and Physiological Optics*, **9**, 139 -142

8. Loveridge, R. (1993) Breaking up is hard to do? *Optometry Today*, Nov 15, 18–24
9. Guillon, J.-P. (1986) Observing and photographing the pre corneal and pre lens tear film. *Contax* (Nov), 15–22
10. Guillon, J.-P. (1997) The Keeler Tearscope-Plus – an improved device for assessing the tear film. *Optician*, **213** (5594), 66–72
11. Craig, J.P. and Tomlinson, A. (1997) Importance of the lipid layer in human tear film stability and evaporation. *Optometry and Vision Science*, **74**(1) 8–13
12. McMonnies, C.W. and Ho, A. (1987) Patient history in screening for dry eye conditions. *Journal of American Optometric Association*, **58**, 296–301

Chapter 6

Lens types and materials

6.1 Hard gas-permeable lenses

Gas-permeable hard lens materials are given the suffix *-focon* and classified according to the chemical groups shown in Table 6.1.[1]

Hard gas-permeable lenses are therefore available in a wide range of materials and *Dk*s. Oxygen considerations, however, must take into account:

- The barrier effect, which reduces the *Dk* on the eye to approximately 55% of that measured in air in the gas/gas situation.[2]
- Centre and average lens thickness.[3,4]

Table 6.1 Chemical Group classification of hard lens (focon) materials (By courtesy of the Association of Contact Lens Manufacturers)

Group 1a
Essentially pure polymethyl methacrylate (99.0%). *Dk* essentially zero

Group 1b
Copolymers of PMMA with not more than 10% max. of other monomers that may alter hardness, wettability and stability. *Dk* essentially zero

Group 2a
Essentially pure cellulose acetate butyrate (90%). *Dk* range typically of 2–8

Group 2b
Copolymers of mixtures of cellulose acetate butyrate and other monomers.

Group 3
Copolymers of one or more alkyl methacrylates with one or more siloxanylmethacrylates, plus other water active monomers and cross-linking agents. Typical *Dk* of more than 6

Group 4
Hard lens material formed from polysiloxanes

Group 5
Copolymers of one or more alkyl methacrylates and/or siloxanylmethacrylates, plus other water active monomers, cross-linking agents, and at least 5% by weight of a fluoroalkyl methacrylate or other fluorine containing monomers. Typical *Dk* of more than 20

For physiological reasons, lenses should be as thin as possible, although in practical terms making them too thin is counter-productive since they are very likely to distort throughout the power range and also become too brittle. In most cases, a realistic minimum centre thickness is 0.14 mm, even for high minus powers.

Although *Dk* is important, there are several other considerations which affect comfort, vision and life span. These include:

- Surface wetting properties.
- Lens design.
- Fitting method.
- Manufacturing technique.
- Mechanical stability.
- Optical quality.

6.1.1 Cellulose acetate butyrate

Cellulose acetate butyrate (CAB) was one of the first non-PMMA materials, introduced in 1977. By modern standards, its *Dk* (between 4 and 8×10^{-11}) is low, and it is now fitted infrequently. Its main difficulty when manufactured by traditional lathing methods is dimensional instability. However, when manufactured by moulding, this problem was largely overcome, and lenses such as Conflex and Persecon E have given very good clinical results.

ADVANTAGES OF CAB

- Good wettability.
- Relatively inert.
- Does not attract protein.
- Low breakage rate.
- Very low incidence of CLIPC.
- Relatively good for 3 and 9 o'clock staining.

DISADVANTAGES OF CAB

- Low *Dk*.
- Moulding necessary for dimensional stability.

- Limited range of lens designs.
- Scratches easily.
- Attracts lipids from the tears.
- Corneal adhesion in some cases.
- Lens flexure and distortion on toric corneas with tight lids.

Practical advice

CAB can be very useful as a problem solver:
- With CLIPC, where contact lens wear can generally be maintained while the condition resolves.
- Where other materials with different wetting properties cause severe 3 and 9 o'clock staining.

6.1.2 Silicon acrylates (siloxanes)

Silicon acrylates are copolymers in varying proportions of acrylate (PMMA), which provides lens rigidity, and silicon, which controls the degree of oxygen permeability. Also included are cross-linking agents to improve the strength of the material and wetting agents such as methacrylic acid to improve the naturally hydrophobic properties of silicon. A good range of materials is now available with widely different physical properties and Dk values (Table 6.2). They give a superior oxygen and physiological performance compared with CAB and most have stood the test of time in terms of dimensional stability and optical and mechanical results. They are routinely fitted for daily wear and to a limited degree have been used for extended wear.

Table 6.2 Silicon acrylates

Lens	Dk at 35°C
Polycon II	12
Boston II	15
Paraperm O2	15
Boston IV	26.7
Dk43	43
Paraperm EW	56

ADVANTAGES OF SILICON ACRYLATES

- Wide range of materials available.
- Wide range of designs with practitioner control.
- Low to medium *Dk*s available.
- Good dimensional stability.
- Good vision with limited lens flexure.
- Good scratch resistance.

DISADVANTAGES OF SILICON ACRYLATES

- Attract protein from the tears.
- Some materials are brittle with a breakage problem.
- High incidence of 3 and 9 o'clock staining.
- Some incidence of CLIPC.

6.1.3 Fluorosilicon acrylates

Fluorosilicon acrylates (sometimes loosely described as *fluoro-carbons*) are composed of fluoromonomers and siloxy acrylate

Table 6.3 Fluorosilicon acrylates

Lens	Dk at 35°C
Fluoroperm 30 (Fluorocon 30)	30
Boston ES	31
Fluoroperm 60 (Fluorocon 60)	65
Equalens	71
Fluoroperm 90	95
Quantum	92
Boston 7	73
Equalens 125	125
Aquila	143
Fluoroperm 151	151
Optacryl F	160
Quantum 2	210

monomers. The addition of fluorine atoms to replace some of the hydrogen present in methacrylate monomers improves surface wettability, tear film stability and deposit resistance[5] as well as increasing oxygen permeability. The solubility of oxygen in fluoro-materials is enhanced and so higher Dks can be achieved (Table 6.3). Alternatively, moderate Dks can be achieved with a lower siloxy acrylate content and hence provide improved wettability. The silicon content ranges from 5–7% with Boston 7 to 16–18% with Fluoroperm 90.

ADVANTAGES OF FLUOROSILICON ACRYLATES

- Very high Dks possible.
- Suitable for flexible extended wear.
- Better wettability.
- Fewer deposit problems.
- Lower incidence of CLIPC.
- Easy to modify.

DISADVANTAGES OF FLUOROSILICON ACRYLATES

- Brittle if too thin.
- Require careful manufacture.
- Dimensional stability depends on material and manufacture.
- Corneal adhesion in some cases.

General advice

- Fluorosilicon acrylates are suitable for almost all straightforward patients and resolve many of the problems found with lower Dk materials. They have also proved suitable for flexible extended wear.
- Silicon acrylates are also suitable for most straightforward patients and give good dimensional stability. They are suitable for normal daily wear and for most problem solving with the exception of CLIPC. They are feasible but not ideal for flexible extended wear.
- CAB lenses are suitable where a low Dk is sufficient, and where CLIPC and 3 and 9 o'clock staining are a problem with other materials.

6.1.4 Fluoropolymers

Fluoropolymers contain no silicon and have a fluorine content of up to 50% by weight, several times that incorporated into fluorosilicon acrylates. They have so far found limited application despite their high Dk, good surface wettability, good deposit resistance and lack of brittleness. These advantages have been outweighed by problems associated with lens flexure, high specific gravity and cost.

6.1.5 Soft-coated gas-permeable hard lenses

Silicon acrylate lenses with an improved hydrophilic surface are sometimes used to assist initial comfort, surface wettability and deposit resistance.

The Novalens (Ocutec) has a Dk of 55×10^{-11} and a 'soft' coating of OH groups which gives the surface characteristics of a hydrophilic lens. The lens itself does not absorb water but has good wettability and improved comfort.

Aquaperm (Nissel) and Aquasil (No. 7) have a Dk of 50 and a surface containing OH groups similar to HEMA. The refractive index is 1.463 and water absorption less than 2%. Following manufacture by conventional methods, lenses are immersed for 120 minutes in a 10.6% solution of sulphuric acid which creates a surface layer of OH groups. These hydroxyl groups are permanently bonded to the polymer and are not reactive.

The Millennium Lens (Vista) is produced differently, by the polymeric grafting of hydrophilic polymers onto a fluorosilicon acrylate material with the surface covalently bonded to the entire lens surface.

Surface-treated lenses are fitted according to hard lens criteria and assessed in the normal way with fluorescein. They may be cleaned and soaked in nearly all conventional hard lens systems. Miraflow, which contains alcohol and aggressive cleaning solutions containing particulates (e.g. Boston cleaner), should be avoided.

6.2 Polymethyl methacrylate

Polymethyl methacrylate (PMMA) has been in use since the 1940s, firstly as a replacement for the earlier glass scleral lenses, and subsequently as the material of choice with the development of corneal lenses. There are many patients who have worn

PMMA successfully for 30 years and longer, although it has now largely fallen into disuse with the advent of modern hard lenses, by comparison with which its permeability is negligible. However, its original merits of inertness and stability mean that it may retain a place for very occasional new patients as well as a small minority of existing wearers. There are many long-standing patients who exhibit neither signs nor symptoms and are best left without refitting, although their corneas should be carefully monitored (*see also* Chapter 13).

6.2.1 Modified PMMA

Although PMMA has relatively good surface-wetting properties by comparison with many modern materials, various versions with modified surface properties (e.g. BPflex) were introduced in the mid-1970s. The improved wettability gave moderately better comfort, and the increased tear flow beneath the lens proved beneficial in reducing some of the oedema problems almost inevitable with an impermeable material like PMMA.

6.3 Soft lenses

Soft lenses are given the suffix *-filcon* and are classified according to the chemical groups shown in Table 6.4.[1] Lenses are generally discussed according to the interrelated properties of water content, Dk and material type.

WATER CONTENT AND UPTAKE

The definitions for water content and uptake are given in Section 1.3.2. Care must be exercised when interpreting brand names which include a numerical suffix because these do not always accurately reflect the true water content.

IONIC AND NON-IONIC POLYMERS

Polymers have also been categorized into four groups by the FDA, linking water content to ionic properties. It is a materials rather than a clinical classification and in this context, high water content is defined as greater than 50%. Ionic polymers contain more than 0.2% methacrylic acid and these high water content lenses may therefore contain the negatively charged carboxylic acid. The polymers are more sensitive both to temperature and

Table 6.4 Chemical Group classification of soft lens (filcon) materials (By courtesy of the Association of Contact Lens Manufacturers

---

Group 1a
Essentially pure 2-hydroxyethyl methacrylate (HEMA), containing not more than 0.2% weight of any ionizable chemical (e.g. methacrylic acid)

Group 1b
Essentially pure 2-hydroxyethyl methacrylate, containing more than 0.2% weight of any ionizable chemical

Group 2a
A copolymer of 2-hydroxyethyl methacrylate and/or other hydroxyalkyl methacrylates, dihydroxyalkylmethacrylates and alkyl methacrylates, but not more than 0.2% weight of any ionizable chemicals

Group 2b
As described in Group 2a, but containing more than 0.2% weight of any ionizable chemicals

Group 3a
A copolymer of 2–hydroxyethyl methacrylate with an N-vinyl lactam and/or an alkyl acrylamide, but containing not more than 0.2% weight of any ionizable chemicals

Group 3b
As described in Group 3a, but containing more than 0.2% weight of any ionizable chemicals

Group 4a
A copolymer of alkyl methacrylate and N-vinyl lactam and/or an alkyl acrylamide, but containing not more than 0.2% weight of any ionizable chemicals

Group 4b
As described in Group 4a, but containing more than 0.2% weight of any ionizable chemicals

Group 5
Soft lens materials formed from polysiloxanes

---

the composition of care products, so lens parameters show greater variability with environmental factors. The materials attract higher levels of deposit from the tears, particularly protein, and are generally more suitable for disposable lenses where life span is less important.

The four groups are:

1. Low water content, non-ionic polymers, including HEMA, but excluding those with methacrylic acid, e.g. Crofilcon (CSI), 38.5%, polymacon (B & L HEMA lenses), and Phemfilcon A (Durasoft 55). Materials generally show lower levels of protein deposit.

2. High water content, non-ionic polymers, e.g. Lidofilcon A (B & L 70%), Atlafilcon A (Excelens 64%), Surfilcon A (Permaflex 74%). Heat and sorbic acid should be avoided for disinfection because of the risk of lens discolouration.
3. Low water content, ionic polymers, e.g. Bufilcon A (Hydrocurve II, 45%). Lenses show moderate protein deposition.
4. High water content, ionic polymers, e.g. Etafilcon A (Acuvue, 58%), Perfilcon (Permalens, 71%), Vifilcon A (Focus, 55%). These polymers show the highest level of protein deposition and, as with group 2, heat and sorbic acid should be avoided for lens disinfection.

6.3.1 Clinical implications of soft lens water content

Hydrophilic lenses have been produced with water contents from 18% to 85%. However, many of the lenses currently being used are still HEMA-based in the region of 38–46%.

ADVANTAGES OF LOW WATER CONTENT LENSES

*   Greater tensile strength.
*   Less breakage.
*   Longer life span.
*   Smaller swell factor.
*   Better reproducibility.
*   Easier to manufacture.
*   Can be made thinner.
*   Less dehydration on the eye.
*   Less discolouration with age.
*   Fewer solutions problems.

DISADVANTAGES OF LOW WATER CONTENT LENSES

The disadvantages of low water content lenses relate mainly to their relatively low *Dk* values.

*   A greater tendency to cause corneal oedema.
*   A long-term tendency with thicker lenses to cause vascularization.

ADVANTAGES OF HIGH WATER CONTENT LENSES

Most high water content materials have *Dk*s between three and five times that of HEMA. Apart from their obvious application in oedema cases, they have several other advantages:

- Better comfort because of material softness.
- Faster adaptation.
- Longer wearing time.
- Extended wear.
- Easier to handle because of greater thickness.
- Better vision because of greater thickness.
- Better for intermittent wear.

DISADVANTAGES OF HIGH WATER CONTENT LENSES

Despite these good features, there are nevertheless disadvantages with conventional high water content lenses which preclude their use in some cases. These problems are less significant with disposable lenses.

- Shorter life span.
- Greater fragility.
- More deposits, especially white spots.
- More discolouration.
- Reproducibility less reliable.
- More difficult to manufacture by lathing.
- Greater variation with environment.
- Fitting requires longer settling time.
- Greater variability in vision.
- More solutions problems.
- Lens dehydration.
- Corneal desiccation.

6.3.2 Clinical implications of soft lens thickness

The typical centre thickness for a 'standard' corneal diameter HEMA lens of power –3.00 D is in the region of 0.10 mm–0.14 mm. Lenses below 0.10 mm may be regarded as thin; those below 0.07 mm as ultrathin and thinner than 0.05 mm as superthin or hyperthin. They represent a very satisfactory way of increasing transmissibility (Dk/t) and improving physiological performance as well as giving an inherent safety factor for patients who accidentally fall asleep while wearing their lenses. Low plus and aphakic lenses cannot truly be considered ultrathin because of their necessarily greater centre thickness. Nevertheless, 'thin' plus give a more satisfactory performance.

Oxygen performance for a lens cannot be judged solely in relation to its specified centre thickness but must be considered for the entire lens. If an 'average' or 'mean' thickness is used, this itself requires definition to avoid error and give valid comparison.[6]

ADVANTAGES OF THIN LENSES

- Lower incidence of oedema.
- Reduced lid sensation because of thinner edges.
- Reduced limbal irritation because of thinner edges and larger total diameter.
- Different fitting characteristic may provide better centration than standard lenses.
- Easier to fit because fewer fitting steps are necessary.
- Safer if patients accidentally fall asleep.

DISADVANTAGES OF THIN LENSES

- Handling is more difficult, especially in low minus powers below about –2.00 D.
- Higher breakage rate than standard thickness lenses.
- Life span is shorter, especially with heat disinfection.
- Visual acuity may be less good with toric corneas.
- Greater tendency to dehydrate on the eye and disturb pre-corneal tear film.

6.3.3 Dehydration of soft lenses

One of the main reasons for the clinical success or failure of a particular lens on the eye relates to its dehydration characteristics.

EFFECTS OF LENS DEHYDRATION

- Change in parameters and fitting.
- Reduction in comfort.
- Reduction in Dk.

- Disruption of tear film.
- Corneal desiccation and staining.
- Increased deposits.
- Reduction in vision.

FACTORS INFLUENCING LENS DEHYDRATION

Ocular factors

- Volume of tears.
- Quality and stability of tear film.
- Osmolarity of tears.
- Blinking habits.
- Size of palpebral aperture.

Other factors

- Lens material.
- Lens thickness.
- Temperature changes.
- Relative humidity.
- Drafts and wind.
- Systemic drugs.
- Alcohol.

The water content contained within the polymer matrix consists of *bound* water directly attached to hydrophilic sites by hydrogen bonding Van der Waals forces and *free* water, which is more readily lost by evaporation. The higher the bound water (e.g. with biocompatible polymers), the less any particular material will dehydrate on the eye.[7]

Generally, most water loss occurs within the first few minutes and high water content materials give greater dehydration. Tear film stability is better with thicker lenses and low water contents: it is worse with ultrathin and high water content lenses.

6.4 Biocompatible and biomimetic lenses

BIOCOMPATIBLE LENSES

Biocompatibility has been defined as 'the ability of a material to interface with a natural substance without provoking a biological response'. The advantages of biocompatible materials are their good physiological response with reduced evaporation of tears, corneal desiccation and deposits. Current lenses include Proclear and Vistagel PLUS.

The Proclear materials include phosphorylcholine (PC), a naturally occurring component in the cell membrane of red blood cells, which has a high affinity for water and is resistant to protein adsorption. Similar technology is used for intraocular lenses as well as cardiac, orthopaedic and other health care products. The range of contact lenses includes both conventional, manufactured by lathing, and disposable, produced by cast moulding.

Biomimesis is where the principles of the complex structure and chemistry of nature are emulated by much simpler scientific means, which nevertheless achieve the same results. The Vistagel PLUS material is based on the idea of biomimesis.

In its main features, Vistagel Plus is modelled on the structure of the cornea which experiences no deposit problems within the environment of the tears film. This logic was applied to the composition of the lens material. Two versions of Vistagel PLUS are available with water contents of 40% and 55%.

COLLAGEN LENSES

Collagen lenses are also produced from biological polymers and show good biocompatibility. Their main applications have been therapeutic. They dissolve after a number of days and are therefore never permanent.

6.5 Silicone lenses

6.5.1 Silicone rubber lenses (elastomers)[8,9]

Silicone lenses differ from hard lenses in several ways. They can be flexed, stretched and turned inside out. They have excellent elastic properties, partly conform to the shape of the cornea in wear, and have extremely high Dks in the region of 200×10^{-11}. They are also unlike hydrophilic lenses because their natural state is dry and they are extremely tough. Since they do not absorb water to any significant extent, fluorescein can be used in their fitting and they do not need disinfecting in the same way as soft lenses.

Because of the amorphous nature of the silicone rubber raw materials, lenses are produced by a moulding and vulcanization technique, which also assists in maintaining good reproducibility. The main difficulty with silicone is that its natural surface is extremely hydrophobic, and it has been necessary to devise methods of rendering the surface permanently hydrophilic without interfering with any of its optical or physical properties. The final stage of manufacture is therefore surface treatment by ion bombardment.

Because of the following advantages and disadvantages, silicone has remained very much a minority lens with limited therapeutic applications (*see* Section 32.3).

ADVANTAGES OF SILICONE LENSES

- Very high *Dk*.
- Better and more stable vision than many soft lenses.
- Little variation in comfort or fitting with environmental factors.
- Low risk of loss or damage.

DISADVANTAGES OF SILICONE LENSES

- Difficult to fit, requiring as much precision as hard lenses.
- A negative pressure effect producing lens adhesion, particularly if not correctly fitted.
- Breakdown in surface coating and difficulties with wetting.
- Build-up of deposits.
- Foreign bodies, especially with loose fittings.

6.5.2 Silicone resin lenses

Resin lenses differ from silicone elastomers because they are not flexible, having many of the physical properties of hard lenses. *Dk* values, however, are significantly lower than the elastomers and they have so far found only limited application.

References

1. Parker, J. (1990) The classification of contact lens materials. *Contact Lens Year Book 1990*. Medical and Scientific Publishing, Hythe, Kent, p.54
2. Holden, B.A., La Hood, D. and Sweeney, D.F. (1985) Does Dk/L measurement accurately predict overnight edema response? *American Journal of Physiological Optics*, **62**, 95P

3. Fatt, I. (1986) Some comments on methods used for measuring oxygen permeability (*Dk*) of contact lens materials. *Contact Lens Association of Ophthalmologists Journal*, **11**, 221–226
4. Brennan, N., Efron, N.A. and Holden, B.A. (1986) Oxygen transmissibility of hard gas permeable and hydrophilic contact lenses. *American Journal of Physiological Optics*, **63**, 4P
5. Fatt, I. (1985) A new look at fluoropolymers. *Optician*, **190** (5015), 25–26
6. Sammons, W.A. (1980) Contact lens thickness and all that. *Optician*, **180** (4467), 11–18
7. Hart, D.E. (1987) Surface interactions on hydrogel contact lenses: scanning electron microscopy (SEM). *Journal of the American Optometric Association*, **58**, 962–974
8. Hill, R.M. (1966) Effects of a silicone rubber contact lens on corneal respiration. *Journal of the American Optometric Association*, **37**, 1119–1121
9. Roth, H.W., Iwaski, W., Takayama, M. and Wada, C. (1980) Complications caused by silicone elastomer lenses in West Germany and Japan. *Contacto*, **24**, 28–36

Chapter 7

Principles of hard lens design

7.1 Basic principles of hard lens design

- Lenses may be spherical, aspheric or a combination of both.
- Most corneal lenses have a central zone which is fitted just apically clear or in alignment with the central cornea, combined with a much flatter peripheral zone which is designed to lift away from the cornea.
- Central alignment gives optimum acuity (*see* Section 9.6).
- Peripheral clearance is necessary for adequate tears exchange.
- The transition between the central portion and the periphery is sharp for a spherical bicurve design, becoming smoother as additional curves are added.
- Aspheric lenses have a much smoother transition and for some designs can be compared with very well-blended spherical multicurves (*see* Chapter 11).

7.2 Forces controlling design

Corneal lenses of all materials are affected by a variety of forces when placed on the eye. These factors are both ocular (*see* Chapter 5) and physical in nature.[1]

7.2.1 Centre of gravity

- The centre of gravity of a lens lies somewhere behind the back surface (Figure 7.1).
- It is affected by radius, diameter, thickness and power.
- Steep lenses have the centre of gravity further back than flat lenses and therefore give better centration (Figure 7.2a).

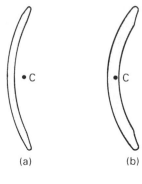

Figure 7.1 Centre of gravity (C) in (a) minus and (b) plus lenses

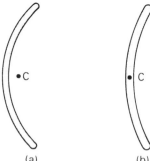

Figure 7.2 Centre of gravity (C) in (a) steep and (b) flat lenses

- Flat lenses have the centre of gravity further forward and give worse centration (Figure 7.2b).
- Large diameter lenses have the centre of gravity further back than small lenses and give better centration.
- Small lenses have the centre of gravity further forward and give worse centration.

7.2.2 Frictional forces

The viscosity of the tear film maintains the lens in a stationary position by means of frictional forces. Thinning of the tear film or an increase in its aqueous content (e.g. during adaptation) reduces the centration ability of these forces.

7.2.3 Capillary attraction

- The closer the lens matches the shape of the cornea, the greater the capillary attraction and stability.

- Since a hard lens cannot ever exactly match the shape of the cornea, a balance has to be found between sufficient capillary attraction for lens stability and sufficient movement for tears exchange.
- An excessively flat fitting gives less capillary attraction and greater movement.
- A steep fitting can create a negative pressure or suction effect.
- The tears meniscus at the edge of the lens also provides forces for centration. The greater the meniscus, the better the adhesion.

7.2.4 Specific gravity

- The clinical significance is demonstrated when two lenses of the same design (and volume) but different specific gravity behave differently on the eye. The lens with the lower specific gravity has less weight.
- A lens that drops because gravitational forces are greater than fluid forces may achieve better centration by using a material of lower specific gravity and vice versa.
- With prism ballast, a high specific gravity material is advantageous as it gives a greater difference in weight between the apex and base of the lens.

7.2.5 Thickness and lenticulation

Thickness depends on back vertex power (BVP), design and material. Centre thickness (t_c) and edge thickness (t_e) are both important (Tables 7.1 and 7.2).

Table 7.1 Typical thickness values assuming a constant TD = 9.60 and BOZD = 7.80 mm

BVP (D)	t_c (mm)	t_e (mm)
−10.00	0.13	0.25
−6.00	0.13	0.22
−3.00	0.15	0.20
−1.00	0.18	0.18
+1.00	0.22	0.12
+3.00	0.26	0.13
+6.00	0.34	0.15
+10.00	0.45	0.16

Table 7.2 Suggested minimum thicknesses for different materials (BVP –3.00 D)

Material	t_c (mm)	t_e (mm)
PMMA	0.10	0.12
CAB	0.16	0.12
Silicon acrylate	0.15	0.13
Fluorosiliconacrylate	0.14	0.15

- BVPs greater than –6.00 D or +4.00 D should be lenticulated to reduce excess thickness and mass.
- Lenticulation reduces thickness in the centre for plus and towards the edge for minus lenses by making the front optic zone diameter (FOZD) smaller (Figure 7.3).
- The FOZD should be approximately 0.50 mm larger than the back optic zone diameter (BOZD).

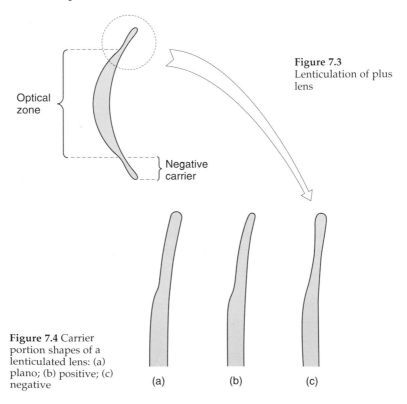

Figure 7.3 Lenticulation of plus lens

Figure 7.4 Carrier portion shapes of a lenticulated lens: (a) plano; (b) positive; (c) negative

(a)   (b)   (c)

- The carrier portion of a lenticulated lens can be plano, negative or positive in shape (Figure 7.4). The choice depends upon the intended effect (e.g. lid attachment techniques) (*see* Section 7.5).

Practical advice

- Do not order centre thickness less than 0.14 mm with most modern materials because of lens flexure, particularly with toric corneas and tight lids.
- Edge thickness should be a minimum of 0.12 mm. A 'knife edge' causes discomfort and is fragile, especially with plus lenses.
- Minus lenses usually give a natural lid attachment.
- A negative carrier helps give lid attachment with a low-riding or plus lens.
- A positive carrier helps reduce a high-riding tendency.

7.2.6 Refractive index of materials

The following are typical examples of refractive index:

PMMA:	1.49
CAB:	1.47
Silicon acrylate:	1.471–1.48
Fluorosiliconacrylate:	1.453–1.471
Silicone:	1.43

- The higher the refractive index, the thinner the lens can be made.
- Modern hard lenses have a lower refractive index than PMMA and are therefore thicker.
- High refractive index plastics are used for bifocal segments. They can incorporate fluorescent dye to assist fitting.
- The refractive index is important in toric lens fitting (*see* Chapter 22).

7.2.7 Edge shape

- Extremely important for comfort.
- Must be smooth and well finished.
- Should blend into the final peripheral curve.
- Can help lens removal.

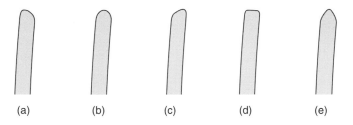

Figure 7.5 Edge shapes of lenses: (a) posterior; (b) central; (c) anterior; (d) blunt; (e) sharp

- Varying degrees of taper and roundness are used, depending on fitting philosophy (*see* Section 7.5) and lid sensitivity. Edges are described as (a) posterior, (b) central, (c) anterior, (d) blunt, and (e) sharp[2] (Figure 7.5).
- Edge thickness depends on BVP (*see* Section 7.2.5).

7.3 Concept of edge lift

The concept of edge lift is related to the lens design off the eye. It embodies the series of curves that lead into the edge shape. Edge lift can be specified in an axial or a radial direction.

Axial edge lift is defined as the distance between a point on the back surface of a lens at a specified diameter and the continuation of the back central optic zone, measured parallel to the lens axis[3] (Figure 7.6). The flatter the BOZR, the greater the degree of peripheral curve flattening that is required to maintain a particular edge lift.

Current lens designs are usually defined in respect of axial edge lift (AEL). Lenses are sometimes designed by deciding on

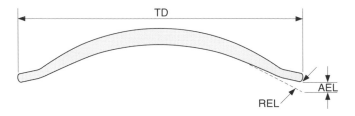

Figure 7.6 Axial edge lift (AEL) and radial edge lift (REL) in a rigid lens design (TD, total diameter)

the AEL required and calculating the peripheral curves needed. The edge lift of each individual curve contributes to the total figure.

Historically, the concept of edge lift has used a variety of terms:

- *Z value*, or axial edge lift.
- Constant axial edge lift (CAEL) (see section 8.3).
- *Z factor*, or radial edge lift.
- Flattening factor

The usual value of axial edge lift varies between 0.09 mm and 0.15 mm. If the same increase is given to the peripheral curves of both steep and flat lenses, the steep lens has, relatively, a greater edge lift.[4]

Example:

r   *r* + 0.5   *r* + 2.2   *r* + 4.7

8.40:7.00/8.90:8.00/10.60:8.50/13.10:9.00 AEL = 0.117 mm

7.20:7.00/7.70:8.00/9.40:8.50/ 11.90:9.00 AEL = 0.172 mm

CAEL lenses[4] are multicurves which for a given TD are designed to give the same AEL throughout the range of radii. The clinical appearance and performance are therefore consistent.

The Z factor[5] or radial edge lift (REL) is defined as the distance between a point on the back surface of the lens at a specified diameter and the continuation of the back central optic zone, measured along the radius of the latter (*see* Figure 7.6).

The ratio of axial to radial edge lift is approximately 5:4.

Example:

7.40:7.00/8.10:7.80/9.30:8.60/10.50:9.00

Taken from 0.15 mm CAEL trial set with a total diameter (TD) of 9.00 mm.[6]

AEL at 7.80 = 0.025; AEL at 8.60 = 0.095; AEL at 9.00 = 0.15
The designated value for the final peripheral curve

REL at 9.00 = 0.12   Ratio REL/AEL = 0.80

The flattening factor (ff) defines the extent to which the peripheral curve flattens in relation to the central radius in an offset lens (*see* Section 8.2).

There are two approaches to calculating the contribution of each peripheral curve of a given lens design:

BAND WIDTH METHOD

The band width method considers the edge lift at the edge of the intermediate curve.[7]

STEP-BY-STEP METHOD

The step-by-step method calculates the AEL of the mid-curve as the AEL produced as if the mid curve were extended out to the Total Diameter (TD) of the lens.

Compared with the band width approach, the step-by-step method produces a larger AEL for the mid-peripheral curve and a smaller AEL for the third curve.

For a tricurve, the mid-curve produces two-thirds of the AEL, with the third curve contributing one-third. For a tetracurve lens, the first peripheral curve provides half of the AEL, the second one-third, and the fourth one-sixth. The contribution of each curve is easily calculated with the aid of a computer program.

7.3.1 Concept of edge clearance

The term *edge clearance* relates to the lens on the eye and is estimated by the fluorescein pattern. The lens periphery must be fitted flatter than the cornea to:

- Provide tears exchange beneath the lens for the maintenance of corneal metabolism.
- Give a tears meniscus so that capillary attraction and lens centration forces can function (*see* Section 7.2).
- Assist lens removal by the lids.
- Avoid pressure and corneal insult at the lens edge.
- Avoid lens adhesion.

Too little edge clearance gives:

- Inadequate tears exchange
- Poor lens movement.
- Pressure at the lens edge and arcuate staining.
- Difficulty with lens removal.
- Lens adhesion.

Too much edge clearance gives:

- Excessive lens movement.

- Bubbles under the lens periphery which can cause frothing or dimpling.
- Poor centration.
- Lens displacement off the cornea.
- 3 and 9 o'clock staining because of tear film disruption.

Practical advice

· AEL relates to the lens design off the eye.
· Edge clearance relates to the lens on the eye.

7.4 Tear layer thickness

- Tear layer thickness (TLT) is the clearance between the back surface of the lens and the cornea, usually in respect of the central area (typical example, Figure 7.7).

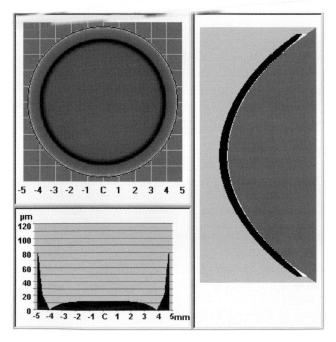

Figure 7.7 Tear layer profile

- The fitting technique and lens design govern the values for apical (and edge) clearance.
- TLT is expressed in microns (µm) (1 µm = 0.001 mm), whereas edge lift is given in millimetres and relates only to the physical dimensions of the lens.
- Fluorescein with a TLT of <20 µm cannot be seen with a Burton lamp.

TYPICAL VALUES[8]

Tear layer thickness = 5–10 µm
Edge clearance (EC) = 75–80 µm

7.5 Lid attachment lenses

Lid attachment (hitch-up) utilizes the edge contour and shape of the anterior peripheral surface of the lens to increase lid–lens adhesion.[9,10]

- Lid attachment occurs when the peripheral lens contour remains in constant contact with the upper lid margin after blinking or eye closure.
- The lens therefore moves with the upper lid and returns to a superior position on the cornea after blinking.
- Minus lenses give a natural lid attachment on most eyes because of their edge shape, but larger diameter lenses are often necessary (Figure 7.8).

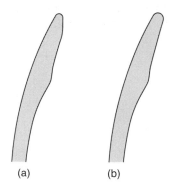

(a)   (b)

Figure 7.8 Korb edge contour (a), compared with a standard edge design (b)

- When the upper lid is in its normal position, its upward retention effect on the lens is greater than the downwards pull of gravity or the centration forces of the tears meniscus.
- Plus lenses give the reverse effect and tend to escape from lid retention because of their edge shape.
- The correct anterior lenticular construction is essential.

ADVANTAGES

- More comfortable.
- Helps maintain normal blinking.
- Counteracts low-riding lenses.
- Helps tears exchange on blinking.
- Lenses can be made thinner with high powers.
- Less 3 and 9 o'clock staining.

DISADVANTAGES

- Flare from lower edge of pupil
- Peripheral curves may need to be individually designed.
- Front surface may require complex construction.

7.6 Interpalpebral lenses

The technique aims to give good centration using very thin lenses with a total diameter smaller than the vertical palpebral aperture. It has mainly been applied to PMMA to improve the physiological performance and where thinner lenses can be more easily manufactured.

FITTING

TD: At least 2.00 mm larger than maximum pupil diameter, i.e. usually 7.50–8.50 mm.

BOZR: Up to 0.15 mm steeper than flattest 'K' to give the appearance of an alignment fit.

BOZD: 5.00–7.00 mm.

Example 1: 7.80:6.50/8.60:7.50/10.40:8.50 $t_c = 0.10$

Example 2: 7.80:7.00/10.50:8.00 $t_c = 0.08$

ADVANTAGES

- Better for narrow lid apertures.
- Less sensation with sensitive lids.
- Better for corneas with irregular periphery.
- Often successful with moderate or even highly toric corneas where a small lens may permit a spherical design.
- Less disturbance of corneal metabolism.
- Lens positions away from the limbus and may help with 3 and 9 o'clock staining or limbal disturbance.

DISADVANTAGES

- More difficult to manufacture because they must be made thinner.
- Difficult to handle.
- Difficult to remove.
- Fragile edges.
- Flare.
- Disincentive to blinking and may give increased 3 and 9 o'clock staining.

References

1. Hayashi, T.T. and Fatt, I. (1980) Forces retaining a contact lens on the eye between blinks. *American Journal of Optometry and Physiological Optics*, **57**, 485–507
2. La Hood, D. (1988) Edge shape and comfort of rigid lenses. *American Journal of Optometry and Physiological Optics*, **65** (8), 613–618
3. Bennett, A.G. (1968) Aspherical contact lens surfaces. *Ophthalmic Optician*, **8**, 1037–1040, 1297–1300, 1311, **9**, 222–230
4. Stone, J. (1975) Corneal lenses with constant axial edge lift. *Ophthalmic Optician*, **15**, 818–824
5. Hodd, F.A.B. (1966) A design study of the back surface of corneal contact lenses. *Ophthalmic Optician*, **6**, 1175–1178, 1187–1190, 1203, 1229–1232, 1235–1238, **7**, 14–16, 19–21, 39
6. Douthwaite, W.A. (1995) *Contact Lens Optics and Lens Design.* 2nd edition, Butterworth-Heinemann, Oxford
7. Rabbetts, R.B. (1993) Spreadsheet programs for contact lens back surface geometry. *Journal of the British Contact Lens Association*, **16**, 129–133
8. Atkinson, T.C.O. (1987) The development of the back surface design of rigid lenses. *Contax* (Nov), 5–18
9. Korb, D.R. and Korb, J.E. (1970) A new concept in contact lens design. *Journal of the American Optometric Association*, **41**, 1023
10. Mackie, I. (1973) Design compensation in corneal lens fitting. In *Symposium on Contact Lenses: Transactions of the New Orleans Academy of Ophthalmology*, Mosby, St. Louis

Chapter 8

Development of hard lens design

8.1 Introduction

The first PMMA corneal lens was designed in 1947.[1] It consisted of a single curve approximately 0.30 mm flatter than 'K' and a total diameter of about 11.00 mm. Limited practical success was achieved for physiological reasons. It was not until practitioners such as Bier in the early 1950s realized that the cornea was more complicated than a simple sphere, that a bicurve construction was introduced. Further improvements were made by adding a flatter, third curve to assist tear circulation. The complex elliptical shape of the cornea was more fully understood by the late 1960s and multicurve lenses evolved together with the first aspheric constructions.[2] Most designs were fitted as:

- Either central alignment or minimal clearance with peripheral clearance.

- Central clearance with peripheral alignment.

The following BSI/ISO terminology, abbreviations and symbols are used:

BOZR (r_0) = back optic zone radius

BOZD $(\varnothing_0)$ = back optic zone diameter

r_1 = first back peripheral radius

$\varnothing_1$ = first back peripheral zone diameter

r_2 = second back peripheral radius

TD$(\varnothing_T)$ = total diameter

In addition, 'K' is used to refer to flattest keratometry reading

8.2 Early lens designs

BIER CONTOUR TECHNIQUE

Developed in the UK by Bier in 1957.[3] A spherical bicurve design, fitted with apical alignment and peripheral clearance. Now rarely used except for refitting existing problem-free wearers.

BOZR = 'K' ± 0.10 mm

r_1 = BOZR + 0.40–0.80 mm

BOZD = 6.50–7.50 mm

TD   = 8.50–10.00 mm

Example: 7.80:6.80/8.60:9.65 –3.00 (Figure 8.1)

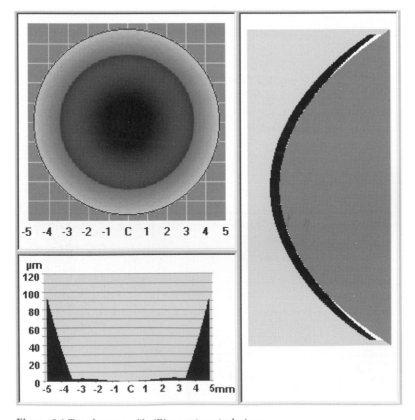

Figure 8.1 Tear layer profile/Bier contour technique

MODIFIED CONTOUR TECHNIQUE

A tricurve, modified version of the Bier contour technique. The fitting is central alignment with the first peripheral curve, giving some degree of corneal alignment; the final curve is small and flat. Occasionally used for refitting and where large edge lift is required with PMMA.

BOZR = 'K' ± 0.50 mm

r_1 = BOZR + 0.30–0.50 mm

r_2 = 9.50–12.50 mm, 0.20–0.40 mm wide

BOZD = 6.00–7.50 mm

TD   = 8.50–9.50 mm

Example: 7.80:6.50/8.30:9.10/12.25:9.50 –3.00 (Figure 8.2)

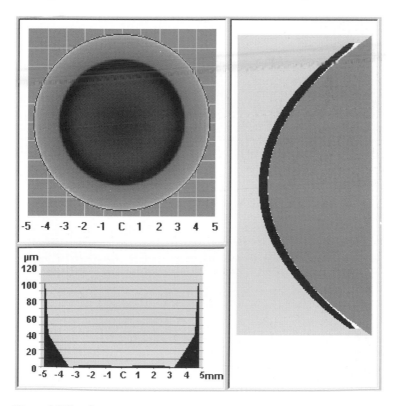

Figure 8.2 Tear layer profile/modified contour technique

BAYSHORE TECHNIQUE

Developed in the USA by Bayshore in 1962.[4] A small tricurve corneal lens, fitted to give central clearance and peripheral alignment. Occasionally used to give a tight interpalpebral fitting.

BOZR ='K' –0.30 mm

BOZD = 5.60–6.60 mm

TD   = 7.00–8.80 mm (0.20 mm less than the vertical palpebral aperture)

r_1 = BOZR + 1.00–1.50 mm (aligned with cornea)

r_2 = 17.00 mm, 0.10–0.30 mm wide

Fenestration = central, 0.20–0.25 mm in diameter

Example: 7.60:6.00/8.80:7.00/17.00:7.60 –3.00
            Single central fenestration, 0.20 mm

CONOID LENS

Developed in Australia by Thomas in 1967.[5] Fitted to give apical clearance, it has a spherical BOZR with a conical periphery commonly tangential to the BOZR.

Comfort is good because of reduced lid sensation, but gross corneal steepening and distortion occurs. Now only used for occasional refitting and where a very tight lens is required for centration.

BOZR   = 'K' –0.30 mm

BOZD   = 6.50 mm

TD   = 9.00 mm

Fenestration = 0.25 mm in diameter, 0.20 mm in from the lens edge, just within the optic zone.

PERCON LENS

Developed in Holland by Stek in 1969[6] and in the UK by Cantor in 1970.[7] It has a spherical BOZR and a conical peripheral zone with a constant axial lift of 0.10 mm. The cone angle is almost exactly tangential to give virtually no transition (see Offset lens, below). The fitting gives central alignment with peripheral clearance and is occasionally used to give large edge lift with PMMA.

BOZR   = 'K' + 0.05 mm

BOZD   = 6.60–7.20 mm (related to cone angle)

TD   = 8.60–9.40 mm

Cone angle = depends on both BOZR and TD

Example: 7.80:6.80/   9.00   Cone angle 130°

OFFSET LENS

Developed in the UK by Ruben in 1966.[8] The centre of curvature of the back peripheral curve is offset to the opposite side of the central axis, virtually eliminating any transition. It has been termed a *continuous bicurve lens*[2] or *contralateral offset* (Figure 8.3). A *homolateral offset* is also possible, where the centre of curvature of the peripheral curve is displaced to the same side of the central axis.

The degree of flattening is referred to as the *axial edge lift*, *Z value* or *flattening factor*. It is usually specified by the distance at the lens edge between the extension of the BOZR and the peripheral curve. The distance in millimetres is measured along a line parallel to the axis of symmetry.

Offset lenses give good comfort because of the minimal transition and are useful for early keratoconus and where large edge lift is required with PMMA. The small optic, however, gives flare and special offset lathes are required for manufacture.

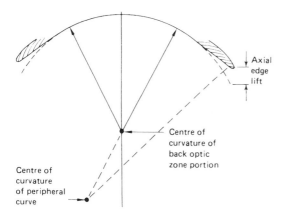

Figure 8.3 Contralateral offset or continuous bicurve lens (from Phillips and Speedwell, *Contact Lenses*, 4th edn, Butterworth-Heinemann, Oxford, by permission)

Offset No 1   BOZD: 6.00 mm   TD: 9.00 mm

Offset No 2   BOZD: 6.90 mm   TD: 10.00 mm

Offset No 3   BOZD: 5.50 mm   TD: 8.50 mm

The above all had a flattening factor (AEL) of 0.10 mm in low minus powers. Nowadays with new computer lathes the BOZD and AEL can both be varied.

Example: 7.00:6.00 AEL 0.1 at 9.00   −5.00

8.3 Current designs: bicurve, tricurve, multicurve

Corneal lenses are now designed with one or more peripheral zones which are deliberately intended to lift away from the cornea. Most modern spherical lenses are based on these designs.

Bicurve (C2)

Consists of a central radius and one flatter peripheral curve (Figure 8.4). There is a sharp transition between the two curves.

Examples: 7.80:7.00/8.70:9.00 (Figure 8.5)
7.80:7.80/10.50:9.00 (Figure 8.6)

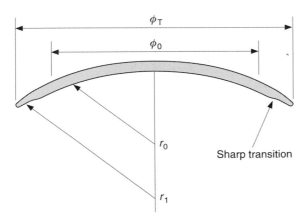

Figure 8.4 Bicurve corneal lens ($\varnothing_T$, total diameter; $\varnothing_0$, back optic zone diameter; r_0, back optic zone radius; r_1, first back peripheral radius)

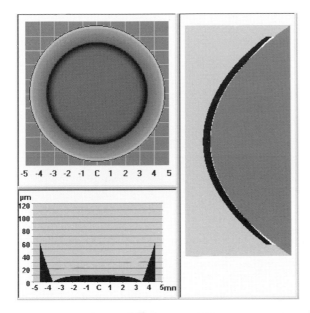

Figure 8.5 Tear layer profile/bicurve (C1)

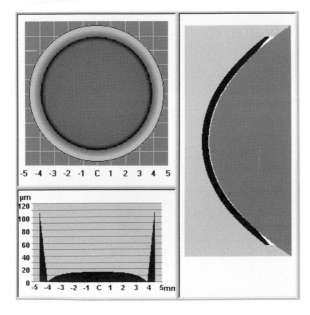

Figure 8.6 Tear layer profile/bicurve (C2)

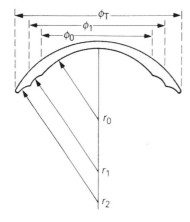

Figure 8.7 Tricurve corneal lens ($\varnothing_T$, total diameter; $\varnothing_1$, first back peripheral zone diameter; $\varnothing_0$, back optic zone diameter; r_0, back optic zone radius; r_1, first back peripheral radius; r_2, second back peripheral radius) (from Phillips and Stone, *Contact Lenses*, 3rd edn, Butterworth-Heinemann, Oxford, by permission)

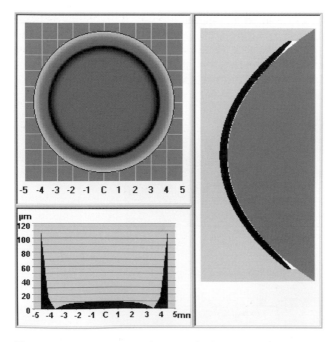

Figure 8.8 Tear layer profile/tricurve (C3)

TRICURVE (C3)

Consists of a central radius and two flatter peripheral curves (Figure 8.7). It is the basic design of most modern hard lenses, where the final curve is much flatter than first peripheral radius.

Example: 7.80:7.00/8.40:8.00/10.50:9.00 (Figure 8.8)

MULTICURVE

Consists of a central radius and three or more peripheral curves (Figure 8.9). It follows the flattening of cornea better than bicurves and tricurves, and when the transitions are well blended, behaves like a continuous curve lens.

Example: 7.80:7.00/8.40:7.90/8.90:8.80/11.25:9.30 (Figure 8.10)

CONSTANT AXIAL EDGE LIFT

CAEL lenses[9] (see Section 7.3) were developed as a further refinement of multicurve lens design to give a constant linear clearance between the edge of the lens and the cornea, over the whole range of radii for a given diameter. The axial edge lift of the peripheral curves is calculated to remain constant for all BOZRs, unlike conventional lenses where the calculated AEL is greater with steeper lenses than with flatter lenses.

N.B. AEL relates to the lens design off the eye.

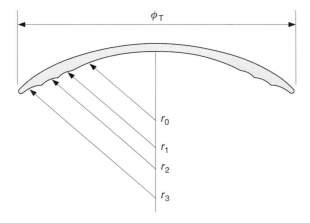

Figure 8.9 Multicurve corneal lens (r_3, third back peripheral radius; other symbols as in Figure 8.4)

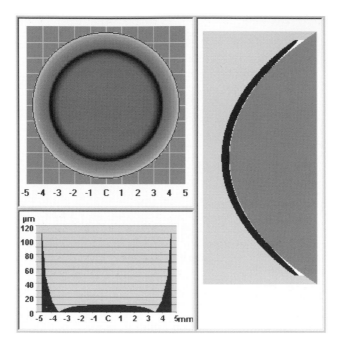

Figure 8.10 Tear layer profile/multicurve

Average CAEL for a TD of 8.60 mm ≡ 0.105 mm
Average CAEL for a TD of 9.20 mm ≡ 0.11 mm
Average CAEL for a TD of 9.60 mm ≡ 0.14 mm

8.4 Aspheric lenses

Aspheric lenses have one or both surfaces of a non-spherical construction. Aspherics usually take the form of a parabola, ellipse or hyperbola and are defined by eccentricity.

DEFINITIONS

Eccentricity (e):   Defines mathematically the departure of an aspheric curve from a circle. Used to describe both a lens form and the curvature of the cornea.

P value: Defines the rate of flattening with eccentricity: $p = 1 - e^2$.

The closest mathematical approximation to the topography of the human cornea is an ellipse. Mean eccentricity = 0.45; p = 0.8.

Circle: Completely symmetrical. Eccentricity = 0; p = 1.
Ellipse: Symmetrical about two axes, but has two diameters – one long and one short. Eccentricity = 0 < e < 1; p = < 1.
Parabola: Symmetrical about one axis. Eccentricity = 1; p = 0.
Hyperbola: Eccentricity > 1; p = <0.

8.4.1 Aspheric designs

NISSEL ASPHERIC

The Nissel design (1967)[10], now rarely used, was based on the US Volk lens. It had a central aspheric portion with a 7.80 mm diameter, two spherical zones at diameters of 8.40 mm and 8.80 mm, and an 0.50 mm wide bevel of radius 10.00–12.00 mm to assist tear flow. It was fitted 0.10 mm steeper than 'K' to give central alignment with the appearance of a multicurve.

CONFLEX (WOHLK, 1982)

Moulded from Anduran material (CAB + ethyl vinyl acetate), this lens[11] consists of a spherical optic with three aspheric peripheral zones. The edge shape is termed *ski-tip*. The lens is fitted 2.00 mm less than the horizontal visible iris diameter (HVID) to give central alignment, or just flatter than 'K' with slight superior decentration.

TD   = 9.40 mm, 9.90 mm, 10.20 mm
BOZR   = 'K' + 0.00–0.10 mm
Aspheric periphery = 0.80 mm, 1.60 mm, 3.50 mm flatter than
                      BOZR

CONFLEX AIR (WOHLK, 1989)

A fully aspheric design in a fluoropolymer material, fitted with central alignment.

TD   = 9.30 mm, 9.80 mm, 10.30 mm
BOZR   = 7.20–8.60 mm
Aspheric periphery = (e = 0.4)

PERSECON E (CIBA, 1981)

The aspheric version of an earlier spherical design, both in CAB. The back surface gradually flattens to the periphery with e = 0.40

and $p = 0.84$. There is a spherical edge curve to assist tears exchange. It is fitted to give minimum edge clearance either with central alignment or slightly flat to ensure adequate movement and tears exchange.

BOZR	= 'K' + 0.10 mm
Spherical edge width	= 0.20–0.30 mm
Spherical peripheral radius	= 10.00–12.00 mm
TD	= 8.80 mm, 9.30 mm, 9.80 mm, 10.30 mm
Edge clearance	= 20–60 µm

TD (mm)	AEL (mm)
8.80	0.016–0.030
9.30	0.020–0.041
9.80	0.025–0.053
10.30	0.033–0.069

ASPHERICON (Wesley Jessen.PBH, 1998)

The design consists of a progressive aspheric back surface with a spherical ski-tip periphery 0.40 mm wide. The lens has a standard eccentricity of e = 0.55 (p value = 0.7) which gives a constant edge clearance equivalent to an axial edge lift of 0.12 mm. There are also flatter and steeper eccentricities available. The front surface is spherical and lenticulated where necessary.

The optimum fluorescein pattern shows central alignment or slight apical clearance and gives the appearance of a well fitted multicurve. The ski-tip edge should be 0.40 mm to 0.70 mm wide with an edge clearance between 0.10 mm and 0.12 mm. The fitting can be adjusted by selecting either the larger or smaller eccentricity. The 9.30 mm diameter is selected first, except for large corneas or tight lids which would cause lens decentration.

BOZR	Aspheric equivalent to 7.20 to 8.30 mm in 0.1 mm steps
Total Diameters	9.30 mm and 9.80 mm
Eccentricities	0.55 (p = 0.70), 0.70 (p = 0.50), 0.40 (p = 0.84)
Centre thickness	At –3.00 D, 0.13 mm for 9.30 TD, 0.12 mm for 9.8 mm
Edge thickness	0.12 mm

QUASAR (NO. 7, 1994)

The lens is designed to be a progressive eccentric aspheric, based on a corneal model with $e = 0.458$. The eccentricity value at the lens apex = 0 and increases with the semi-diameter from the centre outwards. The back surface consists of a modified conic profile giving a central, differentially flattening aspheric geometry. An aspheric 'ski-bevel' peripheral band and a specially lathed edge curve are added to generate edge clearance and edge form respectively. The central lens geometry aims for a TLT of 6.5 μm with a fluorescein pattern showing no obvious bearing area. There is also an even band of peripheral clearance about 0.50 mm wide, increasing in intensity towards the lens edge.[12]

BOZR	= flattest 'K', with up to 1.50 DC
Diameter of central zone	= 6.00 mm
FOZD	= 8.00 to 6.80 mm depending on BVP
TD	= 9.20 mm, 9.60 mm, 10.00 mm
Edge thickness	= 0.10 mm (radial)
Centre thickness	= 0.17 mm at –3.00 D

8.5 Use of corneal topography in lens design

Videokeratoscopy (*see* Section 2.3) can be used in the design of contact lenses to fit individual corneal topography. This can often be more satisfactory than using a conventional fitting set and has the added advantage that simulated fluorescein patterns can be generated to accompany any change in lens design (*see also* Section 9.7).

8.6 Reverse geometry lenses

Reverse geometry lenses differ from conventional designs in that the intermediate curve is *steeper* than the base curve. Such lenses are used to improve centration (e.g. with corneal flattening procedures such as orthokeratology, *see* Chapter 14) and for some therapeutic applications (*see* Section 31.3.1).

The secondary curve is between 1.00 D and 9.00 D steeper than the BOZR. This maintains a tear reservoir (TR) as an annulus over the mid-peripheral cornea. The peripheral curve (PC) is a flat aspheric, usually 0.50 mm wide. As the TD of the lens is increased, the BOZD and PC remain constant and the width of the TR is increased. There are different edge lifts available. The standard AEL is 0.12 mm, but this can be increased or reduced in 0.02 mm steps.

Practical advice

- Altering the BOZR of a reverse geometry lens can cause a marked change in both TLT and fluorescein appearance. It is not necessarily the first parameter to change in attempting to improve the fitting.
- Changing the diameter rather than the BOZR gives a smaller alteration in lens sag and may well be preferable.
- Increasing the TD often improves centration and fitting response.

Reverse geometry lenses are fitted by a combination of corneal sag calculation and careful fluorescein evaluation. The required tear layer thickness (TLT) is added to the sag value and the nearest matching radius selected from the trial set (*see* Section 14.2). The correct lens is significantly flatter than 'K' (0.30–0.40 mm) and chosen to maintain a TLT of at least 10 µm.

The fluorescein pattern consists of central touch over the central 3 mm surrounded by an annulus of fluorescein representing the steeper tear reservoir. The TR is in turn surrounded by an area of peripheral touch and a band of edge clearance. This gives a typical 'bulls-eye' pattern.

References

1. Dickenson, F. and Hall, K.G.C. (1946) *An Introduction to the Prescribing and Fitting of Contact Lenses*, Hammond and Hammond, London
2. Bennett, A.G. (1968) Aspherical contact lens surfaces. *Ophthalmic Optician*, **8**, 1037–1040, 1297–1300, 1311, **9**, 222–230
3. Bier, N. (1957) The contour lens. *Journal of the American Optometric Association*, **28**, 394–396
4. Bayshore, C.A. (1962) Report on 276 patients fitted with microcorneal lenses apical clearance and central ventilation. *American Journal of Optometry*, **39**, 552–553
5. Thomas, P.F. (1967) *Conoid Contact Lenses*. Corneal Lens Corporation, Australia
6. Stek, A.W. (1969) The Percon contact lens – design and fitting technique. *Contact Lens*, **2**, 12–14
7. Cantor, D. (1970) The Percon lens – design and fitting techniques. In *Fitting Manual*, Darling and Cantor Ltd, Brackley, Northants
8. Ruben, M. (1966) Use of conoidal curves in corneal contact lenses. *British Journal of Ophthalmology*, **50**, 642–645
9. Stone, J. (1975) Corneal lenses with constant axial edge lift. *Ophthalmic Optician*, **15**, 818–824
10. Nissel, G. (1967) Aspheric contact lenses. *Ophthalmic Optician*, **7**, 1007–1010
11. Gasson, A.P. (1982) Conflex, a new gas permeable hard lens. *Optician*, **184**, 25–29
12. Meyler, J. and Ruston, D. (1995) The development of a new aspheric RGP contact lens. *Optician*, **209** (5487), 30–37

Chapter 9

Hard lens selection and fitting

9.1 Introduction

Compared with PMMA, modern hard lenses can employ different fitting criteria because of:

- The physical properties of the materials (e.g. flexibility).
- Oxygen transmission and the improved physiological response of the cornea.
- The problems it is hoped they will solve (e.g. flare).

9.2 Back optic zone radius (BOZR)

- Trial sets usually have steps of 0.10 mm, although prescription lenses can normally be ordered in 0.05 mm steps.
- The preferred fitting for most corneal lenses is alignment or very slightly flatter.
- Trial lens selection is based on keratometry.
- The initial lens usually has a BOZR nearest to flattest 'K'.
- Toric corneas (1.00–3.00 D of astigmatism) should also be fitted on or near flattest 'K' to minimize flexure and achieve good acuity with a spherical lens.[1]
- The radius must be considered in relation to BOZD. Where a very large optic is required (e.g. 8.40 mm), the radius is usually flatter (e.g. 'K' + 0.10 mm) to achieve an alignment fitting.
- Additional factors such as lid tension, BVP and centre of gravity must also be considered (*see* Section 7.2).
- Right and left eyes generally require radii within 0.05 mm of each other, except in cases of anisometropia.

Example 1   (Alignment): 'K' 8.00 × 7.95
            Initial radius selected: 8.00 mm
Example 2: (Alignment): 'K' 7.97 × 7.83
            Initial radius selected: 8.00 mm
Example 3: (Toric cornea): 'K' 8.00 × 7.50
            Initial radius selected: 7.95 mm

9.3 Total diameter (TD)

- Compared with PMMA, it is possible to err on the large side, since the material and lens design provide the necessary oxygen and tear flow.
- TD is chosen on the basis of corneal size to be approximately 2.0 mm smaller than HVID.
- TD depends on pupil size, especially in low illumination.
- TD depends on the size of vertical palpebral aperture.
- The choice can be regarded as *small* (< 9.20 mm), *medium* (9.20–9.70 mm) or *large* (>9.80 mm).
- Changing to a larger diameter generally stabilizes the fitting, although it does not always have a significant effect on the fluorescein pattern.
- Highly toric corneas need either small lenses to avoid excessive edge stand-off in the steep meridian or large lenses for lid attachment.
- The TD should be evaluated in relation to BVP. High powers require larger diameters for lens stability.
- The final choice of diameter also depends on the method of fitting (e.g. whether lid attachment or interpalpebral).
- Right and left eyes almost always require the same TD.

9.4 Back optic zone diameter (BOZD)

- Often predetermined by the laboratory.
- Depends on pupil size, especially in low illumination.
- The pupil position must be assessed for aphakics.
- BOZD is chosen to be at least 1.50 mm larger than pupil size.
- The choice may be regarded as *small* (< 7.30 mm), *medium* (7.30–7.90 mm) or *large* (>7.90 mm).

- A larger BOZD for a particular radius gives a greater sag and therefore a steeper fitting.

- A smaller BOZD is often chosen with a toric cornea to reduce the area of mismatch.

- A larger BOZD is often chosen to permit a flatter BOZR which gives less flexure on a toric cornea.

- An excessively large BOZD gives a periphery which is very narrow. The peripheral curves must therefore be much flatter than normal for adequate edge clearance. This results in a sharp transition.

- The BOZD should be considered in relation to BVP and lenticulation. High minus lenses frequently require very large BOZDs to avoid flare.

Typical fittings:

Example 1: 7.80:7.50/8.60:8.30/10.50:9.30 (Figure 9.1)

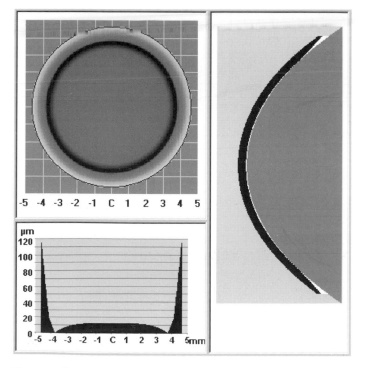

Figure 9.1 Tear layer profile/BOZD

Example 2: 7.80:8.20/8.70:8.90/10.50:9.80 (Figure 9.2)

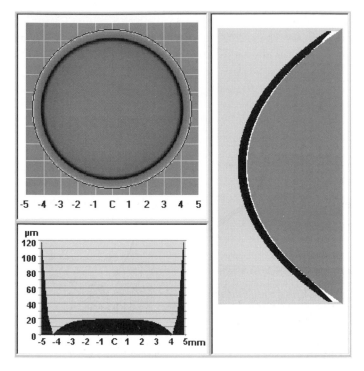

Figure 9.2 Tear layer profile/BOZD

9.5 Peripheral curves

- The first peripheral curve should be at least 0.70 mm flatter than the BOZR and rather more for lenses at the flatter end of the scale.
- For a tricurve, the final peripheral curve is typically chosen as 10.50 mm, with a width of 0.50–1.00 mm.
- A flat peripheral curve gives less corneal irritation but greater lid sensation.
- Compared with PMMA, less peripheral clearance is both feasible and desirable. Hard gas permeable lenses are fitted alignment or slightly flat, so that an excessively wide periphery is unnecessary for adequate tears and oxygen flow.

- Too little peripheral clearance, however, gives unsatisfactory tears exchange because of increased capillary attraction. It can also cause arcuate staining and lens adhesion (*see* Section 7.3).

- Excessive clearance results in an unstable fitting because of an inverted tears meniscus and reduced lens adhesion (*see* Section 7.3). It can also cause peripheral dimpling and 3 and 9 o'clock staining.

Examples:

Tight periphery   7.90:8.00/8.60:8.60/9.15:9.20 (Figure 9.3) AEL = 0.05 mm

Average periphery 7.90:8.00/9.10:8.60/12.30:9.20 (Figure 9.4) AEL = 0.12 mm

Loose periphery   7.90:7.00/8.85:7.80/10.40:8.60/11.50:9.00 AEL = 0.15 mm (Figure 9.5)

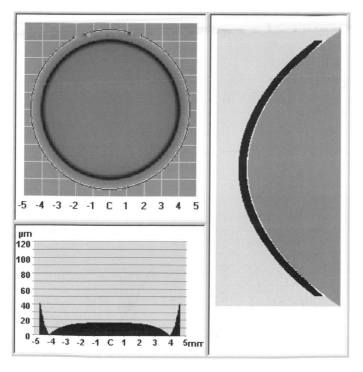

Figure 9.3 Tear layer profile/tight periphery

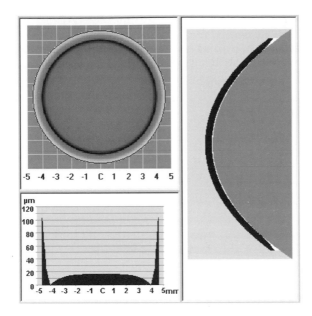

Figure 9.4 Tear layer profile/average periphery

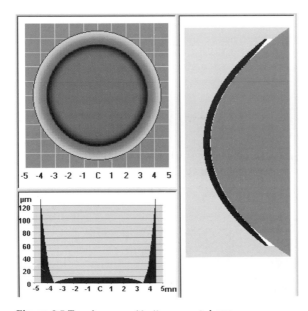

Figure 9.5 Tear layer profile/loose periphery

9.6 Back vertex power (BVP) and over-refraction

- Trial lenses should be as near as possible to the anticipated BVP. Minus trial lenses for hypermetropes should be avoided and *vice versa*.

- If a lens is fitted *steeper* than 'K', a *positive* liquid lens is created, requiring more negative power in the over-refraction (Figure 9.6a).

- If a lens is fitted *flatter* than 'K', a *negative* liquid lens is created, requiring more positive power in the over-refraction (Figure 9.6b).

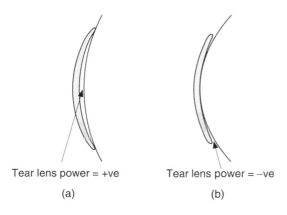

Tear lens power = +ve   Tear lens power = −ve

(a)   (b)

Figure 9.6 (a) Steep contact lens – positive lens power; (b) flat contact lens – negative lens power

- Different BVPs are likely for the same degree of with- and against-the-rule astigmatism.

- The final BVP should correlate with the spectacle *Rx* after taking into account the vertex distance.

Examples: Spectacle *Rx*: –3.00 DS   'K':   8.00 mm @ 180
                                                                    7.95 mm @ 90

(1) BOZR	8.10 mm	over-refraction	= –0.50 D
Trial lens	–2.00 D	liquid lens	= –0.50 D
		final BVP	= –2.50 D
(2) BOZR	8.00 mm	over-refraction	= –1.00 D
Trial lens	–2.00 D	liquid lens	= plano
		final BVP	= –3.00 D

(3) BOZR   7.90 mm   over-refraction $= -1.50$ D
     Trial lens -2.00 D   liquid lens $= +0.50$ D
                              final BVP $= -3.50$ D

Rule of thumb

A change in radius of 0.05 mm $\equiv$ 0.25 D change in power (if the radius is in the region of 7.80 mm).

General advice

- As right and left eyes nearly always require the same TD, use different diameter trial lenses in each eye to observe two fittings at the same time.
- Use a similar technique to evaluate two BOZRs at the same time, as they do not often differ by more than 0.05 mm for similar 'K' readings.
- Check that the BVP from over-refraction correlates with the spectacle *Rx* and astigmatism after allowing for vertex distance. Repeat with a different trial lens in case of doubt.
- Do not over-refract hypermetropes with minus trial lenses and vice versa. The results are nearly always unreliable.
- If the patient was previously a PMMA wearer, order the lenses 0.02 mm thicker than normal to reduce the risk of breakage with more modern materials.

Practical advice

Hard lenses give best vision if:

- The BOZD is relatively large (> 8.00 mm).
- The TD is relatively large (> 9.80 mm).
- The periphery is not too wide (< 1.00 mm).
- The periphery is not too flat (AEL < 0.14 mm).
- Centre thickness is 0.14 mm or greater.
- Fitting is on or near flattest 'K'.

9.7 Lens design by corneal topographers

Videokeratoscopes for corneal topography measurement often include contact lens design programs[2,3] to determine:

- The temporal keratometry reading for the initial BOZR.
- Whether the initial BOZR will allow unobstructed vertical lens movement and redesign curves if necessary.
- The mid-peripheral corneal curvature for superior, temporal and inferior positions.
- The degree and symmetry of any mid-peripheral corneal astigmatism and whether a toric lens is necessary.

Comprehensive computer programs are available to custom design most types of hard gas-permeable lens from C2 to C5. Some programs automatically suggest the optimum lens while others allow the practitioner to insert the BOZR, diameters and AEL in order to compute the intermediate curves.

The value of videokeratoscopy is enhanced by providing simulated fluorescein patterns for the calculated lens design and demonstrating the bearing areas on the cornea. It is also possible to show the effect on the fitting when the various lens parameters are changed. An alternative approach where instruments are able to provide details of AEL and edge clearance (*see* Section 8.5) is to design lenses using the principle of TLT (*see* Section 2.3).

References

1. Stone, J. and Collins, C. (1984) Flexure of gas permeable lenses on toroidal corneas. *Optician*, **188** (4951), 8–10
2. Caroline, P.J., Andre, M.P. and Norman, C.W. (1994) Corneal topography and computerized contact lens-fitting modules. *International Contact Lens Clinic*, **21** (9&10), 185–195
3. Szczotka, L.B., Capretta, D.M. and Lass, J.H. (1994) Clinical evaluation of a computerised topography software method for fitting rigid gas permeable contact lenses. *Journal of the Contact Lens Association of Ophthalmologists*, **20**, 231–236

Chapter 10

Fluorescein patterns and fitting

10.1 Use of fluorescein

10.1.1 Instillation of fluorescein

- A fluorescein strip is moistened with saline and excess removed by shaking.

Practical advice

- *Never* use tap water to wet fluorescein strips. *Pseudomonas aeruginosa* has a strong affinity for fluorescein and may be present together with other micro-organisms such as *Acanthamoeba*.
- Do not apply the strips dry, as they can be very uncomfortable.
- It is usually more comfortable for the patient to look down to reduce lid sensation, especially with an unadapted patient.
- Sometimes, however, with very tight lids and squeamish patients it is better applied in the lower outer canthus, gently pulling down the bottom lid and resting the paper flat against the lower palpebral conjunctiva.
- Insertion of the contact lens with a viscous wetting solution may encourage the fluorescein to spread across the front surface of the lens and mask the posterior fluorescein pattern. Either use saline or give the lens longer to settle.
- Do not paint the wet strip over the conjunctiva, since too much fluorescein masks the true pattern. The excess can also stain skin and clothes.
- *Never* reuse strips on another patient because of the risk of cross-infection. Discard after use to avoid error. Use a different strip for each eye if infection is suspected.
- If a strip is reused for the same patient, fold it as shown in Figure 10.1 to avoid contaminating the tip.

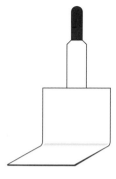

Figure 10.1 Folded fluorescein strip

- The patient is asked to look down while the upper lid is lifted and the wet strip gently touched onto the conjunctiva above the superior limbus, taking care not to instil excess.
- Fluorescein flows beneath the lens with the tears after two or three blinks.
- If a minim of 2% fluorescein is used, one drop only is applied with a glass rod. Some of it is allowed to wash away before inspecting the fit.

10.1.2 Ultraviolet inhibitors

Some materials contain ultraviolet (UV) inhibitors, so that the fluorescein pattern with the Burton lamp shows an apparently black lens with an almost imperceptible green annulus at the periphery.

Additional fluorescein does not change the appearance and it is necessary to use the slit lamp with a blue filter to give a meaningful picture.

10.2 Examination techniques

10.2.1 Burton lamp

BLUE LIGHT

The essential principles in observing fluorescein patterns are:

- The method gives a dynamic assessment of lens fitting.
- Dark blue represents corneal touch.
- Green represents corneal clearance.

- Compared with slit lamp observation, the patient is more relaxed with the Burton lamp, so that both head and eyelids maintain a normal position.
- The Burton lamp uses a UV filter.

Practical advice

- Exercise care with nervous patients. They sometimes feel faint and the UV lamp is often the trigger mechanism. If in doubt, delay fluorescein examination until they are more at ease.
- Despite this, they nearly always make very good contact lens wearers.

WHITE LIGHT

White light with low magnification allows initial investigation of lens position and movement prior to fluorescein assessment, but care is required with a photophobic patient.

10.2.2 Slit lamp

- The cobalt blue filter of the slit lamp permits evaluation of the fluorescein pattern with relatively low magnification ($\times 6$ to $\times 10$).
- A wide beam of 3–5 mm is used for general assessment.
- A narrow slit beam with higher magnification gives a qualitative indication of tear layer thickness and corneal clearance.
- The head and lids are not in a relaxed position on the instrument, so that the assessment of lens centration is not completely reliable.
- The fluorescein pattern appears normal even if the lens material contains a UV inhibitor.
- Contrast is enhanced using a filter, Wratten yellow 6 or 12.

10.3 Fitting

- The central and peripheral fit are independent variables and should always be assessed separately.[1]

- The fitting should be evaluated with the lens both centred on the apex of the cornea and in a decentred position.
- Lens movement during and after a blink should be noted.
- Lens position after a blink is important.
- Lens movement on eye excursions is also significant.

10.4 Correct fitting

10.4.1 Assessment with white light

EXCURSION LAG

With the lids in a normal position, the lens periphery should not extend beyond the limbal area even with wide excursions of the eye.

STATIC LAG

If the lids are held apart and the lens pushed upwards, it should drop slowly of its own accord.

10.4.2 Assessment with fluorescein

ALIGNMENT FITTING (e.g. with modern multicurve designs)

Appearance

The ideal fluorescein pattern should show three fitting areas (Figure 10.2):

- Alignment or the merest hint of apical clearance over the central 7.00 mm.
- Mid-peripheral alignment over about 1.50 mm.
- Edge clearance about 0.5 mm wide.

APICALLY CLEAR FITTING (e.g. with PMMA)

Appearance

Fluorescein pooling over the central 5.00 mm.

- Mid-peripheral alignment.
- Edge clearance about 1.00 wide.

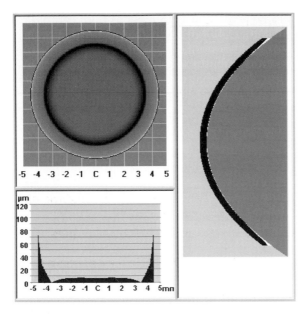

Figure 10.2 Alignment fitting

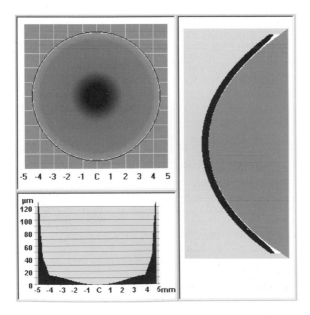

Figure 10.3 Tear layer profile/flat fit

FLATTER THAN 'K' FITTING (e.g. most aspherics)

Appearance

- Alignment or light touch over the central 5.00 mm.
- Mid-peripheral alignment.
- Narrow edge clearance just under 0.5 mm wide.

10.5 Flat fitting

Appearance (Figure 10.3)

- The fitting pattern gives a dense central area of dark blue touch surrounded by fluorescein to the edge of the lens.
- The area of touch is small with an indistinct as opposed to a sharply demarcated border.
- Fluorescein encroaches beneath the periphery of the central portion where alignment would be expected with a correct fit.
- The lens is unstable and decentres.
- If the lens drops, it may show inferior fluorescein pooling. This is not an indication of steepness, since the lens is over-hanging the lower peripheral cornea. If it is repositioned, central touch is observed.
- The entire periphery of the lens shows clearance as a wide area of fluorescein.
- Blinking gives excessive and rapid lens movement which may well be uncomfortable.
- Arcuate movement occurs when dropping between blinks or with static lag.

Practical advice

- Use a steeper BOZR for greatest effect on the fluorescein pattern.
- All other remedies have a lesser effect and the choice of action depends on the degree of flatness.
- Carefully evaluate the TD. If the lens is already large enough, further increase might not be feasible.
- Increasing the BOZD has a greater effect on the fluorescein pattern than making the lens larger.
- Use tighter or narrower peripheries to help the lens centre better.
- All modifications to an existing lens tend to loosen the fit. A flat fitting almost invariably requires a new lens

---

To correct a flat fit

- Use a steeper BOZR to improve centration.
- Increase the TD to stabilize the lens.
- Increase the BOZD to give a larger sag and steepen the fit.
- Use tighter peripheral curves to reduce dynamic forces and the effect of the lids.
- Use a thinner lens to reduce mobility.

10.6 Steep fitting

Appearance (Figure 10.4)

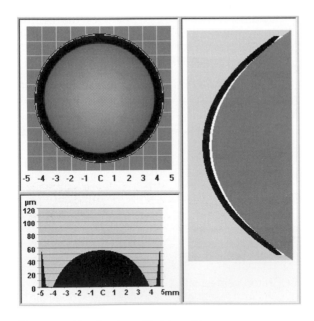

Figure 10.4 Tear layer profile/steep fit

- The fluorescein pattern gives central pooling.
- An air bubble is sometimes present with excessive central clearance.

- Heavy bearing is seen at the transition as an area of dark blue touch beyond the central pooling.
- The smaller the area of central pooling, the greater the degree of steepness.
- The periphery gives only a thin annulus of fluorescein around the lens edge.
- There is little lens movement on blinking.

TO CORRECT A STEEP FIT

- Use a flatter BOZR.
- Decrease the TD to increase lens mobility.
- Decrease the BOZD to give a smaller sag.
- Use flatter peripheral curves to increase the dynamic forces on the lens.
- Use a thicker lens.
- Fenestrate (*see* Section 25.3).

Practical advice

- Use a flatter BOZR to give the greatest effect on the fluorescein pattern.
- Carefully evaluate corneal and pupil sizes before reducing the TD and BOZD.
- Central fenestration is generally a last resort, but encourages tear flow beneath the lens apex and increases mobility.
- All modifications tend to loosen the fit. Several adjustments can therefore be made to improve an existing steep lens.

CLINICAL EQUIVALENTS (*see* Section 16.1)

Rule of thumb
for spherical lenses

An increase in the BOZD of 0.50 mm requires the BOZR to be flattened by 0.05 mm to maintain the same fluorescein pattern.

Example 1 (spherical lens): 7.70:7.00 ≡ 7.75:7.50 ≡ 7.80:8.00

The principle of clinical equivalents still applies to an elliptical lens, but the differences found with tear layer theory are greater.[2]

Example 2 (elliptical lens): 7.70:7.00 ≡ 7.75:7.70 ≡ 7.80:8.50

**Rule of thumb
for elliptical lenses**

An increase in the BOZD of 0.70 mm requires an increase in the BOZR of 0.05 mm to give the same tear layer thickness.

10.7 Peripheral fitting

The ideal peripheral clearance is 60–80 µm, equivalent to an edge lift of 0.12–0.15 mm. It depends on corneal topography and method of fitting. In practical terms, this gives an annulus of fluorescein about 0.50 mm wide at the edge of the lens. The limit of clinical significance is about 10 µm.[3]

TIGHT PERIPHERY

Appearance

- Good centration.
- Periphery presses the limbus on blinking and may cause discomfort.
- Poor tears exchange under the lens and several blinks necessary for fluorescein circulation.

To improve a tight periphery

An increase in edge clearance of at least 10–15 µm is necessary to give a discernible change in fluorescein pattern. Axial edge lift should be increased in increments of 0.03 mm (e.g. from 0.12 mm to 0.15 mm).

- Use a flatter peripheral radius (e.g. 10.75 mm instead of 10.25 mm).
- Add one or more flatter peripheral curves (e.g. 12.25 mm, 0.4 mm wide; or 15.00 mm, 0.2 mm wide).

- Increase the width of the peripheral curves.
- Use a flatter BOZR and smaller BOZD.
- Increase blending of peripheral curves.
- Change the lens design. Centration affects the peripheral interaction with the cornea.

LOOSE PERIPHERY

Appearance

- Lens rides high and does not drop after a blink.
- Bubbles are found at the edge and superior dimpling may occur.
- The edge lifts away from the cornea on blinking.
- The lens is unstable on excursion movements.
- Frequently gives 3 and 9 o'clock staining.

To improve a loose periphery

To improve a loose periphery requires a decrease in edge clearance of at least 10–15 μm. The axial edge lift is decreased in increments of 0.03 mm (e.g. from 0.15 mm to 0.12 mm).

- Use a tighter peripheral radius (e.g. 10.00 mm instead of 10.50 mm).
- Reduce the width of the peripheral curves.
- Use a larger BOZD, possibly with a flatter BOZR to compensate.
- Change the lens design and possibly try an aspheric.

General advice

- Use a negative carrier for low-riding plus lenses.
- Aspheric lenses sometimes give better centration and comfort with plus lenses.
- A displaced corneal apex causes lens decentration even if the fitting is not too flat. Use a larger TD if flare is a problem.
- Tight lids with a toric cornea also cause decentration. Consider a back surface toric lens.

References

1. Phillips, A.J. (1997) Rigid gas permeable corneal lens fitting. In *Contact Lenses* 4th edn, A.J. Phillips and L. Speedwell (eds) Butterworth-Heinemann, Oxford, pp. 313–357
2. Atkinson, T. (1987) The development of the back surface design of rigid lenses. *Contax*, Nov., 5–18
3. Atkinson, T. (1985) A computer assisted and clinical assessment of current trends in gas permeable lens design. *Optician*, **189** (4976), 16–22

Chapter 11

Aspheric lenses

Aspheric lens design has evolved because clinical models have shown the overall form of the cornea to be elliptical.[1-3] The variation in the shape of an ellipse is called the eccentricity (e) and is an important factor in lens design and fitting. Mathematically, it is always less than 1 (*see* Section 8.4).

11.1 Advantages and disadvantages of aspherics

ADVANTAGES OF ASPHERICS

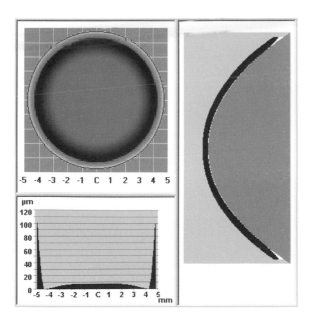

Figure 11.1 Aspheric lens showing close fit to corneal topography

- Fit more closely to the corneal topography (Figure 11.1).

- Distribute pressure more evenly over the cornea.
- Edge lift or Z value is smaller, giving less lid sensation.
- Can sometimes fit up to 4.00 D of astigmatism.
- Some designs can give improved distance vision, others can assist presbyopia (*see* Section 24.4.2).
- Absence of transition zones assists tear flow.

DISADVANTAGES OF ASPHERICS

- Manufacture requires sophisticated lathes.
- Reproducibility and verification more difficult.
- Aberrations with some back surface designs.
- Decentration if fitted flatter than 'K' to obtain movement.
- Decentration with a decentred corneal apex.

11.2 Aspheric designs

11.2.1 Fully aspheric lenses

A completely aspheric back surface can cause problems if the eccentricity chosen fits the corneal topography too closely, resulting in the lens edge pressing into the peripheral cornea. A narrow, spherical bevel or separate aspheric edge is therefore usually incorporated into the design.

If a bi-aspheric lens with fixed high eccentricity decentres, it can induce residual astigmatism because of the differential power effect of the sagittal and tangential radii towards the lens periphery. Conversely, with designs which have differential flattening, there can be a significant reduction in both positive and astigmatic aberration in the optic portion of the lens.

 QUASAR

The Quasar design[4] (No. 7 Laboratory) has a back surface consisting of a conic profile with a central differentially-flattening aspheric geometry. A further aspheric 'ski-bevel' peripheral band ensures adequate edge clearance. The eccentricity value at the lens apex is zero and increases with the semi-diameter from the centre outwards. The reduction in initial flattening results in a more spherical central optic portion. The edge clearance of 80 µm is based on a corneal model with $e = 0.458$ (Figure 11.2).

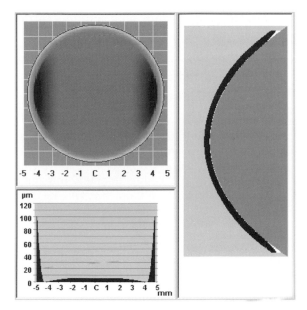

Figure 11.2 Tear layer profile (Quasar)

11.2.2 Mainly aspheric/part sphere

These designs consist of a mainly aspheric back surface with a spherical peripheral curve. The spherical curve is needed to prevent the elliptical edge from pressing into the cornea. It also assists tears exchange and lens removal.

The common designs are the Persecon E (CIBA Vision), Aquila (CIBA Vision) and Asphericon (Wesley Jessen.PBH).

PERSECON E

The Persecon E has an eccentricity of $e = 0.4$ and rate of flattening $p = 0.84$. It has a spherical periphery between 10 mm and 12 mm in radius and between 0.20 mm and 0.30 mm wide, to give an edge clearance of 20–60 μm.

AQUILA

The Aquila and Persecon 92E designs (CIBAVision) have an aspheric back surface design which is bi-elliptic with an integrated tangential bevel. The eccentricity has an average value of $e =$

0.4. TDs are 9.3 mm, 9.8 mm and 10.3 mm with a minus carrier available for powers of +2.00 D or greater with the two larger diameters. The optic zone varies with the TD, ranging from 7.50 mm to 8.00 mm with BVPs over ±8.00 D. The lens geometry is calculated using computer assisted design (CAD).

ASPHERICON

The Asphericon (Wesley Jessen.PBH) has an aspheric back surface with a spherical periphery 0.40 mm wide. It is available in three eccentricities: standard (e = 0.55, p value = 0.7) which gives a constant edge clearance equivalent to an axial edge lift of 0.12 mm; high (e = 0.70, p value = 0.50); and low (e = 0.40, p value = 0.84). The front surface is spherical and lenticulated where necessary (Figure 11.3).

11.2.3 Mainly spherical/part asphere

These consist of a central spherical portion with an aspheric peripheral zone area and are termed *polynomial asphenc designs*. The aspheric zone is, in turn, surrounded by a small spherical edge bevel.

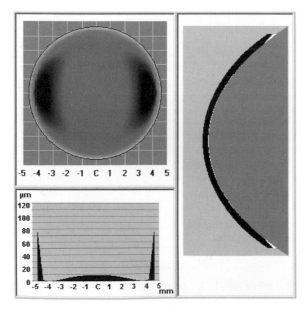

Figure 11.3 Tear layer profile Asphericon

Quantum

The Quantum lens (Bausch & Lomb) has a 3.50–4.00 mm central spherical portion with an aspheric periphery. The edge has a radius of 11.25 mm, 0.3 mm wide.[5]

Reflex 60

The back surface design of Reflex 60 (Hydron) has a spherical central curve tangentially connected to a conic 'mid-section' which is in turn tangentially connected to a ski-bevel peripheral radius.[6] The aspheric/conic section starts at the junction of the BOZD and varies with BOZR. In all cases it has a constant chord diameter of 8.40 mm. The ski-bevel extends from 8.40 mm out to the TDs of 9.00 mm, 9.30 mm, 9.70 mm or 10.00 mm. Both the eccentricity of the conic section and the total AEL of the lens vary with BOZR. They range from 1.16 to 2.26 and from 0.109 mm to 0.186 mm, respectively.

11.3 Principles of fitting

11.3.1 Fully aspheric lenses

Progressive eccentric aspheric lenses (e.g. Quasar) are generally fitted on flattest 'K'. The fluorescein pattern shows no obvious area of bearing over the central and mid-peripheral area while the lens edge gives a well-defined tears meniscus. The lens position should be central with 1.5 mm–2 mm of movement on blinking. If the TD needs to be ordered larger (10.00 mm) or smaller (9.20 mm) than the 9.60 mm trial lenses, there is no need to change either the BOZR or BVP.

With toric corneas, the central radius is chosen 0.10 mm steeper than flattest 'K'. The lens should still give good centration but will show greater peripheral clearance along the vertical rather than horizontal meridian. Mid-peripheral bearing indicates the need for a flatter lens, whereas hard central touch or decentration requires a steeper fitting.

11.3.2 Mainly aspheric/part sphere

Persecon E

The Persecon E design is manufactured from CAB (see Section 6.1). It is fitted slightly flatter than flattest 'K'. The total diameter is chosen according to corneal size: 8.80 mm or 9.30 mm for corneas up to 11.0 mm, and 9.80 mm or 10.30 mm for those larger than 11.0 mm.

A correct fitting shows alignment or the suggestion of light central touch. In the case of decentration, a larger lens should be tried before steepening the curvature. The edge bevel is cut with a common tangent to the ellipse to give good comfort.

Examples: 'K' 7.89 mm × 7.83 mm
Persecon E: 8.00:9.30

AQUILA AND PERSECON 92E

Aquila and Persecon 92E are fitted at least 0.05 mm flatter than flattest 'K'. The fluorescein fit is alignment to slightly flat with a small degree of edge clearance. As the elliptical base curve flattens towards the edge of the lens in the same way as the cornea, the TD can be altered without causing any change to the fluorescein pattern. However, if the base curve is altered, the BVP requires compensation in the usual way.

Practical advice

The design of the Aquila and Persecon 92E differs from the earlier Persecon E so that the correct trial set must be used to achieve an optimum fitting.

11.3.3 Mainly spherical/part asphere

QUANTUM

The spherical central radius is selected 0.10 mm steeper than flattest 'K' to allow the aspheric mid-peripheral portion to align with the cornea. The fluorescein pattern gives slight central pooling surrounded by an area of alignment with peripheral edge clearance. The lens design can give excessive edge clearance with steep corneas and too little clearance with flat corneas. Quantum does not ride as high as some of the flatter fitting designs and is useful where it is desirable to avoid lid attachment. The usual total diameter is 9.60 mm. To help centration, 10.20 mm lenses are available, but even 9.60 mm is too large for some small corneas. Only plus lenses are available in a 9.00 mm diameter.

REFLEX 60

The initial trial lens is chosen on flattest 'K' or slightly steeper for up to 1.00 D of astigmatism. This should maintain the appearance of alignment over the central area of the lens with gradually increasing clearance in the periphery. With greater than 1.00 D of astigmatism, the BOZR is selected 0.10–0.15 mm steeper than 'K'. The lens should centre with 1–1.5 mm of movement on blinking.

11.3.4 General fitting considerations

Aspheric lenses:

- Do not require such critical fitting because fewer parameters.
- Need to be fitted slightly flat to give adequate movement and sufficient edge clearance (except designs like Quantum).
- Flat fitting, however, tends to give decentration as a common problem.

SPHERICAL CORNEA

The ideal fit is alignment or slightly flatter than alignment. A slightly flat fit gives light central touch, but because of even pressure distribution any stress to the cornea is kept to a minimum.

A flat fit shows hard central touch surrounded by an excessive annulus of fluorescein. There is increased lid sensation and unstable vision.

A steep fit gives excessive central pooling with a sharp border, surrounded by a peripheral ring of hard touch and a very narrow meniscus of fluorescein at the periphery.

TORIC CORNEA

The ideal fit is also alignment or slightly flatter than flattest 'K' to minimize lens flexure and maintain good acuity.

11.4 Fluorescein patterns compared with spherical lenses

- A much more gradual change in the fluorescein pattern from centre to periphery.

- True alignment can be achieved if the correct eccentricity has been assessed, as the p value of the lens and cornea can be chosen to be the same (e.g. using a videokeratoscope).[7]
- The peripheral tear layer thickness increases more gradually towards the edge.
- Larger lenses have to be used to help centration.

Practical advice

The axial edge lift of an aspheric lens is less than with the equivalent multicurve. It is sometimes possible to fit higher degrees of astigmatism because of the reduced edge stand off in the steeper meridian.

References

1. Bibby, M. (1976) Computer assisted photokeratoscopy and contact lens design. *Optician*, **171** (4423), 37–43, **171** (4424) 11–17, **171** (4425), 15–17
2. Kiely, P.M., Smith, G. and Carney, L.C. (1984) Meridional variations in corneal shape. *American Journal of Optometry and Physiological Optics*, **61**, 619–626
3. Guillon, M., Lydon, D.P.M. and Wilson, C. (1986) Corneal topography: a clinical model. *Ophthalmic and Physiological Optics*, **6**, 47–56
4. Meyler, J. and Ruston, D. (1995) The development of a new aspheric RGP contact lens. *Optician*, **209** (5487), 30–38
5. Atkinson, T.C.O. (1989) Towards a new gas permeable lens geometry. *Optician*, **197** (5181), 13–17
6. Elder Smith, A. (1996) Practical experience with a new RGP lens design. *Optician*, **212** (5571), 32–33
7. Rabbetts, R.B. (1985) The Humphrey auto keratometer. *Ophthalmic and Physiological Optics*, **5**, 451–458

Chapter 12

Hard lens specification and verification

12.1 International Standards

Glossary of Terms and Symbols is a dual publication of International Standard ISO 8320 – 1986. 'Rigid' lens specifications are given in ISO 8321–1:1991.

ISO 9000 covers manufacturers of assessed capability and implies that verification, production, tolerances, quality assurance, and sampling conform to this standard,

12.1.1 International Standard terms

The terminology for a standard tricurve lens in ISO 8320 – 1986 symbols is:

$$r_0 \quad : \quad \varnothing_0 / r_1 \quad : \quad \varnothing_1 / r_2 \quad : \quad \varnothing_T \, t_c \quad F^1 V \; Tint$$

$$BOZR \; : BOZD/BPZR_1 : BPZD_1/BPZR_2 : TD \qquad BVP$$

Example:

7.90:7.80/8.70:8.60/10.75:9.20 t_c 0.15 BVP –3.00 D Tint light blue

7.90	=	*back optic zone radius (BOZR) r_0*
7.80	=	*back optic zone diameter (BOZD) $\varnothing_0$*
8.70	=	*first back peripheral radius r_1*
8.60	=	*first back peripheral zone diameter $\varnothing_1$*
10.75	=	*second back peripheral radius r_2*
9.20	=	*total diameter $\varnothing_T$*
0.15	=	*geometric centre thickness t_c*
–3.00	=	*back vertex power (BVP)*

For a lenticular lens (reduced optic):

7.90:7.80/8.70:8.60/10.75:9.20 t_c 0.45 t_e 0.16   BVP +10.00 D
FOZD 8.30   Tint light blue

0.45   =   geometric centre thickness t_c
0.16   =   edge thickness t_e
+10.00 =   back vertex power (BVP)
8.30   =   front optic zone diameter $\emptyset_{a0}$

The subscript 'a' indicates an anterior surface component and the format is the same for both plus and minus lenses.

12.2 Examples of hard lens types and fittings

(Assuming a spherical 'K' reading of 7.75 mm and low minus power)

INDIVIDUAL DESIGNS

- TD 8.60 mm   CAEL 0.12 mm[1]
  7.80:7.00/9.00:7.80/10.90:8.60
- TD 9 00 mm   CAEL 0.15 mm[1]
  7.80:7.00/8.75:7.80/10.10:8.60/11.30:9.00
- TD 9.20 mm CAEL 0.12 mm[2]
  7.80:8.00/8.80:8.60/12.30:9.20
- TLT 13 µm, EC 60 µm
  7.80:7.70/8.30:8.20/9.20:9.20
- TD 9.50 mm   CAEL 0.175 mm[3]
  7.80:7.50/8.90:8.50/10.00:9.00/11.15:9.50
- TLT 12 µm, EC 60 µm
  7.80:8.30/8.20:8.80/9.00:9.80

PROPRIETARY DESIGNS

- Series II (No. 7 laboratory) 7.80:7.80/8.65:8.70/9.90:9.50
- Quantum (Bausch & Lomb): 7.70/9.60
- Persecon E (CIBA Vision): 7.80/9.30 or 7.80/9.80
- Standard Polycon II (Wesley Jessen.PBH): 7.80:7.80/AEL 0.10 at 9.00
- Asphericon (Wesley Jessen.PBH): 7.80/9.80 standard e

12.3 Hard lens verification

All lenses should ideally be checked before use:

- To ensure the accuracy of trial lenses.
- To ensure prescription lenses are suitable for dispensing.
- To establish the specification of the patient's existing lenses.
- Where lens parameters are thought to have altered.
- Where lenses are thought to have distorted.
- To confirm that lenses are being worn in the correct eyes
- To confirm that current and old lenses have not been confused.
- To ensure records contain full details of lens specification.

12.3.1 Back optic zone radius (BOZR)

RADIUSCOPE

Based on Drysdale's method which measures the distance between the lens surface and the centre of curvature.

Practical advice

- To obtain a good image, ensure the lens is well dried before being placed on a drop of distilled water in the concave holder.
- To help location of the images, ensure the instrument light is at the centre of the lens.
- Travelling from the zero to the second position the image of the bulb filament is seen. The quality of this image gives an indication of any lens distortion.
- Always take two or three readings and average the results.
- The image at the lens surface is usually much larger and brighter than that at the centre of curvature, as well as showing any surface scratches.
- The zero reading with unstable hard lenses can 'creep' and may require several attempts before giving a reliable result. If the creeping does not stop, average the first three readings.

OTHER METHODS

Keratometer

Uses a lens holder with a front surface silvered mirror. 0.03 mm is added to correct for the concave surface.[4] Autokeratometers can also be used.

Radius-checking device

The radius is derived from the focimeter FVP, using refractive index and thick lens formula.[5]

Toposcope

Uses moire fringes.[6]

12.3.2 Peripheral radius (BPZR)

Peripheral radii can be measured with the radiuscope if the lens is tilted and the band width is at least 1 mm.

A qualitative assessment can be made with a Burton lamp by observing the reflection of the white light tube in the lens surface.

12.3.3 Total diameter (TD) and zone diameters (BPZD)

MEASURING MAGNIFIER (BAND MAGNIFIER)

Consists of an engraved graticule plus an adjustable eyepiece with ×7 magnification. The lens is repositioned on the scale for different zones, and measurement is easier with sharp transitions.

V GAUGE

Consists of a V-shaped channel graduated between 6.0 mm and 12.5 mm. Only measures TD.

PROJECTION MAGNIFIER

Projects a magnified image of the entire lens onto a calibrated screen (e.g. Zeiss DL2).

Practical advice

- Ensure that the lens is dry or it can be difficult to remove from a smooth surface because of capillary attraction.
- Avoid wet cell instruments because of difficulty in lens manipulation.

12.3.4 Back and front vertex power (BVP and FVP)

FOCIMETER

- Place focimeter in a vertical position or use a V-slot holder.
- For BVP, place the concave surface towards the focimeter.
- The lens must be placed as close as possible to the focimeter, either by using a very small stop or by removing the stop cover. The reading may still give more plus or less minus than the true BVP because of the steep lens radius.
- For FVP, place the convex surface towards the focimeter stop. FVP reads less than the BVP, with a greater difference in plus powers than minus.

Practical advice

- Note the quality of the image on the focimeter. Distortion indicates a poor optic.
- A good image does not necessarily guarantee a distortion-free optic because a small stop is used and only the centre of the lens is measured.

POWER PROFILE MAPPING (e.g. VC 2000)

An extremely accurate computerized method, mainly used by manufacturers, for the bi-dimensional measurement of the contact lens power map. Hard contact lenses are evaluated in air and soft lenses in a saline wet cell. The power profile of both spherical and toric lenses can be made by computation from thousands of measurement points. Information is obtained on tolerances for all lens designs and provides automatic axis measurement relative to the true optical parameters for toric lenses. It is also possible to achieve accurate results for multifocal lenses.

12.3.5 Centre and edge thickness (t_c and t_e)

THICKNESS GAUGE

Consists of a spring-loaded, ball-ended probe geared to a direct reading scale.

Practical advice

- Take several readings of the lens edge, as the thickness may vary around the circumference.
- Take care not to damage a thin edge.

RADIUSCOPE

The lens holder is left dry and the target focused on each lens surface in turn. The distance between the two images multiplied by the refractive index of the material gives the central lens thickness.

12.3.6 Edge form

Edge form is best examined with about ×20 magnification using either a hand loupe or the slit lamp.

12.3.7 Surface quality

Surface scratches and defects can be assessed in a variety of ways:

- Projection magnifier with a clean dry lens.
- Slit lamp, using transillumination.
- Band magnifier.
- Radiuscope by examining the first image.

12.3.8 Material

Confirming lens material is difficult, although comparison of specific gravity measurements can give an approximate guide. The most reliable indication can sometimes be colour, since certain hard lenses are available in only one distinctive tint (e.g. Conflex, very pale blue; Polycon Il, medium blue).

12.3.9 Other features

- Engravings (e.g. 'R' or a dot for the right lens).
- Laboratory codes.
- Fenestrations: number, position, size and finish.
- Tint.

- Prism ballast: increased edge thickness at the base.
- Truncation.
- Carrier design: assessed by edge measurement.

12.4 Tolerances

See Table 12.1.

Table 12.1 Suggested tolerances

Parameter	BSI/ISO suggested tolerances
BOZR	± 0.05 mm
BPZR	± 0.10 mm
BOZD	± 0.20 mm
TD	± 0.10 mm
Edge and centre thickness	± 0.02 mm
BVP	± 0.12 D up to ± 5.00 D
	± 0.18 D from ± 5.00 D to ± 10.00 D
	± 0.25 D from ± 10.00 D to ± 15.00 D
	± 0.37 D over ± 15.00 D to ± 20.00 D
	± 0.50 D over ± 20.00 D

Practical advice

- The easiest methods for practitioner verification are:

BOZR	Radiuscope
DIAMETERS	Band magnifier
POWER	Focimeter
THICKNESS	Thickness gauge
CONDITION	Projection or band magnifier.

- Hard and PMMA lenses flatten on both front and back surfaces with hydration.[6] Flattening relates to BVP (greater with high minus) and centre thickness.

- New lenses should be hydrated for 24 hours before a reliable measurement can be made.

- Very rapid changes in BOZR also occur on dehydration.[7]

- Hard gas permeable trial lenses should be kept hydrated. PMMA lenses in powers <±10.00 D are reliable if dry.

References

1. Stone, J. (1975) Corneal lenses with constant axial edge lift. *Ophthalmic Optician*, **15**, 818–824
2. Atkinson, T.C.O. (1980) The return of hard times, part II. *Journal of the British Contact Lens Association*, **3**, 105–112
3. Rabbetts, R.B. (1976) Large corneal lenses with constant axial edge lift. *Ophthalmic Optician*, **16**, 236–239
4. Watts, R. (1997) Rigid lens verification procedures. In *Contact Lenses* 4th edn, A.J. Phillips and L. Speedwell (eds), Butterworth-Heinemann, Oxford, pp. 407–425
5. Sarver, M.D. and Kerr, K. (1964) A radius of curvature measuring device for contact lenses. *American Journal of Optometry*, **41**, 481–489
6. Phillips, A.J. (1969) Alterations in curvature of the finished corneal lens. *Ophthalmic Optician*, **9**, 980–1110
7. Pearson, R.M. (1977) Dimensional stability of several hard contact lens materials. *American Journal of Optometry and Physiological Optics* **54**, 826–833

Chapter 13

PMMA corneal lens fitting

13.1 Physiological problems caused by PMMA

PMMA lenses have in many cases now been worn for over 30 years.[1] Patients are very often quite happy with their lenses, and it is only at an aftercare examination that the practitioner may detect corneal changes. In other cases, patients seek advice because of reduced wearing time, red eyes or depressed vision. The common changes found with long-term PMMA wear are.

- Epithelial oedema.
- Reduced corneal sensitivity.
- Central punctate epithelial staining.
- Chronic 3 and 9 o'clock staining.
- Stromal oedema.
- Folds in Descemet's membrane.
- Endothelial distortion.
- Endothelial polymegathism.

These changes are due to chronic lack of oxygen, drying of the corneal tissue and the mechanical action of the lens. The combination of these long-term effects produces the loss of tolerance known as *corneal exhaustion syndrome*.

Also found, although less commonly, are:

- Dellen.
- Opacification and vascularization at 3 and 9 o'clock.
- Vertical striae.
- Fischer–Schweitzer mosaic pattern.
- Hyperaemic lids.
- CLIPC.

13.2 When PMMA might still be fitted

There is a very small minority of cases where PMMA may still be considered:

- Flexure problems with modern hard lenses give unsatisfactory acuity, especially where a thin lens is necessary.
- Where a trial lens is needed to check the fluorescein pattern of a complicated fitting (e.g. keratoconus or opaque cosmetic) and PMMA is significantly cheaper.
- Children or clumsy patients who may break modern hard lenses too easily.
- Deposit problems with all other hard lens materials.
- Myopia control (*see* Section 30.2.1).
- Where an inert material is required because of allergies (e.g. with CLIPC).
- To give better surface wetting and improved comfort.

13.3 Fitting considerations for PMMA compared with hard gas-permeable lenses

- Fitted with slight apical clearance to encourage good tears exchange, whereas hard gas-permeable lenses are usually fitted in alignment.
- Edge clearance is also greater to allow good tears exchange.
- BOZD is usually smaller to cover less corneal area. Hard gas-permeable lenses have relatively large BOZDs to avoid flare.
- PMMA must be very well blended to avoid oedema and arcuate staining.
- PMMA can be ultrathin (0.10 mm or less) to avoid corneal distortion. Very thin hard gas-permeable lenses flex and cause visual problems.
- High minus powers in PMMA can avoid the lens distortion which occurs with some dimensionally less stable modern materials.
- PMMA is more easily modified and polished than many modern materials because of their surface characteristics and brittleness.

13.4 Modern PMMA fitting

Because of its impermeability, PMMA is fitted according to the following different criteria:

- The BOZR is chosen 0.05–0.10 mm steeper than flattest 'K'.
- For a toric cornea, the BOZR is chosen one-half to two-thirds between flattest and steepest 'K'.
- Where possible, TDs smaller than 9.50 mm are used for low powers. 9.20 mm is a good average diameter.
- A BOZD of approximately 7.00 mm is used for a TD of 9.20 mm; 7.50 mm for a 9.50 mm lens; and 7.80 where a 10.00 mm TD is required by a large palpebral aperture.
- Edges should be well rounded.
- Centre thickness should be $\geqq 0.10$ mm for dimensional stability.

Practical advice

- Give a slower wearing schedule (see Section 27.3).
- Laboratory instructions should always state 'very well blended', as modern hard lens blending is inadequate. Younger technicians will have had little or no experience with PMMA manufacture.
- Where it is essential to fit PMMA and oedema occurs, reduce BOZD or TD and increase edge lift or blending.
- Consider fenestration with the original lens order (*see* Section 25.3).

13.5 Refitting PMMA wearers

Refitting long-term PMMA wearers represents one of the more difficult aspects of modern practice, especially where there are no previous details available. The procedure is further complicated because, however carefully measurement and fitting are carried out, changes are likely to occur as the cornea comes 'off the influence' of PMMA. The correct course of action in nearly all cases is to refit with modern hard lenses. It is not generally feasible to move directly from PMMA to soft lenses (*see* Section 13.6.3).

13.5.1 Problems at initial refitting

- The cornea may show considerable signs of oedema and distortion.
- 'K' readings may be very different from the measurements when fitting has ultimately been completed.
- 'K' readings may exhibit considerable distortion.
- Accurate refraction may be very difficult if not impossible with poor retinoscopy reflex.
- Visual acuity may be depressed because of corneal oedema.
- It is frequently impossible to measure accurately the BOZR of old, distorted lenses.

13.5.2 Problems as refitting progresses

- 'K' readings change, possibly making the initial fitting unsatisfactory. This may occur as long as 6 months later.
- The degree of corneal astigmatism alters.
- The BVP often requires more minus power after 1–3 weeks.
- Patients may experience greater difficulty with foreign bodies as well as greater lens awareness when corneal sensitivity gradually recovers.

13.6 Refitting procedures

13.6.1 General points

- Patients should understand the possible difficulties and that refitting requires careful follow-up.
- Patients should come for their refitting appointment wearing the existing PMMA lenses, as with spectacle prescribing (*see* Section 29.4).
- If they exist, old pre-contact lens spectacles should be examined. They are unlikely to be accurate but offer clues to the original *Rx* and degree of astigmatism.
- Measure the old lenses where possible.

13.6.2 Refitting with hard gas-permeable lenses

FITTING

- The slit lamp is used to observe the extent of any corneal oedema or lens-induced staining.

- The PMMA lenses are assessed with white light and fluorescein, noting where improvements to the physical fitting may be made.
- The PMMA lenses are removed and measured.
- 'K' readings are taken as carefully as possible but they may be distorted, unreliably flat and show an artificial degree of astigmatism.
- An assessment of the refraction is made.
- The initial trial lenses are based on 'K' readings but measurements of old lenses are taken into account. Much more reliance is placed on the fluorescein appearance than 'K's, although this is also difficult because central oedema may give a conus-like fitting.

CHOICE OF DESIGN

- Hard gas-permeable lenses give better vision if steep fittings are avoided.
- PMMA difficulties such as poor centration or flare can often be solved by fitting both a larger optic and total diameter.
- There is less 3 and 9 o'clock staining with narrower edge clearance.
- For patients with very tight lids, designs are avoided with narrow edge lift, especially aspherics. There an increased possibility of lens adhesion (*see* Section 28.3.6).
- If both practitioner and patient are perfectly happy with the existing PMMA design it can be duplicated in a hard gas-permeable material.

CHOICE OF MATERIAL

- A low to medium *Dk* material can be used if the patient is asymptomatic and there are no particular signs of oedema.
- A medium to high *Dk* should be considered where there are more obvious corneal changes.
- Use fluorosilicon acrylates (or possibly CAB), and avoid silicon acrylates, where protein deposits are likely to be a problem (e.g. hay fever sufferers, vernal catarrh).
- Avoid CAB and other less rigid materials with tight lids and toric corneas since lenses may flex or distort.

- Avoid CAB and other easily scratched materials with patients prone to surface damage.
- Avoid brittle materials for initial refitting. Patients used to handling relatively robust PMMA are likely to have breakage problems.
- Consider moulded CAB where there is a strong predisposition to 3 and 9 o'clock staining.

ORDERING LENSES

- More confidence can be placed on the final fitting if it correlates with 'K' readings, old lens measurements, refraction or calculated lens BVP.
- Refraction frequently shows an increase in minus of 0.25–0.50 D after about 2 weeks. Myopes should therefore be fully corrected and binocular adds are not usually given. Take into account the BVP of the old lenses and for non-presbyopes possibly even overcorrect by –0.25 D.
- Carefully specify centre and edge thickness where possible.

Practical advice

- Use a laboratory where lenses can be returned for exchange, modification or credit.
- Fees should take into account the extra time and lens costs that may be required in refitting PMMA.

FOLLOW-UP

- The first check-up should be after about 2 weeks to reassess the fitting, corneas and lens powers.
- Reconsider the lens material.
- Unless there is a gross change in fitting or power, lenses should not be modified for another 4–6 weeks. By this time most corneal changes will have stabilized and a spectacle *Rx* may also be feasible.
- In some cases, further minor changes may be found up to 12 months later.

PROBLEMS

A minority of patients cannot adapt to gas-permeable hard lenses because of:

- Physical discomfort, relating to surface wetting properties and increased corneal sensitivity.
- Poor visual acuity, relating to lens flexure or distortion.
- Greasing and deposits problems.
- CLIPC.

If these problems cannot be resolved, the practitioner may be obliged to return to an improved design of PMMA or change to soft lenses after a further 6–8 weeks.

PATIENT ADVICE

On lens collection, patients should be carefully advised about:

- The importance of using the recommended solutions, and enzyme tablets where necessary.
- The shorter life span compared with PMMA.
- The increased risk of scratching and breakage.
- To note any lens adherence or difficulty with removal.
- Increased discomfort with foreign bodies.

13.6.3 Refitting with soft lenses

Except in very special circumstances, it is not generally feasible to refit PMMA wearers directly with soft lenses.

- The problems listed at initial fitting and as the fitting progresses are much more significant with soft lenses.
- As the 'K' readings change, the degree of astigmatism may alter in an unpredictable fashion. Initially good acuity may deteriorate as corneal toricity changes.
- Some PMMA wearers find the gelatinous feel of a soft lens quite unpleasant on the eye.
- Many PMMA wearers have solutions difficulties, both with allergic response and the additional complexities of soft lens disinfection.

Practical advice

- Do not refit PMMA wearers directly with soft lenses.
- Where it is essential to provide PMMA wearers with soft lenses, it is generally better to refit first with hard gas-permeable lenses as an intermediate step. After about 6–8 weeks, the cornea and refraction may have stabilized sufficiently to make soft lens fitting feasible.
- Disposable lenses have a place in coping with a continuously altering corneal curvature and refraction.

Reference

1.   Boyd, H. (1971) Analysis of 1,000 consecutive contact lens cases. *First Scientific Congress of the European Contact Lens Society of Ophthalmologists*, London (June)

Chapter 14

Orthokeratology and reverse geometry lenses

It has been observed for many years that conventionally fitted PMMA lenses appear to reduce the rate of increase of myopia.[1,2]. Modern gas-permeable lenses seem to produce a similar effect but to a lesser extent.[3] A more active approach to myopia control is orthokeratology, defined as 'the reduction, modification or elimination of a visual defect by the programmed application of contact lenses'.[4]

In practical terms, orthokeratology applies to myopic eyes and aims to eliminate the refractive error or to reduce it to a sufficiently small degree that the patient can function without spectacles or contact lenses for most of the waking day. The result is achieved by flattening the cornea in a controlled fashion by wearing contact lenses with the BOZR significantly flatter than the corneal radius. When the desired result has been achieved, the new corneal shape is maintained by means of retainer lenses.

14.1 Historical

It is only recently that orthokeratology has begun to achieve any scientific acceptability. The procedure has been practised in the USA for over 30 years,[5,6] but with controversial and mainly anecdotal results. It developed from the clinical observation that wearing PMMA lenses flattened the cornea and reduced myopia. Early techniques such as the May–Grant method (named after its originators) used a series of progressively flatter lenses with a TD of about 10.00 mm and BOZD of about 8.50 mm. Results proved unpredictable and lens decentration frequently induced significant corneal distortion. Despite claims of a large reduction in myopia, results were limited to a decrease of approximately 1.25 D.

Orthokeratology has now achieved a degree of clinical reliability with the advent of:

- Hard gas-permeable materials to improve corneal physiology.
- Reverse geometry lenses.
- Corneal topography measurement so that changes in corneal curvature can be carefully monitored.

14.2 Current approach

The success of orthokeratology depends on:

- Lid forces.
- Duration of lens wear.
- Type of fitting.
- The corneal rheology of the individual patient.

The cornea is defined mathematically by its apical radius (Ro), eccentricity or e value (*see* Section 8.4), and chord diameter. The shape is in almost all cases that of a prolate elipse. As the myopia lessens, the e value reduces and the cornea becomes more spherical. The theoretical limit of myopia reduction is achieved when the eccentricity is reduced to zero, although in some cases the cornea may become slightly oblate to give a further small but unpredictable reduction in myopia.

Rule of thumb

A change in e value of 0.21 is approximately equivalent to 1.00 D.

It is therefore feasible to expect a cornea with Rx –2.50 D and e = 0.5 to reduce to emmetropia. If the Rx is –4.50 and e = 0.4, a reduction to only –2.50 D would be anticipated.

ADVANTAGES OF ORTHOKERATOLOGY

- Good vision without spectacles or contact lenses for most of the day.
- It is not a surgical procedure.
- It is reversible.
- It is not painful.

- The technique uses established contact lens procedures with a minimal risk of problems.

Compared with laser surgery, orthokeratology

- Treats both eyes at the same time.
- Does not involve post operative pain.
- Does not incur the risk of corneal haze.
- Is less expensive.

DISADVANTAGES OF ORTHOKERATOLOGY

- It can treat only low degrees of myopia.
- Several visits are required over the first few months.
- Patients must use retainer lenses or the cornea will revert to its original shape.
- The precise reduction of myopia cannot be guaranteed as it varies from one patient to another.
- For the best results, careful patient compliance is necessary.

INDICATIONS

- Young, early myopes.
- Myopia up to –3.00 D.
- Low degrees of astimatism.
- High corneal e value, over 0.50.
- Occasional spectacle wearers.

CONTRAINDICATIONS

- Myopia greater than –3.50 D to –4.00 D.
- With-the-rule astigmatism over –1.00 D.
- Against-the-rule astigmatism.
- Residual astigmatism.
- Low corneal e values.
- Where proper centration cannot be achieved.
- Loose lids where there is minimum force to mould the corneal shape.
- A history of lens adhesion.

- Long-term hard lens wearers of spherical designs, where the corneal asphericity has already been reduced.
- Unrealistic patient expectations.

14.3 Reverse geometry lenses

Reverse geometry lenses have been introduced since the advent of computer-controlled lathes where it is feasible to manufacture the secondary curve steeper than the BZOR (*see* Section 1.4). Reverse geometry lenses are used in orthokeratology to achieve good centration and optimum pressure distribution under the lens. They also give a more rapid corneal response, and the term *accelerated orthokeratology* is sometimes used.

14.3.1 Fitting theory and radius selection for reverse geometry lenses

Unlike most hard lens fitting, which is based on flattest 'K' and lens design, reverse geometry lenses are fitted according to:

- The sagittal depth of the cornea.
- Tear layer thickness (TLT) (*see* Section 7.4).

    The ideal lens has the same sag as the cornea with a compensation of 10 μm for TLT. It gives minimal central clearance with touch at the outer edge of the steep second curve. Lenses are therefore calculated on the basis of the chord which represents the TD minus the width of the peripheral curve (Figure 14.1).

Corneal sag $(z) = Ro - \sqrt{(Ro^2 - y^2p)p}$

where Ro = corneal apical radius
p = $1 - e^2$
y = 1/2 chord diameter

Contact lens sag =

$BOZR - \sqrt{(BOZR^2 - (BOZD/2)^2}$

$+ \sqrt{(BOZR - BPR1)^2 - (BOZD/2)^2}$

$- \sqrt{(BOZR - BPR2)^2 - ((TD-1)/2)^2}$

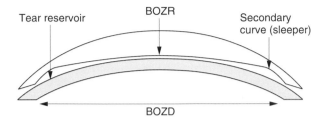

Figure 14.1 Diagram of reverse geometry lens

The radius of the first trial lens can be calculated using these two formulae:

1. Determine effective chord diameter = (TD of lens minus peripheral curve width).
2. Calculate corneal sag using effective chord diameter and e value.
3. Calculate required lens sag (= corneal sag plus TLT compensation of 0.010 mm).
4. Select trial lens with nearest sag to this required value over the same effective chord diameter.

In practice, the first trial lens is generally determined using a computer program which can rapidly calculate the radius required for different lens diameters. With average corneal eccentricity and a lens diameter of 10.60 mm, the correct radius is usually about 0.35–0.45 mm flatter than flattest 'K'.

14.3.2 BOZD

The most commonly used BOZDs are 7.00 mm and 6.00 mm, respectively, although the range is from 6.00 mm to 8.00 mm in steps of 0.50 mm.

14.3.3 Second curve or tear reservoir

The tear reservoir (TR) is responsible for creating the negative pressure, which in turn causes the corneal flattening. The curve is specified in dioptres, between 1.00 D and 9.00 D steeper than the BOZR. The tear reservoir is usually spherical but can be made aspheric for non-orthokeratology use.

- The most commonly used TRs are 4.00 D, usually optimum with a 7.00 mm BOZD (designated 704) and 3.00 D, usually optimum with a 6.00 mm BOZD (designated 603).
- TRs of 5.00 D and over permit only small areas of central touch, less than 3.00 mm.
- TRs less than 3.00 D give too large an area of central touch, more than 3.50 mm.

14.3.4 Peripheral curve

The first choice of peripheral curve is usually tangential and 1 mm wide. This is designated a *C edge*. Sometimes either narrower or aspheric peripheries are used.
- The AEL is standard at 0.12 mm, but is available from approximately 0.08 mm to 0.16 mm.
- Reducing the edge lift gives an overall tighter fitting.
- Increasing the edge lift gives an overall looser fitting.

14.3.5 Total diameter

Lenses are fitted with large TDs to achieve better comfort and centration.
- The first choice is 10.60 mm, but 11.20 mm lenses are sometimes more successful.
- Small corneas may require TDs of 9.80 mm.
- Lenses are sometimes fenestrated to improve tears flow.

14.3.6 Lens specification

Companies such as Contex in the USA produce a very wide range of lenses, but those most commonly used are clinical equivalents and designated the 704 and 603 Series. They achieve the best balance between central touch and depth of TR. The 704 has a 30% greater TR volume than the 603 and is generally the design of first choice. A full specification is recorded as:

8.35:10.60 OK704C −0.75 where

8.35   = BOZR
10.60 = TD
OK   = a reverse geometry lens for orthokeratology
70   = BOZD of 7.00 mm
4   = a TR of 4.00 D

C   = a tangential peripheral curve 1.00 mm wide
−0.75 = BVP (usually plano or low minus because of the flat fitting)

14.4 Clinical appearance of reverse geometry lenses

14.4.1 Fluorescein pattern

The suitability of the lens fitting is determined with fluorescein. The appearance is quite unlike that found with a conventional hard lens and similar in some respects to that seen with silicone elastomer lenses (*see* Section 32.3). The pattern consists of central touch over the central 3 mm surrounded by an annulus of fluorescein representing the steeper TR. The TR is in turn surrounded by an area of peripheral touch, which further supports the lens, and leads into a 1 mm band of edge clearance (Figure 14.2).

Practical advice

Fluorescein only becomes visible when the TLT approaches 20 μm. The central area has been calculated for a TLT of 10 μm and only gives the *appearance* of touch.

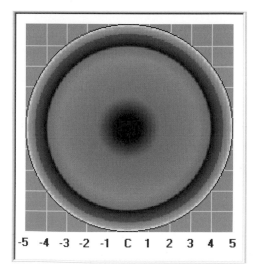

Figure 14.2 Fluorescein pattern of reverse geometry lens

14.4.2 Other fitting points

- The lens must give good centration.
- The area of central touch should be 3.0 mm–3.5 mm wide.
- The TR should have sharply defined edges.
- TLT must not be less than 10 μm. A lens which is too flat may cause central abrasion and staining. When in doubt, fit steep.
- Flat lenses ride high.
- Steep lenses ride low.
- Steep lenses often trap small bubbles in the TR.
- Increase TD to improve centration but any change in parameters must be recalculated to give optimum TLT.
- Changing TD will therefore require a change in BOZR.
- A change in TD gives a smaller change to lens sag than a change in radius.

14.5 Corneal topography

Modern instrumentation enables the mapping of corneal topography over most of its surface (*see* Section 2.3). Those corneal plots most useful in orthokeratology are the tangential, subtractive and numeric. The measurement of corneal topography is essential because:

- It can help predict potential failures by providing values for the apical radius and eccentricity prior to fitting.
- It can provide a permanent record of corneal shape and power at all stages of the procedure.
- It demonstrates graphically any unacceptable degree of corneal distortion.
- The subtractive plot gives a record of progress.
- The type of distortion gives indications as to whether the fit is flat or steep.

14.6 Fitting and aftercare procedures

14.6.1 Fitting

- Full ocular and slit lamp examination.

- Refraction including unaided vision before commencing orthokeratology.
- Corneal topography measurement.
- Numeric plots to establish apical radius and e value.
- Calculation of the first trial lens.
- Trial wear period of 6–8 hours.

A lengthy trial is necessary to provide the following information:

- The new unaided vision.
- Degree of refractive change.
- Extent of shape change.
- Movement and centration of trial lens after settling.
- Corneal response in terms of staining.
- Whether the patient wishes to continue with the procedure.

A satisfactory response usually gives:

- A significant improvement in unaided vision.
- A reduction in myopia of at least 0.75 D.
- No corneal staining or other adverse signs.
- Maintained lens centration and mobility.
- Minimal, if any, corneal distortion.

An unsatisfactory response gives:

- No improvement in unaided vision.
- An insignificant reduction in myopia.
- Corneal staining even with a well-fitting lens.
- Poor patient tolerance.

In some cases it is preferable to repeat the trial because of an unsatisfactory fitting at the end of several hours. This may have caused:

- Lens decentration.
- Lens adhesion.
- Corneal staining.
- Corneal distortion.
- Borderline improvement in refractive error.
- Borderline improvement in unaided vision.

14.6.2 Overnight wear

Lenses for orthokeratology were originally worn during the day, but more recent experience has shown that overnight wear (sometimes called *night therapy*) has several advantages. There is no discomfort from dust, foreign bodies, dry eyes or other environmental factors. Lenses are less likely to be lost or damaged, and gradually the waking day becomes increasingly free of both contact lenses and spectacles. Overnight use is not the same as extended wear because the orthokeratology lenses are removed during the day. Nevertheless, materials should have a high *Dk* of at least 90 and a *Dk/t* greater than 40.

Patients should be warned of the possibility of lens adhesion on waking. They should be advised how to free the lens with careful massage to avoid any risk of corneal abrasion. Fenestration can also be used to facilitate tears flow but may cause dimpling. The first check-up is carried out before the lenses are removed.

14.6.3 Subsequent aftercare visits

If the trial has given a positive response, lenses are then ordered. Because most patients are low myopes and there is a significant minus liquid lens, powers are usually fairly close to plano.

Patients should be checked at the end of 1 and 2 weeks and subsequently monitored on a regular basis. It is important that examinations should take place at the same time of day for each visit, to maintain a consistent record of refraction and unaided vision.

14.6.4 Retainer lenses

Orthokeratology is a reversible procedure. When the optimum result has been achieved, a final pair of *retainer lenses* is used to maintain the new corneal shape and stabilize the improvement in visual acuity. The lenses are worn either overnight or for limited periods during the day, the required time depending on the individual patient. Mountford suggests that, ultimately, 70% of patients require lens wear every second night and 15% every third night.

References

1.   Stone, J. (1976) The possible influence of contact lenses on myopia. *British Journal of Physiological Optics*, **31**, 89–114

2. Black-Kelly, T.S.B. and Butler, D. (1971) The present position of contact lenses in relation to myopia. *British Journal of Physiological Optics*, **27**, 33–48
3. Perrigin, J., Perrigin, D., Quintero, S. and Grosvenor, T. (1990) Silicone/acrylate contact lenses for myopia control: 3-year results. *Optometry and Vision Science*, **67**, 764–765
4. Mountford, J. (1996) *Accelerated Orthokeratology*. Brisbane
5. Jessen, G.N. (1962) Orthofocus techniques. *Contacto*, **6** (7), 200–204
6. *Orthokeratology* (1972) Vol 1. International Orthokeratology Section of N.E.R.F publication
7. *Orthokeratology* (1974) Vol 2. International Orthokeratology Section of N.E.R.F. publication

Chapter 15

Scleral lens fitting

15.1 When scleral lenses should still be fitted

ADVANTAGES OF SCLERAL LENSES

- Almost never lost because they are held in place by the eyelids; capillary attraction is to the sclera rather than the cornea.
- Robust and dimensionally stable.
- Do not deteriorate.
- Handling may be easier for less dextrous patients, e.g. aphakes.
- Dry storage is usually preferable.
- Less expensive to maintain.
- Lid sensation is much less than with corneal lenses.
- Foreign bodies are uncommon except on insertion.
- Extensive power range possible, in excess of ±40.00 D.
- It is possible to encapsulate a realistic painted iris.

INDICATIONS

Irregular corneal topography

- High astigmatism.
- Primary corneal ectasia, i.e. keratoconus and related conditions.
- Corneal transplants.
- Traumatized eyes.

High refractive errors

- High ametropia when high-power corneal lenses lead to centration difficulties.

Encapsulated iris lenses

- Unsightly blind eyes.
- Aniridia
- Microphthalmos.

Therapeutic or protective applications

The large size of a scleral lens protects the anterior eye and enables the retention of a tears reservoir in abnormal conditions, including:

- Corneal exposure.
- Dry eyes.
- Trichiasis or lid margin keratinization.

Other applications

- Ptosis.
- Intermittent use where short-term adaptation may be easier than with corneal lenses (e.g. contact sports).
- Dusty environments.
- Water sports.

15.2 Preformed fitting

15.2.1 Preformed designs

A preformed scleral lens is fitted from trial sets of predetermined shape (Figure 15.1), without taking an impression of the eye.

Conical lenses

Developed by Feinbloom in 1936.[1] The design consists of a spherical optic portion (BOZR), a scleral zone (BSR) of which the major part is conical, and a crescent on the temporal side which has a spherical curve.

WIDE ANGLE LENSES

Introduced by Nissel in 1947.[2] The design is a combination of spherical optic and scleral portions with a conical transition

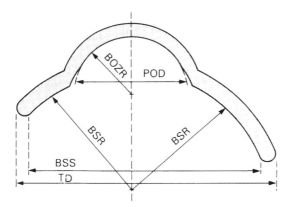

Figure 15.1 Preformed scleral lens. BOZR, back optic zone radius; BOZD, back optic zone diameter; SZR, scleral zone radius; TD, total diameter (from Phillips and Speedwell, *Contact Lenses*, 4th edn, Butterworth-Heinemann, Oxford, by permission)

designed to give a tangential junction between the optic and transition zones. Trial sets are extensive because they require sufficient variables for the fitting of both major parts of the lens. Range required:

SZR (scleral zone radius) 12.50–14.50 mm in 0.25 mm steps
BOZR 8.00–9.00 in 0.25 mm steps.

Transcurve lenses

Redesigned in their present form by Bier in 1948.[3] Lenses have a spherical optic and back scleral surface. The transition is 2.00 mm wide, with a spherical radius of curvature approximately halfway between the back optic and scleral zone. Usual range:

TD 22.50–24.50 mm
SZR 12.50–15.00 mm.

15.2.2 Traditional PMMA preformed scleral lens fitting

Four variables must be considered:

- Back optic zone radius.
- Back optic zone diameter.
- Scleral zone radius.
- Total diameter.

There are two possible approaches:

• Separate fitting of the scleral and optic portions.
• Fitting both parts at the same time.

INDEPENDENT OPTIC AND SCLERAL FITTING

The scleral zone is fitted using scleral fitting sets and the optic zone with a fenestrated lens for optic measurement (FLOM). The method enables some assessment of the independent portions. The disadvantage is that the practitioner never sees the complete and final fitting until the lens is dispensed.

SCLERAL PORTION

Trial sets vary both in scleral zone radius (SZR) and total diameter (TD). A full set consists of 12 lenses in steps of 0.50 mm for radius and diameter, but a useful minimum range is:

   TD: 22.50 mm and 24.50 mm
   SZR: 12.50 mm and 14.50 mm

It is important that the scleral portion does not interfere with the optic fitting, hence the optic radius should be no flatter than 7.50 mm at a chord width of 12.50 mm to ensure that the optic portion is clear of the cornea at all times during fitting. With experience, it is possible to judge by how much to alter the size without necessarily inspecting a second lens in situ . This does not apply to the radius where it is essential to observe the next lens.[4]

Practical advice

• Aim for a minimum clearance fitting, not more than 0.1 mm for a fenestrated scleral lens.
• An optimum fitting scleral radius minimizes conjunctival blood vessel blanching.
• A steep scleral fit bears excessively on the peripheral sclera and constricts the vessels in that area. A flat radius constricts the vessels around the limbus.
• The horizontal sclera is asymmetrical. It is not always possible to eliminate blanching completely so that a 75% 'glove fit' is acceptable.
• Avoid constricting the limbus wherever possible.
• Any modification to a scleral lens, especially the scleral zone, has an unpredictable outcome. Making a cast of the lens before proceeding is a sensible precaution.

The optic zone

The optic zone is fitted using FLOMs, first described by Bier in 1948.[5] They consist of an optic portion with a narrow scleral rim approximately 2 mm wide, and usually have a 13.00 mm radius. This is flatter than the limbal region it covers so that it does not interfere with the corneal fit. To assist fitting, the transition is deliberately left sharp. This can cause discomfort, so topical anaesthetic may be used. The lenses are identified by the back optic zone radius and optic zone diameter. They are optically worked to enable refraction when the correct corneal fitting has been found. FLOMs have a 1.50 mm, peripheral fenestration. The normal range of parameters is:

Radius: 8.00–9.50 mm in 0.25 mm steps
Diameter: 13.00–14.75 mm in 0.25 mm steps
Generally, smaller lenses and optic diameters suit steep corneas

The fitting is assessed with fluorescein and is varied by altering either the radius or diameter. The optimum fit gives clearance over the whole cornea, extending 2–3 mm beyond the limbus. A crescent-shaped air bubble should remain at the limbus (Figure 15.2).

Figure 15.2 Crescent-shaped air bubble in FLOM fitting

Clinical equivalents

Two lenses giving identical fitting characteristics of apical clearance with different but related parameters are known as clinical equivalents.

Rule of thumb

If the BOZR is flattened by 0.25 mm, the BOZD must be increased by 0.50 mm to give the same apical clearance.

Example: $8.00/13.00 \equiv 8.25/13.50$

SIMULTANEOUS OPTIC AND SCLERAL FITTING

The main advantage of simultaneous fitting is that the appearance of the trial lens is similar to that of the final lens. It also avoids the discomfort of a FLOM, and topical anaesthesia is unnecessary. However, a large trial set is required to cover all the permutations. Wide angle lenses have been commonly used for simultaneous fitting because the design eliminates the variable of the BOZD. The permutations are reduced, but the fitting process is simplified. Preformed fitting is ideally carried out with a combination of simultaneous and separate systems.

15.3 Moulded (impression) fitting

Fitting sclerals from eye impressions is much better for dealing with irregular anterior ocular topography. The impression gives a negative shape of the cornea from which the scleral lens is made.[6]

15.3.1 Impression materials

ALGINATES

- Usually Orthoprint (the recommended material).
- The normal mixture is 2 g to 7 ml water, or equal volumes.
- Setting is faster with a higher temperature or humidity.

POLYVINYL SILOXANES

- Panasil *light body*, consisting of a base paste and hardener, is the product in most common use.
- Longer shelf-life if used occasionally.
- Impression does not dehydrate because no water is used.
- Retains dimensional stability after use.

15.3.2 Moulding procedure

- The eye must be anaesthetized with at least three drops of benoxinate, one instilled from above the cornea.
- One drop may also be instilled in the alternate eye to inhibit the blink if necessary.
- The eye to be moulded should look slightly down and in from the primary position. This can be achieved by dissociating the

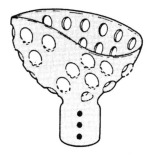

Figure 15.3 Moulding tray. The trays are colour coded (red = right; blue = left) and a system of dots denotes the size (3 dots = large; 2 dots = medium; 1 dot = small)

two eyes and marking the position of the cornea on the lower lid of the alternate eye.

- The moulding shell or tray is chosen as (a) small, medium or large; and (b) left or right, since nasal and temporal sizes are different (Figure 15.3).
- The impression material is mixed and spatulated to eliminate air bubbles.
- The average setting time of the impression material is about 30 seconds at normal room temperature.

INJECTION METHOD

- More time is available to finish mixing the impression material.
- Larger fitting trays can be used.
- The impression material is injected through a tube on the front of the moulding tray when placed on the eye.
- Care should be taken to ensure that the cornea is not distorted by the injection process.
- The tray is gently lifted at its sides to ensure complete coverage of the globe.

INSERTION METHOD

- The moulding tray is filled with material before being placed on the eye with the head in a horizontal position.
- The patient's head remains horizontal until the material has set.
- Insertion method may be preferable for use with polyvinyl siloxanes because they often do not flow as easily as alginates.

15.3.3 Producing the lens or shell

The impression is cast in dental stone to give a permanent positive cast of the eye.

SETTING AND MAKING PROCEDURE

- A PMMA sheet is heat moulded over the cast, trimmed to size and edged.
- The optic zone clearance is worked using diamond-coated lapping tools.
- The substance removed from the centre to give minimum clearance is normally 0.15 mm, whereas 0.22 mm is taken from the limbal area.
- The optic zone is polished with wax tools or cloth-covered spherical brass tools.

LABORATORY METHOD

The cast is sent to a laboratory with the following specifications:

- BOZR. A competent scleral lens laboratory can decide on the optimum BOZR without specific directions and cut according to the cast. If the laboratory cannot make this judgement, the practitioner is advised to find another laboratory that can.
- If necessary to specify, 0.20 mm flatter than flattest 'K' is a guide.[6]
- Total diameter. Usually marked on the cast so that the optimum size is cut.
- The transition is blended.
- Specifying centre thickness is inappropriate since it is determined from the BVP and FOZD.

15.3.4 Back vertex power

Over-refraction is carried out with a lens of known BOZR and BVP, preferably fitted slightly flat. A FLOM can be used if available, or a large diameter corneal lens. The front optic radius is calculated to give the required power and cut with a lathe. If the laboratory has determined the BOZR, an appropriate liquid lens allowance is necessary.

15.3.5 Ventilation of PMMA scleral lenses

Most patients can only wear a sealed PMMA lens for a few minutes before corneal hypoxia causes oedema. Ventilation allows fresh oxygenated tears to reach the cornea and is effected by:

- Fenestration, about 1 mm in diameter.
- Cutting a slot, usually 2 mm wide and one-quarter of the diameter of the limbus in length. It can be thinner if there is too much lid sensation.
- A channel of clearance connecting the optic zone to the lens. In therapeutic fitting, however, scleral lenses are sometimes left sealed (i.e. not ventilated). This helps fluid retention.

15.3.6 Scleral lenses with modern hard gas permeable lens materials

The first preformed hard gas permeable scleral lenses were described by Ezekiel in 1983.[6] The materials are not sufficiently thermoplastic to heat mould, but two methods by which impressions can be used as a starting point for hard gas permeable scleral lens fitting have been described, either by duplicating a fitted PMMA shape using an individualized cast moulding system,[7] or using a button inserted into a PMMA scleral zone with adhesives.[8] Experimental trial results show that there is a distinct improvement in corneal physiology compared with PMMA.[9–14] The use of hard gas-permeable sclerals has increased steadily since the introduction of modern materials and it has become evident that patient tolerance has improved considerably.[15–21] Hard gas-permeable scleral lenses can be lathe cut from large diameter blanks,[6] or produced with a range of moulded back surfaces.[4]

The improved gas permeability has enabled the use of sealed lens designs which simplify fitting processes.[15–19] Sealed lenses are simpler and more predictable to fit because they do not settle back as much as ventilated lenses, hence it is possible to control the apical clearance to a greater extent.[4] They can usually be fitted without the intrusion of an air bubble into the tears reservoir, irrespective of the corneal topography. The main limitation of hard gas-permable sealed preformed lenses is when the sclera is excessively toric or irregular, which is the principal indication for using either of the two methods for manufacturing hard gas-permeable scleral lenses from impressions.The potential for therapeutic uses of scleral lenses to aid corneal coverage is greatly enhanced by hard gas-permeable materials because sealed lenses retain the best possible fluid reservoir where there is a tears deficiency.

15.4 Scleral lens specification

The British Standards relating to sclerals are BS 5562:1978 and BS 3521:1988 Part 3 based on ISO 8320 – 1986.
For spherical preformed lenses:

BOZR = Back optic zone radius
BOZD = Back optic zone diameter
BPOZR = Back peripheral optic zone radius of optic, if present
SZR   = Scleral zone radius
TD   = Total diameter
BSS   = Back scleral size where specified is preceded by the letter B; otherwise TD is assumed
L   = Orientation of long axis in standard notation
D   = Displacement of optic and direction

Example (mm):

R/BOZR:BOZD/BSR:BSS/L/D/transition
R/8.40. 11.00/13.00: B23.50/L10/D 1.00 in/sharp transition

Some fitting sets still use the 1962 British Standards which gives a different specification:

Example (mm): 14.25/8.75/13.75/B23.50 D1 in

Radius of back scleral surface   = 14.25
Radius of back optic zone   = 8.75
Primary optic diameter   = 13.75
Back scleral size or total diameter = B23.50
Displacement   = D1 in

References

1. Feinbloom, W. (1936) A plastic contact lens. *Transactions of 15th Congress of the American Academy of Optometry*, **10**, 44
2. Cowan, J.M. (1948) The wide angle contact lens. *Optician*, **115**, 359
3. Bier, N. and Cole, P.J. (1948) The transcurve contact lens fitting shell. *Optician*, **115**, 605–610
4. Pullum, K.W. (1997) The role of scleral lenses in modern contact lens practice. In *Contact Lenses* A.J. Phillips and L. Speedwell (eds), Butterworth-Heinemann, Oxford, pp. 566–608
5. Bier, N. (1948) The practice of ventilated contact lenses. *Optician*, **116**, 497–501
6. Ezekiel, D. (1983) Gas permeable haptic lenses. *Journal of the British Contact Lens Association*, **6** (4), 158–161

7. Pullum, K.W. (1987) Feasibility study for the production of gas permeable scleral lenses using ocular impression techniques. *Transactions of the British Contact Lens Association Annual Clinical Conference*, 35–39

8. Lyons, C.J., Buckley, R.J., Pullum, K.W. and Sapp, N. (1989) Development of gas permeable impression-moulded scleral contact lenses. A preliminary report. *Acta Ophthalmology*, **67** (Suppl 192), 162–164

9. Ruben, C.M. and Benjamin, W.J. (1985) Scleral contact lenses: preliminary report on oxygen-permeable materials. *Contact Lens*, **13** (2), 5–10

10. Bleshoy, H. and Pullum, K.W. (1988) Corneal response to gas permeable impression scleral lenses. *Journal of the British Contact Lens Association*, **11** (2), 31–34

11. Pullum, K.W., Hobley, A.J. and Parker, J.H. (1990) Dallos award lecture part two: Hypoxic corneal changes following sealed gas permeable impression scleral lens wear. *Journal of the British Contact Lens Association*, **13** (1), 83–87

12. Pullum, K.W., Hobley, A.J. and Davison, C. (1991) 100 + *Dk*. Does thickness make a difference? *Journal of the British Contact Lens Association*, **6**, 158–161

13. Mountford, J., Carkeet, N. and Carney, L. (1994) Corneal thickness changes during scleral lens wear. Effect of gas permeability. *International Contact Lens Clinic*, **21**, 19–21

14. Pullum, K.W. and Stapleton, F.J. (1997) What is the effect of varying *Dk* and lens thickness in scleral lenses? *The Contact Lens Association of Ophthalmologists*. IN PRESS

15. Pullum, K.W., Parker, J.H. and Hobley, A.J. (1989) Development of gas permeable scleral lenses produced from impressions of the eye. Joseph Dallos Award Lecture 1989. *Transactions of the British Contact Lens Association Annual Clinical Conference*, **6**, 77–81

16. Visser, R. (1990) Een nieuwe toekomst hoogzuurtofdoorlatende scleralenzen bij verschillende pathologie. *Nederlands Tijdschrift voor Optometrie en Contactologie*, **3**, 10–14

17. Schein, O.D., Rosenthal, P. and Ducharme, C. (1990) A gas permeable scleral contact lens for visual rehabilitation. *American Journal of Ophthalmology*, **109**, 318–322

18. Ezekiel, D. (1991) Gas permeable scleral lenses. *Spectrum*, July, 19–24

19. Kok, J.H.C. and Visser, R. (1992) Treatment of ocular surface disorders and dry eyes with high gas-permeable scleral lenses. *Cornea*, **11**, 518–522

20. Tan, D.T.H., Pullum, K.W. and Buckley, R.J. (1995) Medical applications of scleral contact lenses: 2. Gas-permeable scleral contact lenses. *Cornea*, **14** (2), 130–137

21. Pullum, K.W. and Buckley, R.J. (1997) A study of 530 patients referred for RGP scleral contact lens assessment. *Cornea*, IN PRESS

Chapter 16

Soft lens design and fitting

The most appropriate design has to be selected from the very wide range of lens forms now available. Several factors must be taken into account:

- Size (corneal or semi-scleral).
- Water content (low, medium or high).
- Thickness (standard or thin) (*see* Section 17.4).
- Geometric and optic design (spherical or aspheric).
- Manufacturing method (lathed or moulded).
- Lens flexibility (*see* Section 17.2).
- Lens power (*see* Section 17.1).
- Conventional or disposable (*see* Chapter 19).

All of these factors have some influence on vision, comfort and fitting characteristics, but the predominant factor which determines the method of fitting is usually the total diameter. The two main fitting philosophies into which soft lenses may be divided are therefore *corneal* and *semi-scleral*, although there is now considerable overlap, especially with single diameter lenses, between these two approaches.

16.1 Corneal diameter lenses

The majority of corneal diameter lenses are still manufactured from low to medium water materials to give reproducible lenses of good durability. The thinner varieties, in particular, cause minimum interference with corneal metabolism and give excellent cosmetic appearance.

INDICATIONS

- Most straightforward cases.
- Small corneas.

- Patients with small palpebral apertures and difficulty in handling.
- Cosmetic reasons

CONTRAINDICATIONS

- Very large corneas.
- Shallow corneoscleral junction allowing decentration.
- Tight lids causing lens decentration.
- Sensitive lid margin.
- Sensitive limbus.

FITTING

Radius

- Radius selection is based on keratometry
- Most radii are between 7.90 mm and 8.90 mm.
- Less flexible low water content materials may require radii 0.70 mm or more flatter than 'K'.
- The radius for standard HEMA lenses is usually between 0.30 mm and 0.60 mm flatter than 'K'.
- High water content lenses are fitted closer to alignment.
- Fitting steps are usually between 0.20 mm and 0.40 mm.
- Most corneal lenses have a single curve back surface.

Total diameter

- Lenses should be just slightly larger than the horizontal visible iris diameter (HVID). They should extend beyond the limbus by up to 0.50–0.75 mm to avoid irritation.
- Most corneal lenses vary in size from 12.50 to 13.50 mm, with the possible range from 12.00 to 14.00 mm.
- High water content lenses are fitted approximately 0.50 mm larger than HEMA.
- High plus and high minus lenses are fitted approximately 0.50 mm larger than low powers in order to achieve stability on the cornea.
- Fitting steps are usually 0.50 mm.

Power

After allowing for vertex distance considerations, the lens power is usually within 0.25 D of the spectacle *Rx*. Thicker designs require about 0.25 D less minus than thin lenses.

Fitting appearance

Fitting characteristics are mainly as described in Chapter 18, but it is essential for a correctly fitting lens to give complete corneal coverage with proper centration to avoid the risk of epithelial dehydration and arcuate staining of any exposed area. The slit lamp should be used for careful observation of centration and movement, since these can be significantly influenced by factors such as:

- Corneal topography.
- Limbal topography.
- Lid pressure.
- Size of palpebral aperture.
- Position of cornea within palpebral aperture.

Figure 16.1 shows the four common ways in which a lens may position on the cornea with the eye in the primary position:

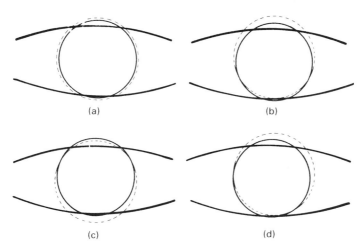

(a)   (b)

(c)   (d)

Figure 16.1 The four common positions (*see* text) taken up by soft lenses of corneal size, on an eye in the primary position: (a) correctly centred; (b) slightly high; (c) slightly low; (d) laterally decentred

(a) An optimum fitting is shown. The lens is perfectly centred and there should be 0.25–0.50 mm of vertical movement on blinking.
(b) The lens is riding high, influenced perhaps by a tight upper lid. This may prove acceptable, provided that the decentration is no more than about 0.50 mm. An attempt should be made to improve the fitting by selecting a larger diameter.
(c) The lens is riding in a low position. It generally represents an unsatisfactory fitting which is either too small or too flat and the patient is likely to complain of unacceptable lid sensation. It can also occur with the downwards pressure of a relatively heavy upper lid. This creates a fitting which is too tight, although initially quite comfortable. There is the possibility, after several hours of wear, of arcuate staining at the superior limbus together with oedema from insufficient tears exchange.
(d) The lens is eccentrically located. This may also be due to a fitting which is too small or too flat, or because of lid pressure with a shallow corneoscleral junction. It represents an unsatisfactory fitting and a larger total diameter should be tried. However, if the decentration is limited to 0.50 mm, it may occasionally prove acceptable. An attempt should always be made to improve the fitting characteristics of a decentred lens by selecting a larger diameter. Where this fails, it may be necessary to consider a semi-scleral lens.

Clinical equivalents

The principle of clinical equivalents applies where two lenses of the same design and material, with different but related parameters, give similar fitting characteristics on the eye.

Rule of thumb

A change in diameter of 0.50 mm ≡ a change in radius of 0.20 mm.

Examples: 7.90:12.50 ≡ 8.10:13.00
8.30:13.00 ≡ 8.50:13.50

To improve a loose fitting

• Select a larger total diameter.

- Select a steeper radius.
- Use a more rigid or lower water content material.
- Use a different lens thickness.

To improve a tight fitting

- Select a flatter radius.
- Select a smaller total diameter.
- Use a less rigid or higher water content material.
- Use a different lens thickness.

16.1.1 Examples of corneal diameter lenses

HYDRON MINI (HYDRON)

A standard thickness, corneal diameter lens for daily wear; manufactured by lathing.

Material properties

Chemical nature	HEMA cross-linked polymer. Non-ionic
Water content	38.6% at 20°C
Dk	8.0×10^{-11} at 20°C
	10.0×10^{-11} at 35°C
Refractive index	1.513 (dry), 1.43 (wet)

Lens geometry

- Centre thickness is 0.12 mm at −3.00 D and 0.21 mm at +2.00 D.
- Back surface is a single curve.
- Front surface is lenticulated.

Parameters available

See Table 16.1.

Fitting technique

- Total diameter should be at least 1.00 mm larger than the HVID.
- Lenses of 13.00 mm diameter are used in about 90% of cases.

Table 16.1 Parameters available for Hydron Mini lenses

Radius (mm)	7.90–8.90 in 0.20 steps	8.10–9.30 in 0.20 steps
Diameter (mm)	12.50	13.00
Power (D)	±10.00 in 0.25 steps	
	±10.50 to ±30.00 in 0.50 steps	

- Initial radius is selected approximately 0.70 mm flatter than 'K'.

Typical lens specification

8.70:13.00   −3.00

LUNELLE ES 70 (ESSILOR)

A high water content mainly corneal diameter lens for daily or flexible extended wear, manufactured by lathing. One of the few high water content lenses available in a small diameter.

Material properties

Chemical properties	Copolymer of PMMA and polyvinyl pyrrolidone. Non-ionic
Water content	70%
Dk	35.0×10^{-11} at 25°C
Refractive index	1.38

Lens geometry

- Centre thickness is 0.12 mm at −3.00 D; average thickness is 0.15 mm.
- Back surface is a single curve.
- Front surface is lenticulated.

Parameters available

See Table 16.2.

Fitting technique

- The 14.00 mm diameter is selected for corneas larger than 11.25 mm; the 13.00 mm diameter for corneas 11.25 mm or smaller.

Table 16.2 Parameters available for Lunelle ES 70 lenses

Radius (mm)	7.70–8.30 in 0.30 steps	8.00–9.20 in 0.30 steps
Diameter (mm)	13.00	14.00
Power (D)	+8.00 to –12.00	±20.00

- The radius is selected to be at least 0.60 mm flatter than 'K' for 14.00 mm lenses and 0.30 mm flatter than 'K' for 13.00 mm lenses.
- Lens movement should be 0.50–0.75 mm.
- The relative stiffness of the material gives an advantage in correcting low to medium degrees of astigmatism (0.75–1.25 D).
- A low rate of lens dehydration is claimed to assist or avoid dry eye problems.

Typical lens specification

8.00:13.00   –3.00
8.90:14.00   –3.00

RELATED LENSES

- Standard front surface toric.
- Toric *Rx* TDI, a back surface toric.
- A range of four colour enhancers.
- Lunelle Solaire, with sun filter and UV inhibitor.
- Standard UV; and Aphakic UV, with powers from +10.00 to +20.00.
- Lunelle Therapeutic, plano lenses for bandage use.

16.2 Semi-scleral lenses

The majority of lathed semi-sclerals are significantly larger and thicker than corneal soft lenses, giving better stability of both vision and fitting. In order to provide good physiological response, they are now mostly manufactured from medium to high water content materials with high *Dk* values.

INDICATIONS

- Most straightforward cases.

- Large corneas.
- Large palpebral apertures.
- Sensitive lid margin.
- Sensitive limbus.
- Hyperopes and high powers, if high water content.
- Moderate degrees of astigmatism (0.75–1.25 D).

CONTRAINDICATIONS

- Very small corneas.
- Small palpebral apertures, and tight lids if handling difficult.
- Corneas prone to oedema, if low water content.
- Where cosmetic appearance is important.

FITTING

Radius

- Radius selection is based on keratometry.
- Most radii are fitted between 8.30 mm and 9.20 mm.
- High water content lenses are fitted between 0.30 mm and 1.00 mm flatter than 'K'.
- Low water content lenses are fitted flatter, between 0.70 mm and 1.30 mm flatter than 'K'.
- Fitting steps are usually 0.30 mm or 0.40 mm.
- Most semi-scleral lenses are of bicurve construction, with a relatively flat but narrow peripheral curve.

Total diameter

- Lenses are fitted significantly larger than the visible iris diameter, to give deliberate apical touch with further support beyond the limbus where they overlap onto the sclera. This type of three-point touch is shown in Figure 16.2.
- The total diameter is selected to be 2.00–3.00 mm larger than the horizontal visible iris diameter. However, many semi-scleral lenses are manufactured in only one size.
- The majority of semi-scleral lenses are fitted with total diameters of 14.20–14.80 mm; the possible range is from 13.50 to 16.00 mm.

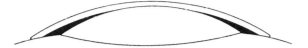

Figure 16.2 Semi-scleral lens giving three-point touch

- High and low water content lenses are both fitted with very similar diameters.
- Fitting steps are usually 0.50 mm.

Power

Mainly because of flexure effects, the power of a correctly fitting lens often shows approximately 0.25–0.50 D less minus than the spectacle *Rx*, after allowing for any vertex distance considerations. With more rigid low water content lenses, this difference can be as great as 0.75 D.

Fitting appearance and lens movement

Fitting characteristics are mainly as described in Chapter 18 and Table 18.1. It is essential that a correctly fitting lens should be sufficiently large to span the limbus and not interfere with the blood vessels in this region.

Soft lens fittings are assessed in relation to lens movement with

- Blinking.
- Upwards and lateral gaze.
- The 'push-up test'.

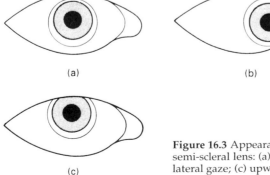

(a)

(b)

(c)

Figure 16.3 Appearance of a correctly fitting semi-scleral lens: (a) primary position; (b) lateral gaze; (c) upward gaze

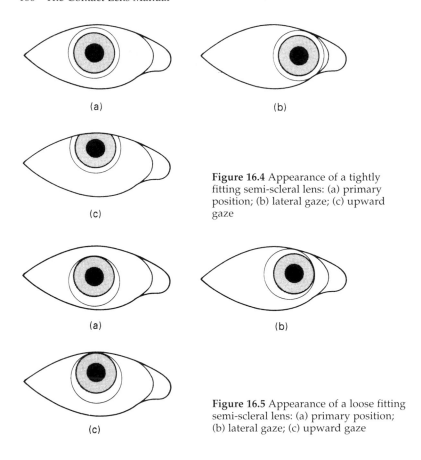

Figure 16.4 Appearance of a tightly fitting semi-scleral lens: (a) primary position; (b) lateral gaze; (c) upward gaze

Figure 16.5 Appearance of a loose fitting semi-scleral lens: (a) primary position; (b) lateral gaze; (c) upward gaze

Figure 16.3(a–c) shows diagrammatically the limits of acceptable movement and position for semi-scleral lenses with the eye in the primary position and in lateral and upward gaze. Figure 16.4(a-c) indicates the lack of movement with a tight lens, whereas Figure 16.5(a-c) shows the excessive mobility of a loose fitting.

The 'push-up' test

This simple test is used to assess the speed of recovery when a soft lens is displaced vertically upwards by the practitioner with the eye in the primary position. A rapid recovery movement suggests a satisfactory fitting, whereas a slow recovery may be indicative of tightness.

Clinical equivalents and altering the fitting

The principle of clinical equivalents also applies so that two lenses of different but related specification behave in the same way on the eye.

Rule of thumb

A change in radius of 0.30 mm ≡ a change of diameter of 0.50 mm.

Examples: 8.10:13.50 ≡ 8.40:14.00
8.70:14.50 ≡ 9.00:15.00

Clinical equivalents have approximately the same ratio of sagittal depth to total diameter. They do not have the same sagittal depth.

To improve a loose fitting

- Select a steeper radius.
- Select a larger total diameter.
- Use a more rigid or lower water content material.
- Use a different lens thickness.

A lens of specification 8.70:14.00 may be progressively tightened with the following steps: 8.70:14.50; 8.40:14.00; 8.40:14.50.

To improve a tight fitting

- Select a flatter radius.
- Select a smaller total diameter.
- Use a less rigid or higher water content material.
- Use a different lens thickness.

A lens of specification 8.70:14.50 may be progressively loosened with the following steps: 8.70:14.00; 9.00:14.50; 9.00:14.00.

16.2.1 Examples of semi-scleral lenses

DURASOFT 3 LITE TINT (WESLEY JESSEN. PBH)

A medium water content semi-scleral lens for daily or flexible extended wear, manufactured by lathing.

Material properties

Chemical nature	Copolymer of HEMA and 2-ethoxyethyl methacrylate. Non-ionic
Water content	55%
Dk	16×10^{-11} at 35°C
Refractive index	1.412

Lens geometry

- Back surface is of monocurve construction.
- Front surface is lenticulated.
- Centre thickness is 0.05 mm for a lens of BVP –3.00 D

Parameters available

See Table 16.3

Table 16.3 Parameters available for Durasoft 3 Lite Tint lenses

Radius (mm)	8.30, 8.60, 9.00
Diameter (mm)	14.50
Power (D)	±20.00 to –20.00

Fitting set

Lenses are provided in a three-lens trial set consisting of the three radii with powers of –3.00 D.

Fitting method

- The 8.60 radius (designated *median*) is used in the great majority of cases and is selected first unless the cornea is very steep or flat.
- The total diameter should be 1.5–2.0 mm larger than the HVID.

Typical specification

8.60:14.50 –3.00

Related lenses

- Durasoft 3 Optifit Toric: a back surface toric stabilized with front surface thin zones.
- Durasoft 3 Colours: a range of nine cosmetic tinted lenses.
- Durasoft Complements: a range of five cosmetic tinted lenses.

OMNIFLEX (HYDRON)

A high water content, semi-scleral lens for daily wear, manufactured by lathing.

Material properties

Chemical nature	A copolymer of methyl methacrylate and vinyl pyrrolidone. Non-ionic.
Water content	70%
Dk	32×10^{-11} at 35°C
Refractive index	1.39
Geometry	Spherical bicurve back surface; spherical lenticulated front surface. Centre thickness 0.12 mm for −3.00 D and 0.23 mm for +3.00 D.

Parameters available

See Table 16.4.

Table 16.4 Parameters available for Omniflex lenses

Radius (mm)	8.40, 8.80
Diameter (mm)	14.30
Power (D)	±20.00

Fitting method

- The total diameter is constant at 14.30 mm.
- The 8.40 mm radius fits approximately 80% of eyes.
- The 8.80 mm fitting is required for flat or small diameter corneas.

Typical specification

8.80:14.30 −3.00

Related lenses

- Omniflex toric: a back surface toric with prism free front optic and stabilization zones.
- Omniflex Softints: a range of four colour enhancers in 10% and 20% densities.

General advice

- Select the flatter of two possible fittings where there is a choice because:

  (a) It is easier to see the movement of a lens which is too loose rather than the relative lack of movement of a steep fitting.
  (b) A sharper end-point is obtained with over-refraction.
  (c) Soft lenses become steeper and therefore tighter after initial settling.

- Steep corneas require lens selection to be relatively much flatter than flat corneas where the optimum result is likely to be much closer to 'K'. This applies to both corneal and semi-scleral lenses. Thus a radius of 8.10 mm may be necessary for a 13.00 mm lens on a 7.40 mm cornea, whereas an 8.40 mm cornea might well require a much closer radius of 8.70 mm or perhaps 8.50 mm.
- It is better to achieve a more stable fitting by increasing the size. A steeper radius is likely to give worse acuity.
- It is essential to ensure adequate lens movement to allow proper exchange of tears and the removal of debris.
- It is also important to avoid fitting too tightly because of the risk of oedema. This can occur even with thin or high water content lenses.

Chapter 17

Other soft lens fitting considerations

17.1 Lens power

Power is an important consideration in deciding which type of lens to fit.

Low minus (< –2.00 D)

- Thin lenses should be avoided because of handling difficulties and the greater chance of dehydration.
- A thicker, medium or high water content lens should be selected.

High minus (> –7.00 D) and medium to high plus (> +3.00 D)

- Low water content lenses should be avoided because of the greater thickness and physiological problems.
- Semi-scleral lenses usually give better stability of fitting.

Medium minus (–2.00 D to –7.00 D) and low plus (< +3.00 D)

- Thin or high water content lenses are the probable choice, except where problems arise with fitting characteristics, dehydration or visual acuity.

17.2 Lens flexibility

An important influence on the fitting characteristics of all lenses is the flexibility of the material. This explains why two lenses of apparently the same specification but different material can behave in entirely different ways on the cornea.[1] Permalens, for example, which is very flexible, often requires to be fitted steeper than 'K' compared with other more rigid materials where the more usual flatter than 'K' approach is correct. Similarly, thin spun-cast lenses and moulded lenses with overall a thin cross-section and inherently greater flexibility than their lathed counterparts lend themselves better to a 'one-fit' fitting philosophy which relies on draping the cornea.

Practical advice

- Because of flexibility and manufacturing considerations, the lenses from one laboratory cannot necessarily be duplicated by another, merely by ordering the same nominal specification.
- Fitting must be carried out with trial lenses of the type to be ordered to ensure optimum reliability.

17.3 Additional visual considerations

FLEXURE AND LIQUID LENS POWER

Flexure occurs when a soft lens fitted flatter or steeper than 'K' bends to follow the corneal curvature. The refractive effect with both plus and minus lenses is to add negative power[2,3]

A liquid lens occurs if the posterior surface of the soft lens fails to conform to the front surface of the cornea.[4] This is more likely to be present with semi-scleral designs, whereas there is virtually no liquid lens with ultrathin lenses which completely drape the cornea.

Practical advice

- Any discrepancy between contact lens and spectacle *Rx* (allowing for vertex distance) is caused mainly by flexure but possibly by liquid lens power.
- This is unlikely to be greater than 0.50 D with a satisfactory fitting.
- Thin corneal lenses require more minus power than thick semi-scleral lenses.

ASTIGMATISM

The usual limit for acceptable acuity with a thin spherical lens is about 1.00 DC, but it can be as little as 0.50 DC for critical observers. Very occasionally, acceptable vision is obtained with cylinders as high as 4.00 D and with an amblyopic eye there may be no advantage in the additional complexity and cost of a toric lens.

Soft lenses are generally fitted flatter than 'K' so that less minus is required compared with the best vision sphere used with hard lenses.

Example:

Spectacle Rx –3.50/–1.00 × 180
Likely BVP of spherical soft lens –3.50 D.

ENVIRONMENTAL FACTORS

The power of a soft lens depends on its basic dimensions of radius, diameter, thickness and refractive index which can all vary with environmental factors. These include ocular effects such as temperature, pH, tonicity and volume of tears. Some of these are in turn influenced by external factors such as ambient temperature, humidity, or the degree of lens hydration when placed on the eye. Generally, HEMA undergoes smaller changes than high water content materials and gives less variation in vision.

17.4 Thin lenses

Lenses with a centre thickness less than 0.10 mm may be regarded as *thin* (*see* Section 6.3.2). Lenses in the range 0.05–0.07 mm are *ultrathin* and those less than 0.05 mm have been termed either *superthin* or *hyperthin*.

The fitting characteristics of thin and standard lenses differ even if having otherwise identical specification. Lens thickness may therefore be regarded as an additional fitting variable.

In practical terms, thin lenses generally

- Possess greater flexibility.
- Prove easier to fit because there are fewer fitting steps.
- Drape the cornea more completely and give less mobility.
- Give less lid sensation and are more comfortable.

- Have better transmissibility (*Dk/t*).
- Possess different fitting characteristics and sometimes permit better centration.
- Give less satisfactory acuity on toric corneas.
- Dehydrate to a greater extent on the eye after settling.

HYDRON ZERO 6 (HYDRON)

Thin HEMA, semi-scleral lenses for daily wear; manufactured by lathing.

Material properties

HEMA 38.6% (*see* Section 16.1).

Lens geometry

- Centre thickness is 0.06 mm for all minus lenses of power −3.00 D or greater.
- The mid-periphery is deliberately thickened to make handling easier.
- Zero 6 plus lenses have an average thickness of of 0.10 mm.
- The back surface is a bicurve with a constant BOZD of 13.28 mm and peripheral curve width of 0.36 mm (13.28 mm + 0.36 mm + 0.36 mm = 14.00 mm).
- The front surface is lenticulated with BOZDs of 6.70 mm at −10.00 D and 8.3 mm at +10.00 D.

Parameters available

See Table 17.1.

Fitting technique

- Approximately 70% of minus lenses are fitted with the 8.70 mm radius.

Table 17.1 Parameters available for Hydron Zero 6 and Z Plus lenses

Radius (mm)	8.10, 8.40, 8.70, 9.00, 9.30
Diameter (mm)	14.00
Power (D)	±20.00

- The most common radius for plus lenses is 9.00 mm.
- There is no very firm relationship between 'K' and radius because of greater lens flexibility.
- 14.00 mm is the only available diameter. Lenses may prove unsuitable if the cornea is either very large or very small.

Typical specification

Zero 6: 8.70:14.00   –3.00

Related lenses

- Zero 6T: a front surface toric with prism-free optic zone.
- A range of five colour enhancer tints with densities of 10% and 20%.

17.5 Aspheric lenses

BACK SURFACE ASPHERICS

A minority of soft lenses have an aspheric back surface designed to match the aspheric nature of the cornea. A correctly fitting lens behaves in the main as described in Section 18.1, but compared with spherical lenses:

- Aspherics do not have a true radius but are designated in some other way such as by 'fitting value' or posterior apical radius (PAR).
- Changing the total diameter does not necessarily alter the fitting characteristics.
- Lens mobility of between 0.25 mm and 0.75 mm can be acceptable.
- With some corneal geometries, proper centration cannot be achieved and a spherical lens is required, although the reverse is also true.

WEICON CE (60%) (CIBA VISION)

A back surface aspheric, corneal diameter lens for daily or extended wear, manufactured by CNC lathes.

Material properties

Chemical nature	Methyl methacrylate/vinyl pyrrolidone (MMA/VP) copolymer. Ionic
Water content	60%
Dk	28×10^{-11} at 35°C
Refractive index	1.4037

Lens geometry

- Centre thickness of a –3.00 D lens is 0.09 mm.
- All lenses have an elliptical back surface with a flat (FL) or steep (ST) fitting value instead of a radius.
- Radius and eccentricity are varied to give a consistent performance throughout the power range.
- Lenses feature a *tangential bevel* to give a continuous transition between back surface and ski-shaped edge.

Parameters available

See Table 17.2.

Table 17.2 Parameters available for Weicon CE lenses

Fitting value (eccentricity)	Flat (FL) or steep (ST)
Diameter (mm)	13.00, 13.80, 14.60
Power (D)	±25.00

Fitting technique

- The 13.80 mm diameter is most commonly used.
- The FL fitting value is generally selected.
- The ST fitting value is tried only if the FL is excessively mobile after complete settling.
- The 13.00 mm fitting can be used as a high water content corneal diameter lens.

Typical specification

Weicon CE: FL 13.80   –3.00

Related lenses

- The Weicon CE Toric: a high water content back surface toric stabilized by dynamic stabilization.
- The Weicon 38E. The original HEMA version of the Weicon CE.

Front surface aspherics

A front surface aspheric (e.g. Nissel EV38) can give improved acuity in cases of low to medium astigmatism (0.75–1.50 D) by the correction of optical aberrations.

17.6 Spun-cast lenses

ADVANTAGES OF SPIN-CASTING

- Better surface quality and edge shape.
- Mass production ensures better reproducibility and consistency of manufacture.

DISADVANTAGES OF SPIN CASTING

- Limitations on the variety of back surface forms which may be conveniently obtained.
- The full power range is not obtainable for each series of lens.

SOFLENS (BAUSCH & LOMB)

Corneal and semi-scleral lenses for daily wear; manufactured by spin-casting in open moulds.

Material properties

Chemical nature	HEMA cross-linked polymer. Non-ionic
Water content	38.6%
Dk	8.0×10^{-11} at 20°C
Refractive index	1.43

Lens geometry

- The front surface gives the 'series' or 'base curve', determined by the constant curvature of the mould during manufacture.

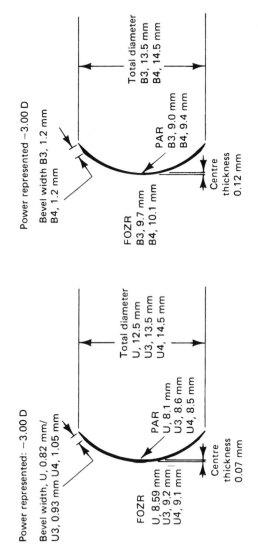

Power represented: −3.00 D

Bevel width, U, 0.82 mm/
U3, 0.93 mm U4, 1.05 mm

Total diameter
U, 12.5 mm
U3, 13.5 mm
U4, 14.5 mm

PAR
U, 8.1 mm
U3, 8.6 mm
U4, 8.5 mm

FOZR
U, 8.59 mm
U3, 9.2 mm
U4, 9.1 mm

Centre
thickness
0.07 mm

Power represented −3.00 D

Bevel width B3, 1.2 mm
B4, 1.2 mm

Total diameter
B3, 13.5 mm
B4, 14.5 mm

PAR
B3, 9.0 mm
B4, 9.4 mm

FOZR
B3, 9.7 mm
B4, 10.1 mm

Centre
thickness
0.12 mm

Figure 17.1 Two typical series of the Bausch & Lomb Soflens (from Phillips and Speedwell, *Contact Lenses*, 4th edn, Butterworth-Heinemann, Oxford, by permission)

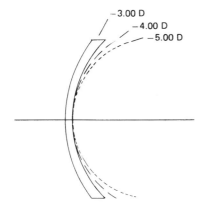

Figure 17.2 Bausch & Lomb Soflens. The front surface radius is constant. Variation in power is achieved by altering the posterior apical radius: the steeper the radius, the higher the negative power

This is the opposite of conventional lathed lenses (typical series are shown in Figure 17.1).

- The back surface is aspheric and governs the power (Figure 17.2).
- Most of the minus series have constant sag and centre thickness, irrespective of power (*see* Table 17.4).
- The higher the minus power, the tighter the fitting.
- Series are designated according to thickness and size. The suffix '4' denotes a 14.50 mm diameter; the suffix '3' a 13.50 mm diameter; and where there is no numerical suffix (e.g. U and the original F series), a 12.50 mm diameter.

Parameters available

See Table 17.3.

Fitting technique

- The constant sag and the greater flexibility of spun lenses effectively give a one-fit approach for each particular series.
- Fitting characteristics depend upon total diameter, thickness and power.
- Diameter is chosen on the basis of corneal size. 13.50 mm lenses (3 series) are used where HVID is less than 11.75 mm, and 14.50 mm (4 series) where it is greater.
- Series and thickness are selected according to physiological and handling considerations.

Table 17.3 Parameters available for Bausch & Lomb conventional lenses

Lens series	Power range (D)	Diameter (mm)	Centre thickness (mm)	Sag (mm)
Sofspin	−0.25 to −12.00	14.00	0.05–0.09	
U	−0.25 to −9.00	12.50	0.07	2.89
U3	−9.00 to +6.00	13.50	0.07–0.18	3.09
U4	−9.00 to +6.00	14.50	0.07–0.18	4.05
B4	−9.00 to +6.00	14.50	0.12–0.30	3.59
O3	−1.00 to −9.00	13.50	0.035	3.18 (3.12†)
O4	−1.00 to −9.00	14.50	0.035	4.10 (3.68‡)
H3	+10.00 to +20.00	13.50	0.48–0.61	3.40–3.47
H4	+10.00 to +20.00	14.50	0.48–0.61	3.69–3.80
HO3	−8.00 to −20.00	13.50	0.035	3.61
HO4	−8.00 to −20.00	14.50	0.035	3.67
Optima 38	−0.25 to −6.00	14.00	0.06	3.60/3.82

Except: *−12.50 to −20.00; †−1.00 to −1.25; ‡−1.00 to −1.75.

- Power is based on spectacle *Rx* and vertex distance.

- If adequate centration cannot be achieved with the initial diameter, the next larger lens with the same letter series should be tried (e.g. if U3 is too small, change to U4).

- It is particularly important to achieve complete corneal coverage or there is a likelihood of arcuate staining at the limbus from corneal drying and edge abrasion.

- Lens decentration is likely to give poor vision because of the aspheric optics.

- Decentration can occur with either a loose or a tight fitting, but in the latter case there is no recovery movement on blinking.

- Movement on blinking is only about 0.25 mm (i.e. less than most other lenses).

- Other fitting characteristics are mainly as described in Chapter 18.

- Plus lenses are selected according to similar principles, although centre thickness varies according to power.

Using the different series

U3 and U4 ($t_c = 0.07$ mm)

The most commonly used series.

Typical specification

Soflens: –3.00 U4

O series ($t_c = 0.035$ mm)

Where greater transmissibility is required for extended wear. However, they are extremely difficult to handle and have a tendency to dehydrate more readily on the eye (*see* Sections 6.3.3 and 21.4.2).

B series ($t_c = 0.12$ mm)

For easier handling and to provide an extension to the power range.

HO series ($t_c = 0.035$ mm)

For high minus powers. The large FOZD, despite lenticulation, gives a relatively thick periphery, so these lenses are not always ideal for cases prone to vascularization.

Sofspin ($t_c = 0.05$–0.09 mm)

Where a variable centre thickness is required with a single diameter (14.00 mm) for ease of fitting.

Optima ($t_c = 0.06$ mm)

Where greater rigidity and ease of handling are required. The back surface is lathed and there are two possible sags. Sag I (3.60 mm) gives greater movement and is fitted with flatter corneas; Sag II (3.82 mm) gives better centration and is used with steeper corneas.

Related lenses

- The Optima Toric: a 45% water content front surface toric stabilized by prism ballast.

- A range of enhancer tints in the Optima Series.
- The Soflens 38, Soflens 66 and Soflens One Day range of disposable lenses (*see* Chapter 19).

17.7 One-fit lenses

Most one-fit lenses are semi-scleral in type. They can give a satisfactory result in a high percentage of cases because of their large diameter, thinness and flexibility.

- Because no fitting adjustment is possible, it is important to recognize early those cases for which the fitting characteristics fail to meet the criteria given in Chapter 18.
- With thinner varieties, especially spun-cast lenses, limited lens mobility of only 0.25 mm may be acceptable.
- To assess the fitting reliably, trial lenses should be as near as possible to the correct power.
- Particular care is required with corneas which are unusually small, large, steep or flat.
- Several disposable lenses are designed to be one-fit, to simplify fitting and reduce the number of parameters required (*see* Chapter 19).

PERMAFLEX (WESLEY JESSEN. PBH)

A single fitting high water content, semi-scleral lens for daily or extended wear, manufactured by cast moulding.

Material properties

Chemical nature	A cross-linked polymer of methyl methacrylate, vinyl pyrrolidone and other methacrylates. Non-ionic
Water content	74%
Dk	38×10^{-11} at 36°C
Refractive index	1.385

Lens geometry

- Centre thickness varies from 0.08 mm to 0.22 mm for minus powers; 0.14 mm for a –3.00 D lens.

- The back surface is of spherical bicurve construction.
- The front surface is lenticulated where necessary to give a minimum FOZD of 7.50 mm.

Parameters available

See Table 17.4.

Table 17.4 Parameters available for Permaflex lenses

Radius (mm)	8.70
Diameter (mm)	14.40
Power (D)	−10.00 to +8.00

Fitting technique

- Fitting is assessed with lenses as near as possible to the correct power
- The spherical 8.70 mm radius fits a very high percentage of corneas. It is sometimes found to be too mobile and, less frequently, too tight.
- Because of the high water content, sufficient time must be allowed for lenses to settle, or an apparently correct fitting may subsequently become tight.

Typical specification

Permaflex: 8.70:14.40   −3.00

Related lenses

Precision UV: monthly disposable lenses available with an additional radius of 8.40 mm. Lenses have a handling tint and UV inhibitor provided by a chromophore known as UVAM.

17.8 Unusual lens performance

Fitting sometimes gives unexpected or unreliable results. If the lens is:

Too tight

- Stored in *hypo*tonic solution, giving temporary osmotic adhesion.
- Causing initial irritation with excessive lacrimation and a hypotonic shift in the patient's tears.
- Ultra-thin with a temporarily distorted shape because it has adhered to the base, neck or lid of the storage vial.
- Disinfected by heat without sufficient time to cool and revert to its proper dimensions.

Too loose

- Stored in *hyper*tonic solution.
- Inserted inside out.
- Damaged.

References

1. Gasson, A.P. (1989) Soft (hydrogel) lens fitting. In *Contact Lenses*, A.J. Phillips and J. Stone (eds), Butterworths, London, pp. 382–439
2. Bennett, A.G. (1976) Power changes in soft lenses due to bending. *Ophthalmic Optician*, **16**, 939–945
3. Sarver, M.D., Ashley, D. and Van Every, J. (1974) Supplemental power effect of Bausch and Lomb Softlens contact lenses. *International Contact Lens Clinic*, **1**, 100–109
4. Wichterle, O. (1967) Changes of refracting power of a soft lens caused by its flattening. In *Corneal and Scleral Contact Lenses*, Proceedings of the International Congress, L.J. Girard (ed.), paper 29, Mosby, St. Louis, pp. 247–256.

Chapter 18

Soft lens fitting characteristics

Every make of lens has, to some extent, its own fitting characteristics. Most of the more general points, however, are summarized below, although the rather greater differences between corneal and semi-scleral lenses have been covered in Chapter 16.

18.1 Characteristics of a correct fitting

The general principles for a good fitting are complete corneal coverage, correct lens movement, good vision and comfort.

- Good centration.
- Complete corneal coverage.
- Approximately 0.5 mm of vertical movement on blinking in primary position.
- Lag of up to 1 mm on upwards gaze or lateral eye movements.
- Rapid recovery on vertical displacement (push-up test).
- Comfortable in all directions of gaze.
- Good visual acuity.
- Retinoscopy reflex crisp and sharp before and after blinking.
- Vision remains stable on blinking.
- Refraction gives a precise end-point.
- Refraction correlates with spectacle BVP.
- Keratometer mires stable and undistorted.
- No irritation of limbal vessels.
- No compression of bulbar conjunctiva.

18.2 Characteristics of a tight fitting

The obvious feature of a tight lens is insufficient movement. Initial comfort is therefore good and sometimes better than a correct fitting. Centration is also usually good, although a corneal diameter lens may sometimes assume a decentred position. This is easily differentiated from a decentred flat fitting because of the lack of movement. A steep lens vaults the corneal apex, but is momentarily pressed onto the eye by blinking to give a transient improvement in vision.

- Little or no movement on blinking (less than 0.25 mm).
- Little or no movement on upwards or lateral gaze (less than 0.25 mm).
- Good centration.
- Slow recovery with push-up test.
- Good initial comfort.
- Subsequent symptoms of discomfort such as heat or stinging.
- Poor visual acuity.
- Retinoscopy reflex shows irregular distortion.
- Unstable vision with temporary improvement on blinking.
- Refraction difficult with poor end-point.
- More negative power required than anticipated because of flexure or possible liquid lens.
- Keratometer mires give irregular distortion.
- Irritation of limbal or conjunctival vessels.
- Compression ring in bulbar conjunctiva (scleral indentation), often seen after the lens is removed.

18.3 Characteristics of a loose fitting

The obvious feature of a loose lens is excessive movement. On looking upwards it may catch against the top lid and cause noticeable discomfort. In the primary position, lower lid sensation is experienced if the lens sags, and the discomfort is accentuated if the fitting is so flat that the periphery buckles to give edge stand-off (Figure 18.1). This is not uncommon on steep corneas with single fitting and disposable lenses with a limited range of parameters.

- Excessive movement on blinking (over 1 mm).
- Excessive lag on lateral or upwards eye movements (over 2 mm).

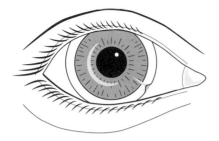

Figure 18.1 Very loose fitting showing buckling of lens edge

- Poor centration.
- Poor comfort because of lid sensation.
- Visual acuity variable.
- Retinoscopy reflex clear centrally with peripheral distortion.
- Variable vision.
- Refraction variable because of lens movement.
- Keratometer mires vary with lens movement, giving peripheral distortion.
- Buckling of lens edge.

18.4 Summary of soft lens fitting characteristics

The general fitting characteristics for soft lenses are summarized in Table 18.1.

Table 18.1 Fitting characteristics of soft lenses

Characteristic	Good fit	Steep fit	Flat fit
Comfort	Good	Good, initially	Poor
Centration	Good, with complete corneal coverage	Usually good, may be decentred, no recovery on blinking	Poor
Movement on blinking	Up to 0.5 mm	Less than 0.25 mm	Excessive, over 1.0 mm
Movement on upwards gaze	Up to 1.0 mm	Little or none	Excessive, over 2.0 mm
Movement on lateral gaze	Up to 1.0 mm	Little or none	Excessive, over 2.0 mm
Vision	Good	Poor and variable, momentary improvement on blinking	Variable, may improve on staring after blinking
Over-refraction	Precise end-point, power correlates with BVP of spectacle Rx	Poorly defined end-point, positive liquid lens	Variable, negative liquid lens
Retinoscopy reflex	Clear reflex, before and after blinking	Poor and distorted, central shadow, momentarily improved on blinking	Variable, may be clear centrally with peripheral distortion
Slit lamp after settling	No limbal injection or scleral indentation	Conjunctival or limbal injection, scleral indentation	Localized limbal injection, possible edge stand-off
Keratometer mires	Sharp, stable before and after blinking	Irregular, momentary improvement on blinking	Variable and eccentric, changing on blinking
Placido disc	Regular image	Irregular image anywhere but at the edge of the lens	Irregular image, more often peripheral only but occasionally central as well

Chapter 19

Disposable lenses and frequent (planned) replacements

19.1 Frequent replacement lenses

Considerably fewer clinical difficulties arise when lenses are replaced on a regular basis[1]. Deposits are avoided and there are much reduced risks of discomfort, CLIPC, infections and red eyes. The distinction is imprecise but *disposable* is generally used to describe lenses replaced monthly or more often, and *frequent replacement* for lenses disposed of on a planned basis of over 1 month.

It has always been difficult to define the life span of a soft lens, since it depends on a variety of factors:

- Water content and material.
- Lens thickness.
- Method of disinfection and cleaning.
- Wearing time.
- Daily or extended wear.
- Tear chemistry.
- Handling ability.
- Environment.

A reasonable average time after which lenses needed either replacement or thorough professional cleaning used to be considered about 12 months. This projected life span is now reduced, with the greater emphasis on high water content lenses and modern solutions, which are easier to use but less efficient at cleaning than peroxide systems. Many practitioners have therefore devised schemes that encourage patients to replace lenses on a frequent and planned basis before they reach the troublesome stage. The time interval is usually 3, 6 or, occasionally, 12 months.

Conventional lenses are easily adapted for frequent replacement where laboratories supply lenses at reduced costs. Large companies such as Bausch & Lomb (Fresh Vision), Hydron (Advantage) and Wesley Jessen.PBH (Continuum) have created schemes which include some or all of their standard range of lens types. They also assist the practitioner with paperwork and computer reminders.

The advent of modern production techniques, particularly moulding, has reduced manufacturing costs so that some lenses are produced specifically for planned disposal. Wesley Jessen. PBH recommend 3-monthly replacement for the Gentle Touch, 65% water content lens and Zeiss suggest the same time interval for their G-72/D ReContact.

The replacement interval should be controlled by the practitioner but depends upon the make of lens and individual patient requirements. If new lenses are exchanged with the patient, there is the additional advantage of removing the older lenses from circulation.

19.2 Disposable lenses

The ultimate frequent replacement lens is the disposable lens, which is discarded and replaced on a much more frequent basis, usually monthly, weekly or daily.

Disposable lenses were originally recommended for weekly extended wear because they avoided most patient handling and eliminated the need for solutions and disinfection. In theory, they should have proved safer but several studies have implicated ionic lenses, and in particular extended wear lenses, with a significant increase in microbial keratitis.[2,3]

Disposable lenses are now used much less frequently for extended wear but have assumed an increasingly important place in routine contact lens practice for daily wear. They offer several clinical advantages over their conventional counterparts.

ADVANTAGES

- Lenses rarely reach the stage where they build up deposits.
- Reduced risk of allergies and infections.
- Reduced incidence of CLIPC.
- Spare lenses are always available.
- Replacement cost is significantly less if lost or damaged.
- Less time and effort required with lens cleaning.

- Cost savings on solutions.
- Patients like the regular fresh feeling of new lenses.
- Easy to fit since fitting parameters are limited.
- Ideal for children requiring soft lenses.
- Theoretically better for most extended wear (*see* Section 21).

DISADVANTAGES

- Restricted range of fittings and powers.
- Restricted availablity for complex lenses such as torics or bifocals.
- Increased cost on an annual basis.
- Uncertain control over patient compliance.
- In the event of a clinical problem, patients may merely replace lenses rather than seek professional advice.
- Not feasible to check every lens.
- Administrative complexities because of the volume of lenses

19.3 Types of disposable lens

MONTHLY AND WEEKLY

There is now a wide range of disposable lenses available in terms of design, water content, material, fitting, power range and wearing schedule. Just some of these are shown in Table 19.1. The majority of lens systems are designed for monthly use which represents a good compromise between life span, convenience and cost. Most are of medium to high water content and manufactured by moulding. Several have a handling tint, UV filter or both.

Although the Bausch & Lomb Soflens 38 was originally available on a weekly basis, the most commonly used weekly lens is now Acuvue (58%), which is available in a wide range of parameters (+6.00 to –11.00D). Acuvue can also be prescribed on a 2-weekly basis.

DAILY DISPOSABLES

Lenses include 1-Day Acuvue (58%), Bausch & Lomb Soflens One Day (70%) and CibaVision Dailies (69%). Since daily disposables are never reused, they represent the only lens form that genuinely requires no disinfection by the patient. Saline is sometimes

Table 19.1 Examples of monthly disposable lenses

Manufacturer	Lens	Water content (%)	Power range (D)	Radii (mm)	Diameter (mm)
Aspect	Frequency 38	38	–0.25 to –8.00	8.6	14
Aspect	Frequency 55	55	–0.25 to –10.00	8.6	14.2
			–0.25 to –8.00	8.90	
			+0.25 to +8.00	8.80	
Bausch & Lomb	Soflens 38	38	+4.00 to –9.00	Aspheric	14.00
Bausch & Lomb	Soflens 66	66	+6.00 to –9.00	8.40, 8.70	14.2
Biocompatibles	Compatibles	60	Plano to –6.00	8.60	14.20
CIBA Vision	Focus	55	+6.00 to –8.00	8.60, 8.90	14.00
Essilor	Rhythmic UV	73	+8.00 to –8.00	8.60, 8.90	14.20
				8.90	14.40
Hydron	Actifresh	73	10.00 to –15.00	8.40, 8.80	14.20
Ocular Sciences	Biomedics 38	38	–0.25 to –10.00	8.6	14.00
Ocular Sciences	Biomedics	55	–0.25 to –8.00	8.6	14.20
			+0.25 to +8.00	8.8	14.20
Johnson & Johnson	Surevue	58	Plano to –9.00	8.40, 8.80	14.00
			Plano to +6.00	9.10	14.40
Johnson & Johnson	Vistavue	48	–0.50 to –9.00	8.60	14.00
Wesley Jessen PBH	Freshlook	55	+6.00 to –8.00	8.6	14.50
Wesley Jessen PBH	Precision UV	74	+10 to –16	8.40, 8.70	14.50

N.B. Fitting parameters, lens names and wearing schedules may vary in different countries.

employed for rinsing while handling. Lenses are significantly more expensive when used on a regular basis and tend to be thin and difficult to insert. Nevertheless, they provide certain important advantages:

- No risk of solutions allergy.
- They avoid patient mistakes in using an incorrect solution.
- A lens case is not required and therefore no contamination from this source is possible.
- No build-up of surface deposits.
- Ideal for patients who wish to use lenses intermittently.

TORIC LENSES

Toric disposables are provided by the major manufacturers with a simplified range of parameters. Lenses are fitted according to the principles of stock torics, described in Section 23.4, and most laboratories provide diagnostic lenses for trial fitting.

The CIBA Vision Focus (55%) and Bausch & Lomb Soflens 66 are available with two radii in both plus and minus powers. Axes are restricted to within 20° of horizontal and vertical. The Hydron Actitoric is based on the Ultra-T (38%) and provides a full range of axes.

BIFOCALS

The Bausch & Lomb Occasions is a multifocal based on their original PA1 design (*see* Chapter 24). It has a 38.6% water content and an equivalent add of +1.25 D.

Vistakon have introduced an innovative simultaneous multi-concentric design for weekly or two weekly replacement based on their standard 58% material.

19.4 Fitting disposable lenses

The selection of lens type and fitting methods follow the principles described in Chapters 16, 17 and 18. Most lenses are either one-fit or have a limited range of parameters with the TD fixed for a given power range at approximately 14.0 mm or greater. The TD cannot therefore be used as a fitting variable, and disposable lenses are often too large for small corneas.

It is important to recognize when a satisfactory fitting cannot be achieved and to prescribe more than one type of disposable lens. In this way an improvement to the centration, fit or comfort can often be managed by changing from one brand to another. It is essential to avoid tight lenses if they are to be used for extended wear.

Disposables are generally fitted from a stock bank and it is a simple matter to supply patients with temporary lenses for an extended tolerance trial of a week or more. Where there is some doubt concerning the ideal fitting or water content, patients can be given either a mixed set of lenses or two different pairs and instructed to wear the more comfortable combination at the first aftercare examination.

19.5 Aftercare with disposable lenses

LENS HANDLING

Many disposable lenses rely on a thin, flexible draping design in order to fit the widest cross-section of corneal curvatures.

Handling is often more difficult than with conventional lenses, particularly in low powers of less than –2.00 D. This applies even to experienced wearers of conventional lenses, who sometimes discontinue for this reason.

SOLUTIONS

Except in cases of known allergy or sensitivity, the modern generation of multipurpose solutions (Section 26.4.1) is generally recommended for use with disposable lenses. Many solutions systems now include new cases, and monthly patients should be encouraged to replace the case at the same time as the lenses. Despite the simplicity of use for one-bottle systems, it is essential to stress the importance of proper lens cleaning and disinfection. Patients often assume that disposability equals minimal lens care.

AFTERCARE

- Aftercare follows the normal principles described in Chapters 28 and 29 for both daily and extended wear.
- Careful observation is required where fittings may be marginal due to limitations in lens parameters.
- Intervals for routine aftercare visits are arranged to coincide with the dispensing of lens supplies, every 3 or 6 months.
- A full aftercare examination is required every 12 months.
- Aftercare visits represent a good opportunity to improve marginally successful fittings with newly introduced parameters or different makes of lens.

19.6 Practice management

The main disadvantage of disposable lenses is the need for careful management of lens supplies.

- For patient simplicity, the replacement interval should be 1, whether this is 1 day, 1 week or 1 month.
- Where possible, supply lenses in units of 6 rather than 3 months. This means that administrative dealings with patients and laboratories occur twice instead of four times a year.
- Computer systems can be used to deal with automatic supplies from laboratories and to select patients from the practice

database, but it is frequently difficult to ensure that dates coincide. There are, in fact, three time scales to correlate, determined by: (1) the laboratory, which may well work on only a 12-week quarter; (2) the practice, which should depend on the practitioner's recommendations to the patient; and (3) the patient, who may be accurate with lens usage, behind schedule by extending the lens life span, or ahead because of lens breakage or loss.

- Consider supplying lenses from a practice stock rather than relying on an inflexible laboratory computer system.
- Consider using standing orders or direct debits to control patient fees.

19.7 Other uses for disposable lenses

The low unit cost of disposables means that they have other very useful clinical applications apart from normal daily and extended wear.

- Low-cost temporary replacement in an emergency.
- Maintaining soft lens wear when CLIPC is causing rapid deposits.
- Short-term use in the hay fever season to avoid CLIPC.
- Periodic use for patients working with VDUs intensively but intermittently.
- To give a lengthy tolerance trial for contact lenses in general (e.g. can the patient cope with handling and disinfection?).
- To give an extended assessment of contact lens vision (e.g. can uncorrected astigmatism or monovision be tolerated?).
- To assess a patient's reaction to the lens material over several days in terms of dehydration and comfort prior to ordering in conventional lens form.
- Temporary lenses for patients undergoing orthokeratology (*see* Section 14).
- As a means of assessing children who require soft lenses.

References

1. Matthews T.D., Frazer D.G., Minassian D.C. *et al.* (1992) Risks of keratitis and patterns of use with disposable contact lenses. *Archives of Ophthalmology*, **110**, 1559–1562.

2. Poggio E.C., Glynn R.J., Schein O.D., Seddon J.M., Shannon M.J., Scardino V.A. *et al.* (1989) The incidence of ulcerative keratitis among users of daily wear and extended wear soft contact lenses. *New England Journal of Medicine*, **321**(12), 779–783.
3. Schein O.D., Glynn R.J., Poggio E.C., Seddon J.C. and Kenyon K.R. (1989). The relative risk of ulcerative keratitis among users of daily wear and extended wear soft contact lenses. *New England Journal of Medicine*, **321**(12), 773–779.

Chapter 20

Soft lens specification and verification

20.1 International Standards and tolerances

The original British Standards document on soft lenses (3521: Part 3:1988) covered only terminology. It derived from the international standard ISO 8320 (1986) which also covers hard lenses. There is no published international standard on product specification for soft lenses because the validity of test methods for soft lens measurement has yet to be established. Recommended tolerances are based on the draft document ISO/CD 8321–2 (1995) *Optics and optical instruments – Contact Lenses – Part 2: Specification for hydrogel contact lenses.*

20.2 Soft lens specification

Table 20.1 Recommended tolerances for soft lenses

BOZR	± 0.20 mm
Total diameter	± 0.20 mm
Central optic zone diameter	± 0.20 mm
Sag at specified diameter	± 0.05 mm
Thickness	
≤ 0.10 mm	± 0.01 mm + 10%
>0.10 mm	± 0.015 mm + 5%
BVP in weaker meridian	
Plano to ± 10.00 D	± 0.25 D
± 10.00 D to ± 20.00 D	± 0.50 D
Over ± 20.00 D	± 1.00 D
Cylinder power	
Plano to 2.00 D	± 0.25 D
2.25 D to 4.00 D	± 0.37 D
Over 4.00 D	± 0.50 D
Cylinder axis	± 5°

A typical soft lens specification takes the following abbreviated form:

8.70:14.50   –3.00   HEMA   38% water content

where   8.70 = back optic zone radius (BOZR)
        14.50 = total diameter (TD)
        –3.00 = BVP

The majority of lenses are made according to predetermined laboratory designs and it is neither necessary nor feasible to specify parameters such as thickness, lenticulation and peripheral curves.

20.3 Soft lens verification

Soft lenses require verification for the same reasons as hard (*see* Section 12.3), although checking is considerably more difficult because parameters vary with:

- Degree of hydration.
- Temperature.
- pH and tonicity of storage solution.
- Nature of the storage solution.
- Time taken if measurement is in air.
- Method of supporting lens.

20.3.1 Back optic zone radius

SPHEROMETERS

Many common methods of radius checking rely on the principle of spherometry, where the sagittal depth is measured for a given chord diameter. The majority of instruments employ a wet cell, but this is not essential.

Wet cell instruments (e.g. Optimec)

- The lens is rinsed and placed in a wet cell containing 0.9% saline solution.
- The lens is centred on a support device.
- A probe is advanced towards the concave surface until it just touches (established by viewing lens movement or electric contact) and the radius is read from the instrument scale.

Measurement in air (e.g. Zeiss spherometer)

- The lens is rinsed in saline; surplus fluid is removed by shaking and rapid superficial drying.
- The lens is centred on a 10 mm support ring, concave side down.
- The central probe is observed from above through a magnifying lens until the first point of contact is made and the radius is read from instrument scale.

OTHER METHODS

Base curve comparator

A simple device consisting of a series of spheres of known radius on which the contact lens is placed and compared by straightforward observation in air.

A much more sophisticated wet cell instrument by Söhnges allowed the profile of the lens to be matched with known radii on a projection screen.

Keratometer

This can be used in conjunction with a wet cell.[1] Measured radius, however, requires conversion to actual radius and observation is difficult because the light intensity is considerably reduced.[2]

20.3.2 Total diameter

PROJECTION MAGNIFIERS

An optical system projects a magnified image of the lens on to a calibrated screen. Instruments may use a wet cell (e.g. Optimec) or support the lens in air on a microscope stage (e.g. Zeiss DL2).

COMPARISON

Comparators consisting of a series of annuli of known diameter can be used as a rapid in-air method.

20.3.3 Power

The most accurate method of measuring power is by power profile mapping (*see* Chapter 12). This is generally only employed by manufacturers. The most usual methods used by practitioners are as follows:

AIR MEASUREMENT

- Rinse the lens with saline.
- Shake off surplus fluid and dry carefully with a lint-free tissue.
- Place lens concave surface down on a reduced aperture focimeter stop.
- Read power directly from focimeter scale.

WET CELL MEASUREMENT

- Place lens in wet cell.
- Mount on focimeter.
- Read power from focimeter scale.
- Convert to approximate power in air by multiplying by 4.[3]

Practical advice

- Power is more easily and more accurately measured in air.
- Any error in wet cell measurement is magnified fourfold (an error of 0.25 D ≡ 1.00 D in air).
- Power in air is reasonably constant for up to about 1 min.
- Best results are obtained with a projection focimeter.

20.3.4 Thickness

PROJECTION MAGNIFIERS

The easiest method of measuring thickness is by means of a millimetre scale calibrated for the screen of a projection magnifier (e.g. Optimec).

DRYSDALE'S METHOD

A hard lens radiuscope can be used to determine lens thickness[4]:

- Place the lens, concave surface down, on a convex sphere (this should have a curvature steeper than the lens to be measured to ensure contact at the centre).

- Focus the target on the surface of the sphere with the lens in place.
- Set the scale to zero.
- Focus the target on the front surface of the lens.
- Read the distance travelled from the scale.
- Multiply by the refractive index of the material to give the actual centre thickness.

20.3.5 Edge form

Edge form and integrity are best observed with projection magnification, but a hand loupe or the slit lamp can also be used.

20.3.6 Surface quality

Surface quality is assessed with the slit lamp or by means of projection magnification. Observation with a wet cell is more difficult because the small difference in the refractive index of the solution largely disguises any surface flaws or cracks.

20.3.7 Water content and material

Water content can be estimated with a refractometer because of its inverse relationship with refractive index. An instrument developed for contact lens measurement is the Atago CL-1 refractometer.[5]

- Rinse the hydrated lens with saline, shake off surplus moisture and blot with a lint-free tissue.
- Flatten lens against prism face, taking care not to cause damage.
- Use an external light source and read directly from the internal scale the water content at the junction between light and dark areas.

Assessing the lens material from the water content alone is far from certain, so identification may depend upon other clues such as style of engraving (see Section 25.1), handling tint or type of edge bevel.

Practical advice

- The easiest methods for practitioner verification are:

BOZR	Wet cell spherometer
DIAMETER	Projection magnifier
POWER	Focimeter in air
THICKNESS	Projection magnifier
CONDITION	Projection magnifier.

- The most useful instrument, which is ideally kept in the consulting room, is a projection magnifier. It is not only used for lens inspection, but also for demonstrating to the patient surface and edge flaws and deposits.
- Wet cells are a source of possible cross-infection and require regular cleaning and disinfection.
- Particular care is required when flattening high water content lenses against a glass surface (e.g. microscope stage or refractometer) because of the difficulty of removal and the risk of damage.

20.3.8 Deposits

Projection magnifiers reveal discrete areas of deposit such as white spots. Films such as protein are more easily observed by looking into the wet cell without magnification. The best method of observing deposits, however, is by dark-field illumination.[6]

High magnification can be achieved with the slit lamp by using an oblique beam and selecting a dark background. In addition, some lens deposits fluoresce with ultraviolet light.

References

1. Loran, D.F.C. (1989) The verification of hydrogel contact lenses. In *Contact Lenses*, A.J. Phillips and J. Stone (eds), Butterworths, London, pp. 463–504
2. Chaston, J. (1973) A method of measuring the radius of curvature of a soft contact lens. *Optician*, **165**, 8–12
3. Poster, M.G. (1971) Hydrated method of determining dioptric power of all hydrophilic lenses. *Journal of the American Optometric Association*, **43**, 287–299
4. Hartstein, J. (1973) *Questions and Answers on Contact Lens Practice*, 2nd edn, Mosby, St. Louis, pp. 155–157
5. Efron, N. and Brennan, N.A. (1987) The soft contact lens refractometer. *Optician*, **94** (5115), 29–41
6. Killpartrick, M.R. (1987) Soft lens contaminant detection by dark field illumination. *Optician*, **193** (5083), 34–37
7. American National Standard (1986) Prescription requirements for first quality soft contact lenses. In *American National Standard Requirements for Soft Contact Lenses 280.8 –1986*, National Standards Institute for Ophthalmics, USA

Chapter 21

Extended wear

Soft lenses have been routinely fitted for extended wear since the early 1970s with the introduction of Permalens and Sauflon PW. Improvements have since occurred not only in lens design but also in the understanding of the physiological requirements of the cornea necessary to achieve extended wear with relative safety. More recently, high Dk hard lenses have also been introduced with some advantage.

21.1 Physiological requirements

21.1.1 Oxygen requirements of the cornea

Limiting any hypoxic effect on the cornea is essential for successful long-term wear of any contact lens. In practical terms for extended wear, the following physiological requirements must be met:[1] (using Fatt units)

First day of extended wear Dk/t for zero swelling $= 24 \times 10^{-9}$
Second day of extended wear Dk/t for zero swelling $= 34 \times 10^{-9}$
For overnight swelling of only 4%, Dk/t $= 87 \times 10^{-9}$

None of the current generation of hydrophilic lenses is able to fulfil these critera, since the theoretically optimum Dk is approximately 40×10^{-11}, limited by the water content of the material. Extended wear, therefore, almost always risks compromising corneal health and should only be undertaken with extreme caution.

New polymers in which the matrix of the lens is siloxane-based (e.g. Lotrafilcon A Dk 140×10^{-11}) and itself highly permeable to oxygen, may well overcome this problem.

Hard lens materials, however, are already available with four or five times the permeability of current high water content soft lenses before taking into account any tears pump effect. Lenses with a Dk in the region of 100 provide approximately 15% EOP. The tears pump adds about 2% oxygen to give a total EOP of 17%

for open eye conditions and 4% for closed eye conditions. This is sufficient to avoid epithelial compromise in extended wear for most patients.[2] A Dk in the region of 150–200 provides an even better physiological performance.

21.1.2 Effects of insufficient oxygen

Extended wear causes chronic cumulative hypoxia to a much greater extent than daily wear because of continuous eye closure during sleep, with sometimes inadequate time for corneal deswelling during the day. Between 10% and 15% oxygen is needed to avoid oedema and measurable corneal changes.[3]

- Epithelial changes include decreased glycolysis,[4] decreased mitosis,[5] decreased cell adhesion[6] and reduced sensitivity.[7]
- The stroma shows oedema which eventually leads to stromal thinning.[4]
- Endothelial cells show distinct polymegathous changes similar to those seen in the *corneal exhaustion syndrome*.[4]

21.1.3 Tears exchange and osmolarity

There is a normal increase in corneal thickness overnight, mainly due to a change in tear osmolarity causing swelling. This rapidly disappears on eye opening. Soft lens materials may become tighter with these changes and lens adhesion may be found in the morning. Lenses usually start moving after a few blinks and this movement is very important to allow tears exchange to eliminate overnight debris from beneath the lens. This might otherwise cause a toxic effect which, when combined with lens adhesion, could precipitate the *acute red eye* response[8] (*see* Section 29.1.2).

21.1.4 Physical and chemical compatibility of lens materials

The physical aspects of materials must be considered to avoid mechanical trauma from friction or surface hardness. Weight distribution is similarly important. Materials should be chemically inert to avoid surface deposits which could irritate the ocular tissues.

21.2 Approaches to extended wear

On a practical level, extended wear lenses can be divided into three possible groups:

FLEXIBLE WEAR (DAILY PLUS)

Many patients requesting extended wear are prepared to accept lenses that they can use safely on an occasional overnight basis, remaining happy to remove them most evenings. This type of lens wear gives maximum flexibility and safety. On a day-to-day basis, they are taking advantage of the excellent physiological properties of either high Dk hard or high water content soft lenses, while at the same time incurring very little risk of adverse ocular response to occasional overnight use.

UP TO 1 WEEK

A maximum of 6 nights' wear followed by 1 night's rest gives a realistic schedule for the majority of patients. Proper lens cleaning and disinfection are maintained by regular removal, and a consistent weekly routine is developed. Disposable lenses fit well into such a routine.

OVER 1 WEEK

Over 1 week may be regarded as continuous wear or long-term extended wear. It is suitable or even essential for many medical cases, poor lens handlers or for some vocational uses. For most normal eyes, wearing schedules beyond 1 week put additional stress on the cornea and must be used with great caution. There is, however, a small group of experienced patients who have learned a 'sixth sense' of when lenses need removal and encounter fewer problems with handling, breakage, solutions and infections by leaving lenses in the eyes for sometimes several months.

21.3 Patient selection

21.3.1 Indications and contraindications

INDICATIONS

The majority of extended wear lenses are fitted at the patient's request for purely cosmetic reasons. With proper supervision, they can work well, but there is always the possibility of problems such as infections, oedema or vascularization (*see* Section 21.7). Great care is required not only by the practitioner but also by the patient, who must be made aware of potential hazards.

The clinical needs must therefore be carefully balanced against the possible risks.

There are, however, many patients for whom extended wear is the most suitable, if not the only possible, form of visual correction:

- Aphakics, where handling and visual difficulties preclude daily wear.
- Other poor lens handlers.
- Therapeutic bandage cases (*see* Section 32.4).
- Young children where daily handling is not feasible (*see* Section 30.1).
- Vocations where good vision is required immediately on wakening.
- Where all soft lens disinfection systems create problems and daily disposables are not feasible.
- Where soft lens patients have no facility for lens disinfection.
- As the rear component of a low vision aid system and handling is impossible.

CONTRAINDICATIONS

- Patients known to be predisposed to corneal oedema.
- Existing corneal vascularization.
- CLIPC.
- Patients unlikely to follow practitioner advice.
- Patients unable to remove lenses.
- Diabetics, where the corneal epithelium is likely to be more fragile.
- Where financial constraints may preclude aftercare and regular lens replacement.
- Where patients are known to be a long way from optometric or medical help in the event of a severe ocular emergency.

21.3.2 Advantages of soft and hard lenses in extended wear

ADVANTAGES OF SOFT LENSES

- More comfortable.
- Easier adaptation.

- Easier to fit.
- No problems with foreign bodies.
- No 3 and 9 o'clock staining.

ADVANTAGES OF HARD LENSES

- Very high *Dk*s possible.
- Tear pump on blinking.
- Avoidance of trapped debris.
- Reduced risk of infection.
- Better vision.
- Fewer corneal changes.
- Lenses do not cover the entire cornea.
- No lens dehydration.
- Fewer deposit problems.
- Easier lens maintenance.
- No solutions sensitivity.
- Longer life span.

21.4 Soft lens fitting and problems

21.4.1 Fitting

The main consideration is to provide the maximum possible oxygen supply to the cornea. This can be achieved in one of two ways:

- By means of high water content (e.g. Permaflex 74% and Incanto 78%). Lenses have high *Dk* values, but the potential problems are lens fragility, deposits and discolouration, and greater likelihood of solutions reaction.
- By making medium or low water content lenses extremely thin (e.g. Acuvue, 58%; Durasoft 3, 55%, Bausch & Lomb O Series, 38%; CSI-Clarity-T, 38%). These rely on good *Dk/t* values but can give problems with handling. Hyperthin lenses also give poor tears exchange on blinking.

Fitting considerations therefore include the following:

- Large refractive errors (both plus and minus) are better fitted with high water content lenses because of average thickness factors.

- Lenses should be as flat as possible consistent with stability of fitting and vision. The exception is the lathed Permalens which is fitted steeper than 'K'.
- Lenses become tighter with wear, particularly overnight because of dehydration.
- Lenses become tighter with age and deposits (*see* Section 29.5).
- Examination during fitting and aftercare must be carried out with the slit lamp, otherwise small degrees of movement cannot be seen.
- Movement should ideally be about 0.50 mm, with a minimum value of 0.25 mm. This ensures proper tears exchange to remove debris from beneath the lens on blinking. It is not always possible with ultrathin lenses because of the way they drape the cornea.
- Some thicker lenses such as aphakics can cause dimpling.

Warning!

Some makes of lens, particularly disposables, are available in only a limited range of parameters. A compromise fitting should never be accepted with extended wear, since lenses are not removed to allow the resolution of otherwise minor difficulties (e.g. arcuate staining from a decentred lens).

21.4.2 Problems

LENS DEHYDRATION AND CORNEAL DESICCATION

Lens dehydration and corneal desiccation can occur with both high water content and ultrathin low water content lenses. The typical result is punctate staining in the mid-periphery of the cornea in the exposed area of the palpebral aperture. With the more rigid materials it can be associated with superior arcuate staining.

Where there is no obvious fault with the fitting, it is usually necessary to change to another make of lens with different dehydration characteristics.[9,10]

(CD)

Acute red eye syndrome (contact lens-induced acute red eye)

The sudden, acute red eye is a serious and unpredictable complication of soft extended wear giving gross conjunctival hyperaemia.[18] It normally occurs on wakening and is usually unilateral, associated with varying degrees of pain, photophobia, lacrimation and limbal infiltrates. The likeliest causes are an inflammatory response to trapped debris and toxins beneath the lens[8,11] and to deposits on the lens surface. The incidence is higher with heat disinfection and is reduced with peroxide systems.[12]

The courses of action are:

- Remove lenses.
- Ensure patient attends for immediate examination.
- Consider referral.
- Wait several days for condition to resolve.
- Change to new lenses.
- Ensure a peroxide disinfection system is used.
- Consider changing to daily wear – essential if the red eye recurs.

Infections

Infections with extended wear lenses tend to be more severe and longer lasting than with daily wear lenses. Immediate medical treatment is absolutely essential for microbial keratitis to minimize the risk of permanent visual loss (*see* Section 29.1). Other actions are as above for red eye.

The risks of infection are reduced with:

- Frequent lens replacement.
- Maximum oxygen supply to the cornea.
- Proper lens mobility.
- Proper lens cleaning and maintenance by the patient.
- Hygienic lens handling by the patient.
- Frequent replacement of lens cases.

Warning!

Chloramphenicol, the only antibiotic currently available to UK optometrists, is ineffective against eye infections caused by Gram-negative bacteria (e.g. *Pseudomonas aeroginosa*) or viruses.

Contact lens-induced papillary conjunctivitis (CLIPC)

The main causes of CLIPC with soft extended wear lenses are deposits and allergic responses during the hay fever season. The incidence is higher with low water content lenses, or where heat disinfection is used with high water content lenses.[12] The courses of action are given in Section 28.3.5.

Oedema

Stromal oedema is the cornea's response to insufficient oxygen under closed eye conditions (*see* Section 28.3.2) and may show in a variety of ways:

- Single stria, indicating 5–6% swelling.
- Several striae, indicating 7–10% swelling.
- Stromal folds, indicating 10–12% swelling.
- Epithelial microcysts.
- Subjective symptoms of cloudy vision.

Epithelial microcysts

Microcysts contain fluid and cellular debris, appearing as small vesicles in the corneal epithelium, seen with high magnification on the slit lamp. They represent an indication of hypoxic corneal stress, although small numbers may be considered sufficiently normal to ignore in the absence of other signs. They are generally seen after 2–3 months of extended wear, but can occur sooner.[13] They can also take several weeks to resolve.

Vascularization

Vascularization is a longer term response of both daily and extended soft lens wear. Vessels may be either superficial, extending from the limbal arcades, or deeper, stromal neovascularization where there is a much greater risk that they may extend into the pupil area. It may be necessary to change from extended to daily wear, from soft to hard lenses, or even (in severe cases) to cease contact lens wear altogether.[14]

Deposits

Because lenses are not removed for cleaning, there is a general predisposition to deposits (*see* Section 29.5). These are kept to a minimum by peroxide and enzyme cleaning and are largely avoided with disposable lenses.

BREAKAGE AND LOSS

Most lenses for extended wear are extremely fragile because of thinness or high water content. This is generally acceptable where handling is infrequent, but causes difficulty with more flexible wearing schedules. Loss is not a great problem, although some of the smaller, thinner lenses are occasionally rubbed out of the eye during sleep.

21.5 Hard lens fitting and problems

21.5.1 Fitting

The main considerations are:

- Sufficient oxygen with a high DK material.
- Adequate edge lift to avoid lens adhesion.
- Avoiding excessive edge lift and 3 and 9 o'clock staining.
- Good centration, particularly avoiding low riding lenses because of the risk of adhesion.
- Sufficient lens movement to provide a good tears pump.
- Avoiding lenses that ride onto or over the limbus.

21.5.2 Problems

Overall, there are fewer problems with hard lenses for extended wear. They do not cover the entire cornea, give a regular tear pump and are easier to remove and clean. By their nature, they avoid absorption, solutions reaction, red eye and vascularization. However, other difficulties can occur, as indicated below.

3 AND 9 O'CLOCK STAINING

3 and 9 o'clock staining is the hard lens equivalent of soft lens dehydration. It rarely causes discomfort, but because patients continue to wear lenses, its effect may becomes cumulative (*see* Section 28.3.2 for possible remedies).

INFECTIONS

(CD) Infection with hard lenses is infrequent. Care, however, is required where lens adhesion occurs because of the possibility of corneal ulceration.[15,16]

CONTACT LENS INDUCED PUPILLARY CONJUNCTIVITIS

(CD) CLIPC can occur with silicon acrylates because of deposits, allergic response or mechanical irritation. It is less common with fluoropolymers.

OEDEMA

(CD) Microcysts and striae occur where materials with insufficient Dk have been used.[1]

VASCULARIZATION

(CD) Vascularization occasionally occurs in the horizontal meridian associated with prolonged 3 and 9 o'clock staining.

BREAKAGE AND LOSS

(CD) Breakage occurs with some of the more brittle high Dk materials and where lenses have crazed or otherwise deteriorated with time. Loss is no worse than with daily wear.

LENS ADHESION

(CD) Most studies report lens adhesion to the cornea in a minimum of 10% of patients immediately on wakening.[15,16] Sticking relates to lens design, material, lid pressure and changes in tear constituents[16] (*see* Section 28.3.6.).

Warning!

Lens adhesion with extended wear increases the risk of corneal ulcers.

21.6 Other lenses for extended wear

21.6.1 Silicon lenses

Silicon lenses (*see* Section 6.5) have extremely high *Dk*s and are occasionally used for extended wear. One of their main applications is with babies to avoid the loss and damage that occur with soft lenses (*see* Section 30.3.1).

21.7 Long-term consequences of extended wear

METABOLIC ACTIVITY

Reduced oxygen supply to the epithelium reduces metabolic rate and therefore cell mitosis. Since the epithelium would not remain intact with decreased cell production and a constant rate of cell death and removal at the anterior epithelial surface, some compensation must occur.

INFECTION

The chances of infection, including microbial keratitis and sterile infiltrates, are significantly greater if the cells at the anterior epithelial surface become functionally less resistant as a result of long-term extended wear[17,18] (*see* Chapter 29).

CORNEAL THINNING

Epithelial thinning occurs as cell production and wastage rates reach a new equilibrium. Stromal thinning results from long-term chronic oedema.[4]

ENDOTHELIAL POLYMEGATHISM

Polymegathism is an irregularity in the cell size of the corneal endothelium caused by a lowering of pH[19] due to increased lactic acid (resulting from lens-induced hypoxia)[20] and/or increased carbonic acid (resulting from lens-induced hypercapnia). There does not seem to be a change in cell density, but a size increase of 27% has been reported.[4] The chances of complications with surgery or trauma are reported to be significantly greater after extended wear.[21]

VASCULARIZATION

The extension of limbal blood vessels into the cornea is a serious indication of chronic hypoxia. The vessels may extend from any position around the limbus, but tend to be further advanced beneath the top lid. Any increase should be monitored, and if the vessels grow more than 2 mm into the cornea, extended wear should be discontinued.

NEOVASCULARIZATION

New vessel growth at a deep stromal level is an unacceptable response to corneal stress caused by hypoxia, limbal compression, tissue damage or an acute infection. If allowed to continue and encroach within the pupil area, vision may be reduced as the surrounding tissue is changed by a lipid keratopathy.

Practical advice

To minimize the risk of potential problems, both short- and long-term patients should:

- Return for regular aftercare visits, not only during the fitting stage but for as long as extended wear continues.
- Replace lenses on a routine basis, at least every 12 months, and preferably much more frequently.
- Use peroxide and enzyme systems with conventional lenses.
- Receive written instructions.
- Receive advice that they *must* remove lenses if they suffer red eyes, discomfort, reduced vision, persistent lacrimation, other abnormal symptoms or illness.
- Know where 24-hour emergency help is available in case of severe infection.

References

1. Holden, B.A. and Mertz, G.W. (1984) Critical oxygen levels to avoid corneal oedema for daily and extended wear contact lenses. *Investigative Ophthalmology and Visual Science*, **25**, 1161
2. Holden, B.A. and Sweeney, D.F. (1987) Ocular requirements for extended wear. *Contax* (May), 13–18
3. Holden, B.A., Sweeney, D.F. and Sanderson, G. (1984) The minimum precorneal oxygen tension to avoid corneal oedema. *Investigative Ophthalmology and Visual Science*, **25**, 476

4. Holden, B.A., Sweeney, D.F., Vannas, A., Nilsson, K.T. and Efron, N. (1985) Effects of long-term extended contact lens wear on the human cornea. *Investigative Ophthalmology and Visual Science*, **26**, 1489
5. Hamano, H., Hori, M., Hamano, T., Kawabe, H., Mikami, M., Mitsunaga, S. *et al.* (1983) Effects of contact lens wear on mitosis of corneal epithelium and lactate content of aqueous humor of rabbit. *Japan Journal of Ophthalmology*, **27**, 451
6. Madigan, M.C., Holden, B.A. and Kwok, L.S. (1986) Extended wear of hydrogel contact lenses can compromise the corneal epithelium. *Investigative Ophthalmology and Visual Science*, **27** (suppl.), 140
7. Millodot, M. (1976) Effect of the length of wear of contact lenses on corneal sensitivity. *Acta Ophthalmologica*, **54**, 721
8. Josephson, J.E. and Caffrey, B.E. (1979) Infiltrative keratitis in hydrogel wearers. *International Contact Lens Clinic*, **6**, 223–242
9. Holden, B.A. (1986) Epithelial erosians caused by thin high water contact lenses. *Clinical and Experimental Optometry*, **69**, 103–107
10. Gasson, A.P. (1987) Aftercare problems with extended wear lenses. *Optician*, **193** (5078), 15–19
11. Zantos, S.G. and Holden, B.A. (1978) Ocular changes associated with continuous wear of contact lenses. *Australian Journal of Optometry*, **61**, 418–426
12. Kotow, M., Grant, T. and Holden, B.A. (1986) Evaluation of current care and maintenance systems for hydrogel extended wear. *Transactions of the British Contact Lens Association Annual Clinical Conference*, **3**, 66–67
13. Efron, N. (1996) Contact lens-induced epithelial microcysts. *Optician*, **211** (5549), 24–29
14. Efron, N. (1996) Contact lens-induced neovascularisation. *Optician*, **211** (5533), 26–35
15. Zabkewicz, K., Swarbrick, H. and Holden, B.A. (1986) Clinical experience with low to moderate *Dk* hard gas permeable lenses for extended wear. *Transactions of the British Contact Lens Association Annual Clinical Conference*, **3**, 101–102
16. Swarbrick, H.A. and Holden, B.A. (1989) Rigid gas-permeable lens binding: significance and contributing factors. *American Journal of Optometry and Physiological Optics*, **64**, 815–823
17. Stapleton, F., Dart, J. and Minassian, D. (1989) Contact lens related infiltrates – risk figures for different lens types and association with lens hygiene and solution contamination. *Transactions of the British Contact Lens Association Annual Clinical Conference*, **6**, 52–55
18. Sweeney, D.F., Grant, T., Chong, M.S., Fleming, C., Wong, R. and Holden, B.A. (1993) Recurrence of acute inflammatory conditions with hydrogel extended wear. *Investigative Ophthalmology and Visual Science*, **34**, S1008
19. Bonanno, J.A. and Polse, K.A. (1987) Measurement of *in vivo* human corneal stromal pH: open and closed eyes. *Investigative Ophthalmology and Visual Science*, **28**, 522–530
20. Holden, B.A., Ross, R. and Jenkins, J. (1987) Hydrogel contact lenses impede carbon dioxide efflux from the human cornea. *Current Eye Research*, **6**, 1283–1290
21. Rao, G.N., Aquavella, J.V., Goldberg, S.H. and Berk, S.L. (1984) Pseudo aphakic bullous keratopathy – relationship to preoperative corneal endothelial status. *Ophthalmology*, **91**, 1135

Chapter 22

Toric hard lenses

Toric hard lenses are used either to improve on the fitting of a spherical lens or to give better visual acuity with an astigmatic eye.

22.1 Residual and induced astigmatism

RESIDUAL ASTIGMATISM

Residual astigmatism is the uncorrected astigmatism found by refraction when a spherical contact lens is placed on the cornea. It derives from the crystalline lens and is usually against-the-rule. It is predictable where the spectacle cylinder and 'K' readings do not correlate. The corneal astigmatism is neutralized by a spherical hard lens leaving the lenticular astigmatism uncorrected.

Residual astigmatism = Ocular astigmatism − Corneal astigmatism

Example 1:
Spectacle *Rx*: −3.00/−1.50 × 95   'K' 7.90 mm × 7.85 mm
Corneal astigmatism = 0.05 mm ≡ 0.25 D
Residual astigmatism = 1.25 D

Example 2:

Spectacle *Rx*: −2.00/−1.00 × 180   'K'   7.60 mm (along 180)
                                              7.80 mm (along 90)
Corneal astigmatism = 0.20 mm ≡ 1.00 D
Residual astigmatism = 2.00 D

INDUCED ASTIGMATISM

The liquid lens beneath a hard contact lens neutralizes nine-tenths of the anterior corneal astigmatism because of the difference in refractive indices.[1] Induced astigmatism is created when a toric back surface is placed on a toric cornea and is against-the-rule if the corneal and spectacle astigmatism is with-the-rule. It is a characteristic of the lens because of the different refractive indices of the lens material and the tears. Modern hard gas-permeable materials tend to give less induced astigmatism than PMMA, which has a higher refractive index.

22.2 Patient selection

22.2.1 Indications and contraindications

INDICATIONS

To improve the physical fit

- The difference between principal meridians is greater than 0.6 mm.
- A spherical lens is unstable.
- A spherical lens decentres, usually along the steeper meridian.
- A spherical lens gives unacceptable bearing areas due to the corneal toricity.
- The bearing areas minimize tears exchange which may give rise to mid-peripheral corneal staining along the flatter meridian.
- A spherical lens produces corneal moulding and unacceptable spectacle blur.
- The cornea becomes significantly more toric towards the periphery.
- Poor comfort with a spherical lens due to rocking.

To give optimum visual acuity

- Residual astigmatism is greater than about 1.00 D.
- Lens flexure due to a steeply fitting spherical lens.
- Induced astigmatism.

CONTRAINDICATIONS

- Where a spherical lens gives a satisfactory result.
- Sensitive eyes where increased thickness causes discomfort or reduces transmissibility to an unacceptable level.

- Critical visual needs where acuity may be unstable.
- With a toric cornea but spherical spectacle *Rx*; a thin spherical soft lens should be the first choice (*see* Section 5.4).
- The greater expense of toric lenses.
- A toric lens is unnecessary with an amblyopic eye.

22.3 Lens designs

There are several possible designs for the correction of astigmatism, of which not all are toroidal.

22.3.1 Non-toric lens forms

SMALL SPHERICAL LENSES

Lenses with very small TDs are often successful. They fit only the central area of the cornea, which may be more spherical than the periphery. Fitting sets with narrow axial edge lift (typically 0.10 mm) are used to avoid excessive edge clearance or stand-off in the steeper meridian.

Practical advice

- Lenses may sometimes be as small as 7.50 mm.
- Centration is important to avoid flare.
- Use a centre thickness in the region of 0.12 mm.

ASPHERIC LENSES

Most aspheric designs also have narrow edge lift and give reduced clearance along the steeper meridian. In some cases they can mask up to about 4.00 D of astigmatism. They are usually fitted in alignment or flatter to avoid flexure.

22.3.2 Toric lenses

FRONT SURFACE TORIC

A spherical back surface with a front surface cylinder to correct *residual astigmatism*. Stabilization is necessary to maintain the correct cylinder axis.

TORIC PERIPHERY

A spherical BOZR with toric back peripheral radii. Used to give stability and to fit corneas where peripheral toricity is significantly greater than central. The front surface is usually spherical.

BACK SURFACE TORIC

Both central and peripheral radii are toric with a spherical front surface. The final peripheral radius is sometimes spherical for ease of manufacture and to assist tear flow. Stabilization is unnecessary since the lens radii should correctly follow the principal meridians of the cornea. The fluorescein appearance should look identical to that of a spherical lens on a spherical eye.

BITORIC

Both central and peripheral back surface radii are toric, combined with a front surface cylinder to correct induced astigmatism. Stabilization is usually needed for correct orientation of the cylinder axis because its position is important.

22.4 Methods of stabilization

PRISM BALLAST

Prism ballast usually employs 1.5^Δ (with an upper limit of about 3.0^Δ). The weight differential between the top and bottom of the lens should cause it to orientate with the prism base downwards. It is usually marked to assist observation. There is a tendency for a 5–10° nasal rotation of the prism base on blinking due to lid tension and eyelid position.

TRUNCATION

Truncation may be used either on its own or in conjunction with prism ballast and can be single or double. A chord of 0.50–1.00 mm is removed from the lens edge and the optimum effect is achieved when the truncation sits on the lower lid. It is therefore ineffective with small diameters and if the lower lid is below the limbus. To assist stability, compared with the optimum trial lens diameter, the TD should be increased by 0.50 mm for single truncation and 1.00 mm for double.

22.5 Fitting front surface torics

METHOD 1

- Use a large spherical trial lens with power as near as possible to the final *Rx* and over-refract.
- Order a lens based on this power, usually with 1.5$^\Delta$.
- Always have the prism base marked so that the lens orientation can be measured on the eye.
- Over-refract and record the cylinder and axis.
- Note the orientation of the prism base.
- If the lens is unstable, consider a truncation of 0.50 mm, increasing the prism, or a larger TD.
- Order the front cylinder, taking into account any rotation of the lens.
- The cylinder can be worked on the initial lens if no other changes are needed.

METHOD 2

- Over-refract with a spherical trial lens and order the final prescription lens directly with the front surface cylinder.
- This procedure is quicker, but an estimate of the final lens rotation is required (usually 5–15° nasal).

Practical advice

- If only one eye requires a toric, there may be problems with tolerance.
- Use truncation if there is a problem with binocular vision because of prism in only one eye.

Example:
Spectacle *Rx*:   –2.75/–1.50 × 80
'K' readings: 7.55 along 80, 7.45 along 170
Lens order: C3 7.55:7.50/9.50 AEL 0.12 *Dk* 60
                 –2.75/–1.00 × 75 1.5$^\Delta$ base down (along 270)
                 Single truncation: 0.50 mm along 180
                 Mark dots at prism base and apex

22.6 Fitting toric peripheries

- Fitted when the cornea is more astigmatic in the periphery and a small lens design fails to work.
- Normally used when the corneal astigmatism is 2.00–3.00 D.
- With a spherical trial set, the fitting should be assessed for central alignment and correct peripheral clearance in the flatter meridian.
- The radius for the steeper peripheral meridian can be determined either from the 'K' readings and looking up axial edge lift tables for each meridian, or from the fluorescein pattern. A minimum toric difference of 0.60 mm is usually required.
- The secondary curves are approximately 0.80–1.20 mm flatter.
- All toric periphery lenses with a spherical BOZR give an oval optic with the smallest diameter along the flattest meridian.
- If there are manufacturing problems with the theoretically designed periphery, an additional spherical edge curve can be used.
- A toric periphery trial set can be used for fitting.
- The prescription lens should give good acuity since the liquid lens neutralizes corneal astigmatism.
- A toric periphery is less expensive than a fully toroidal back surface design but represents a compromise.

Example:
'K'   7.90 mm × 7.50 mm
    C3 7.90:7.00/8.90:8.20/11.30:9.00
             8.30   10.70
    C3 7.90:7.00/8.90:8.20/10.75:9.00
             8.30

22.7 Fitting back surface torics

22.7.1 Toric fitting set

- A trial lens is selected to have the flatter meridian the same as flattest 'K' and the steeper meridian 0.1 mm flatter than the steepest 'K'. The meridians are therefore not exactly matched (e.g. 'K' 8.00 × 7.40; BOZR 8.00 × 7.50).
- The ideal fluorescein pattern should look the same as an alignment spherical fit.

- Over-refraction should be carried out with minus cylinders. The spherical component is the power along the flatter meridian.
- The laboratory will produce the cylinder along the steeper meridian.
- The possibility of induced astigmatism must always be considered.

22.7.2 Spherical fitting set

- A spherical lens is fitted in alignment to establish the flatter meridian
- The steeper radius is determined from the 'K' readings.
- The spherical power is determined by over-refraction with minus cylinders.
- The cylinder is obtained by calculation.

Example:
Ocular refraction: −2.00/−3.00 × 180
Keratometry: 8.00 mm along 180   7.45 mm along 90
The astigmatism is entirely corneal
Trial lens BOZR giving alignment along 180 = 8.00 mm

By fluorescein assessment toric lens needed is:
r_1 = 8.00 mm along 180
r_2 = 7.55 mm along 90

BVP calculation:
$$F = n{-}1/r$$

where refractive index of tears n = 1.336

Along 180 BOZR of 8.00 mm gives anterior surface power to the tear lens in air of:
336/8.00 = +42.00

Along 90 BOZR of 7.55 mm gives anterior surface power to the tear lens in air of:
336/7.55 = +44.50

Along 180 BVP = −2.00 D (from over-refraction with trial lens)
Along 90 BVP = −2.50 D

Final prescription:

8.00:7.00/8.60:8.00/10.50:9.00
7.55   8.15   10.00

$-2.00/-2.50 \times 180$

The rule-of-thumb 0.1 mm $\equiv$ 0.50 D gives useful confirmation, since 8.00 mm -7.55 mm is 0.45 mm $\equiv$ 2.25 D

22.7.3 Fitting by calculation

A lens can also be ordered for the patient by theoretical calculation using the ocular refraction, 'K' readings and refractive index of the material. BOZD, TD and edge clearance are nevertheless determined from clinical assessment. The toric difference of the lens radii can be chosen to neutralize the corneal astigmatism, but the induced astigmatism must also be calculated.[2]

Explanation:
Ocular refraction: Sphere (S)   Cylinder (C)
Induced astigmatism (I):

$$I = \frac{n - n'}{r_1} - \frac{n - n'}{r_2}$$

where
n = refractive index of tears
n' = refractive index of the contact lens material
r_1 = steeper radius of curvature, in metres
r_2 = flatter radius of curvature, in metres

However, other factors have to be calculated.

The lens astigmatism induced by the back surface in air (A)

$$A = \frac{1 - n'}{r_1} - \frac{1 - n'}{r_2}$$

The BVP along the flatter meridian is S.
The BVP along the steeper meridian is S + A
To correct the induced astigmatism this becomes S + A − I along the steeper meridian.

Example:
Spectacle prescription: $-2.00/-3.00 \times 180$
Keratometry: 8.00 mm along 180   7.60 mm along 90
Corneal astigmatism: 0.40 mm = 2.00 D
Residual astigmatism: $(-3.00) - (-2.00) = -1.00$ D
BOZRs chosen: $r_1 = 7.70$ mm, $r_2 = 8.00$ mm
                          $n = 1.336$ $n' = 1.480$

Induced astigmatism: $= \dfrac{-144}{7.70} - \dfrac{-144}{8.00}$

$$= (-18.70) - (-18.00) = -0.70 \text{ D}$$

This almost exactly corrects the residual astigmatism and a front surface cylinder is unnecessary in this case.

BVP along the flatter meridian: $= -2.00$ D
BVP along the steeper meridian needs to be calculated:
  Lens astigmatism in air (back surface lens astigmatism)

$$-1000\,\frac{(1-n')}{r_1} - 1000\,\frac{(1-n')}{r_2} = \frac{-480}{7.70} - \frac{-480}{8.00}$$

$$= (-62.33) - (-60.00) = -2.33 \text{ D}$$

As induced astigmatism is neutralized, the final powers are:
BVP along flatter meridian: $= -2.00$ D
BVP along steeper meridian: $= -2.00 + (-2.33) = -4.33$
Equivalent to: $-2.00 / -2.33$ along flatter meridian

22.8 Fitting bitorics

A bitoric is required when a back surface toric has created suffi-cient induced astigmatism (usually over 0.75 D) to warrant cor-rection with a front surface cylinder.[3]

- If corneal and ocular astigmatism are equal, the induced astig-matism created may require correction.

- If the ocular astigmatism is less that the corneal astigmatism, lenticular astigmatism is revealed by a hard lens and requires neutralizing together with the induced astigmatism. In this case, a large front surface cylinder is needed.

Example:
Spectacle prescription $-2.00 / -3.00 \times 180$
Keratometry   8.00 mm along 180, 7.40 mm along 90
Corneal astigmatism   3.00 D
Residual astigmatism   0.00 D
If we choose BOZRs of: $r_1 = 7.50$ mm, $r_2 = 8.00$ mm
For: $n = 1.336$, $n' = 1.480$

Induced astigmatism $\dfrac{-144}{7.50} - \dfrac{-144}{8.00}$

$$(-19.20) - (-18.00) = -1.20 \text{ D}$$

This degree of induced astigmatism requires correction.
The astigmatism induced by the back surface in air:

$$\frac{-480}{7.50} - \frac{-480}{8.00} = (-64.00) - (-60.00) = -4.00$$

BVP along flatter meridian $= -2.00$ D
BVP along steeper meridian $= (-2.00) + (-4.00) - (-1.20)$
$\qquad\qquad\qquad\qquad\qquad\quad = -4.80$ D

Equivalent to $-2.00/-2.80$ along flatter meridian

22.9 Compromise back surface torics

If the ocular astigmatism is greater than the corneal astigmatism,
a compromise fitting option is worth considering to avoid the use
of a front surface cylinder.[4] In these cases, some of the induced
astigmatism will be neutralized by the residual astigmatism and
the remaining induced astigmatism can be further eliminated by
reducing the difference between the flatter and steeper radii.

* Convert the spectacle prescription to an ocular prescription.
* Calculate the resultant induced astigmatism when the back
  surface toric lens is designed close to alignment.
* Calculate the residual astigmatism or use rule-of-thumb.
* Calculate the difference needed in BOZRs to create induced
  astigmatism that is equal or close to the residual astigmatism.
* Redesign the lens so that the flatter BOZR aligns with the flattest corneal meridian and the steeper BOZR satisfies the above
  calculation.

Rule of thumb

Choosing the lens radii to be approximately 75% of the corneal toric
difference often avoids the need for a bitoric lens.

Example:
Ocular prescription $-4.00/-5.00 \times 180$
Keratometry   8.00 mm along 180   7.20 mm along 90
Corneal astigmatism   4.00 D
Residual astigmatism $(-5.00) - (-4.00) = -1.00$ D

If the BOZRs were chosen to align $r_1 = 7.20$ $r_2 = 8.00$
For $n = 1.336$ $n' = 1.480$

Induced astigmatism = $\dfrac{-144}{7.20} - \dfrac{-144}{8.00}$

$$(-20.00) - (-18.00) = -2.00 \text{ D}$$
Front surface cylinder to compensate = $(-2.00) - (-1.00) = -1.00$ D
However, by flattening the steeper BOZR to 7.40 mm

Induced astigmatism = $\dfrac{-144}{7.40} - \dfrac{-144}{8.00}$

$$(-19.45) - (-18.00) = -1.45 \text{ D}$$
Uncorrected astigmatism = $(-1.45) - (-1.00) = -0.45$ D

The patient would be expected to tolerate this small amount of astigmatism, therefore a bitoric is not needed with a back surface toric of 8.00×7.40 mm.

22.10 Computers in toric lens fitting

Computer programs are now available which help in the design and ordering of bitoric hard gas-permeable contact lenses. The required data are keratometry readings, spectacle Rx, BVD; and possibly the selected BOZR, BOZD and TD. Most programs provide the final lens specification along the flatter and steeper meridians as well as the ocular astigmatism, corneal astigmatism, residual astigmatism and induced astigmatism. From this information it becomes clear whether a front surface cylinder is necessary. Some programs suggest the compromise fit required to avoid a front surface cylinder. Similar information and calculations are provided by corneal topographers (*see* Section 8.5).

References

1. Douthwaite, W.A. (1995) *Contact Lens Optics and Lens Design*, 2nd edn, Butterworth-Heinemann, Oxford
2. Meyler, J.G. (1989) Fitting and calculating toric corneal contact lenses. *Journal of the British Contact Lens Association*, **12** (2), 7–14
3. Edwards, K.H. (1982) The calculation and fitting of toric lenses. *Ophthalmic Optician*, **22**, 106–114
4. Meyler, J.G. and Ruston, D. (1995) Toric RGP contact lenses made easy. *Optician*, **209** (5540), 30–35

Chapter 23

Toric soft lenses

23.1 Patient selection

Toric soft lenses are not prescribed to improve the physical fitting, as with hard lenses (except with very high degrees of astigmatism), but to provide good visual acuity where spherical lenses are unable to achieve this.

INDICATIONS

- Vision is unsatisfactory with a spherical soft lens.
- Astigmatism is 1.00 D or greater (occasionally 0.75 D or 0.50 D cylinders may be fitted).
- Tolerance is poor with a hard gas-permeable lens.
- Keratometry and optical considerations indicate that a hard lens requires a much more complex, bitoric design (*see* Section 22.8).

CONTRAINDICATIONS

- Astigmatism is purely corneal and hard lens tolerance is good.
- Existing hard lens wearers.
- Irregular astigmatism.
- Monocular patients.

23.2 Stabilization

23.2.1 Influences on lens behaviour

The main influences on lens orientation are the method of stabilization and the lids. Eyelids are important in respect of:

- Position of lower lid.
- Size of vertical palpebral aperture.
- Lid tension.
- Force of blink.
- Direction of movement on blinking.

In cases of with-the-rule astigmatism, the thickest portions of the correcting toric lens lie at the top and bottom. The normal action of the lids is to rotate the lens 90° off-axis to bring the thickest parts into the horizontal meridian. The action of the lids on the lens edge has been compared to squeezing a watermelon seed, so that they control the ultimate lens position even with the head inverted.[1]

There are several other factors that have some effect on lens behaviour:[2]

- Gravity.
- Water content.
- Material elasticity.
- Lens thickness.
- Hydrostatic pressure.

23.2.2 Methods of stabilization

Various techniques are possible, either on their own or in combinations.

TRUNCATION

Truncation is now less commonly used with soft lenses. It is usually single, removing a 1.00 to 1.50 mm chord from the lower edge of the lens (e.g. Zeiss Hydroflex-TS, Hydron Rx Toric). Oblique truncations (up to 20°) are feasible and sometimes used with angled lids. Some designs of front surface toric have employed double truncation.

Advantages

- Better stability than other methods.
- Easily observed and measured on the eye.
- Thinner lenses can be used.

Disadvantages

- Less comfortable.
- Buckling of lower edge if too flat or vertical corneal meridian very steep.
- Cosmetically more noticeable.
- Less satisfactory with oblique cylinders.
- Increased deposits along truncated edge.
- Few lens types now available.

PRISM BALLAST

Prism ballast usually employs 1^Δ or 1.5^Δ base down. The upper limit is approximately 3^Δ. Two modern refinements of lens design are able to reduce the thickness previously associated with this method and give improved comfort and physiological response:

- Prism-free optics to incorporate the stabilizing prism only in the peripheral areas of the lens (e.g. Hydron Omniflex toric).
- Slab-off prisms to give equal thickness at both the base and 3 and 9 o'clock positions.

Where a toric is required for only one eye, in theory the spherical lens for the other eye should also include base-down prism to prevent binocular imbalance. This is not often necessary in practice (not at all with prism-free optics) and the spherical lens is usually ordered without prism but with subsequent assessment of binocularity.

Advantages

- More comfortable than truncation.
- Better with oblique cylinders.
- Cosmetically less noticeable.

Disadvantages

- Careful slit lamp observation required to assess lens orientation.
- Lenses may be thicker.
- Greater risk of oedema with low water content.
- Not always successful at stabilization.

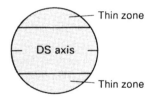

Figure 23.1 Thin zones

THIN ZONES (DYNAMIC STABILIZATION)

Top and bottom portions of the lens are chamfered to reduce the thickness where the stabilization zones fit beneath the lids (Figure 23.1). The optic portion is the central band which lies within the palpebral aperture. Lenses have the *DS axis* marked in the 3 and 9 o'clock positions.

Advantages

- Lens remains thin overall.
- Good comfort with thin edges.
- Good cosmetic appearance.
- Unimportant if lens is upside down.

Disadvantages

- Careful slit lamp observation required to assess lens orientation.
- Limitation to the amount of cylinder (approximately 4.00 D).

TORIC BACK SURFACE

A toric back surface has a natural stabilizing effect when placed in apposition to an equivalently toroidal cornea because least elastic distortion occurs when the lens is correctly aligned. A better result, however, is achieved when used in conjunction with prism ballast or truncation. The toroidal optic zone is ellipsoidal in shape, the dimensions depending upon power and radius. It is larger with a lower cylinder and vice versa.

OTHER METHODS

- Lens elevations (orientation cams) in the 3 and 9 o'clock positions (e.g. Lunelle, Weflex 55).
- Specially shaped, non-circular lenses.

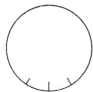

Figure 23.2 Radial engravings

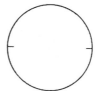

Figure 23.3 Laser lines at 3 and 9 o'clock positions

23.2.3 Assessing lens rotation

LENS MARKINGS

In order to assess any rotation on the eye, it is essential that lenses are marked with reference points except for truncations which are easily measurable. The following methods are commonly used:

- Radial engravings at the base of the lens. These give an assessment of rotation on the eye and are usually separated by either 15° (e.g. Z6T) or 30° (e.g. Hydrocurve III, Optima Toric) (Figure 23.2).
- A single dot usually at the base of the prism (e.g. Sunsoft Toric, Mark Ennovy 5T), but occasionally placed at the apex for identification (e.g. Weflex 55).
- Horizontal lines in the 3 and 9 o'clock positions (e.g. Focus Toric, Hydroflex/m-T) (Figure 23.3).
- Horizontal elevations in the 3 and 9 o'clock positions (e.g. Lunelle).
- A combination of horizontal and base markings (e.g. Proclear)

MEASURING LENS ROTATION

Apart from truncations, engravings can only be clearly observed with the slit lamp. Rotation can be measured by:

- Assessing radial markings by observation alone.
- A graticule, either internal or surrounding the slit lamp eyepiece.
- Rotating a fine slit lamp beam to align with lens engravings and reading the instrument's external protractor scale. Horizontal markings tend to be easier to assess than vertical.
- Using a Javal-type ophthalmometer.[3]

23.3 Lens designs

Several different designs have evolved so that toric soft lenses, apart from stabilization with any of the methods in Section 23.2.2, may be of either corneal or semi-scleral diameter; use a variety of water contents; and have either a front or back toric surface. Disposable torics are also available (e.g. Focus, Soflens 66, Actitoric).

TOTAL DIAMETER

Advantages of corneal diameter torics (e.g. Hydroflex/m-T)

- Less risk of oedema.
- Cosmetically better.
- Less lower lid sensation.

Advantages of semi-scleral torics (e.g. Hydron Z6T, Sunsoft)

- Better stability.
- Less upper lid sensation.
- Wider range of lenses and methods of stabilization.

WATER CONTENT

Advantages of low water content torics (e.g. Hydroflex-TS, Optima, Durasoft 2, Optifit)

- Better stability on the eye.
- More reliable orientation.
- Can be made thinner.
- More reproducible.
- Longer life span.
- Easier to manufacture.
- Wider range of lenses available.

Advantages of high water content torics (e.g. Lunelle, Proclear, Weicon CE)

- Better comfort.
- Less risk of oedema.

FRONT AND BACK SURFACE TORICS

Front surface torics

Front surface torics are capable of correcting both corneal and lenticular astigmatism, up to about 4.50 D. They are successful with a wide variety of geometries, both corneal (e.g. Hydroflex AT) and semi-scleral (e.g. Weicon CE). Stabilization can be by means of prism ballast (e.g. Optima); truncation (e.g. Hydron *Rx* toric); or dynamic stabilization (e.g. Focus). The back surface may be either spherical (e.g. Weflex) or aspheric (e.g. Hydron *Rx* toric).

Back surface torics

Back surface torics have evolved logically from the fact that most of the astigmatism encountered in practice is predominantly corneal. Keratometry and spectacle *Rx* give an immediate prediction of the likelihood of visual success. The back surface of the lens is essentially designed to neutralize the toric cornea by replacing it with a spherical front surface. The radii of the principal meridians may be either predetermined by the laboratory (e.g. Hydrocurve 3) or individually calculated (e.g. Hydroflex/m-T) using a radius to surface power conversion chart (Table 23.1).

Table 23.1 Radius to surface power conversion for $n = 1.4448$

BCOR (mm)	Surface power (D)	BCOR (mm)	Surface power (D)
6.00	74.13	8.00	55.60
6.10	72.92	8.10	54.91
6.20	71.74	8.20	54.24
6.30	70.60	8.30	53.59
6.40	69.50	8.40	52.95
6.50	68.43	8.50	52.33
6.60	67.39	8.60	51.72
6.70	66.39	8.70	51.13
6.80	65.41	8.80	50.55
6.90	64.46	8.90	49.98
7.00	63.54	9.00	49.42
7.10	62.65	9.10	48.88
7.20	61.78	9.20	48.35
7.30	60.93	9.30	47.83
7.40	60.11	9.40	47.32
7.50	59.31	9.50	46.82
7.60	58.53	9.60	46.33
7.70	57.77	9.70	45.86
7.80	57.03	9.80	45.39
7.90	56.30	9.90	44.93

Cylinders as high as 6.00 D can be corrected. Lenticular astigmatism is not theoretically correctable, although in practice reasonable clinical results can often be obtained. The back surface is sometimes stable enough on its own, but is markedly assisted by either prism ballast (e.g. Durasoft 2) or truncation (e.g. Hydroflex TS).

Practical advice

Most back surface torics include only the flatter meridian in the final lens specification (e.g. Hydrocurve 3, Mark Ennovy).

23.4 Fitting

Lenses may be either individually designed and prescribed or selected from a simplified range of parameters predetermined by the laboratory (stock torics).

INDIVIDUALLY DESIGNED LENSES

The design method permits the fitting of most prescriptions which it is technically feasible to manufacture, with a comprehensive range of lens parameters, water contents, spherical and cylinder powers, axis positions and methods of stabilization. The main disadvantages are the greater time required to obtain lenses and additional costs, particularly where changes to the prescription are necessary.

STOCK TORICS

The simplified method enables rapid fitting from either practitioner or laboratory stock, since parameters are carefully restricted. Cylinder powers have an upper range of about 2.50 D (this will cope with 90% of prescriptions[4]), and may be limited to 0.50 D or 0.75 D steps. Axes may be restricted to 20° either side of horizontal or vertical in 10° steps, and oblique cylinders, which are generally more difficult to fit, are frequently omitted. Disposable lenses are necessarily stock torics.

No single make of standard design, even in the common range of astigmatism, can approach the accuracy of a properly calculated practitioner specification.[5] However, by using several makes of stock toric, a standard design can usually be found to match the correction and fitting required. This is then the preferred method of fitting.

FITTING ROUTINE

- Assess spectacle *Rx* and 'K' readings.
- Decide on a back or front surface toric in respect of corneal or lenticular astigmatism.
- Decide on the method of stabilization. A different design placed on each eye usually determines both a preference in comfort by the patient and establishes whether prism, dynamic stabilization or truncation is likely to give best orientation.
- Determine the best fitting trial lens.
- Determine the lens orientation on the eye from the angle at which the lens marking settles. Trial lenses establish at the fitting stage whether compensation is required for the cylinder axis. The most common result is a 5° nasal rotation of the lens base. Success is unlikely if the rotation is more than about 20°, even if consistent, and it is usually better to try a different fitting or lens type. Oblique cylinders generally give less reliable results.
- Over-refract with a fully settled spherical trial lens of power as near as possible to the spectacle *Rx*. Apart from any vertex distance considerations, this is always worthwhile to ensure that the results correlate, particularly in respect of cylinder power and axis. If there is any discrepancy, repeat with a different trial lens.
- There is little value in over-refracting with a toric trial lens, since the result will be that of obliquely crossed cylinders and only indirect information may be gained (*see* Table 23.2). However, the dynamics of a toric lens on the eye are likely to be more reliable than a spherical lens because a correcting cylinder has been incorporated.
- If axis compensation has been made because of lens rotation at the initial fitting, the prescription lens should also settle with exactly the same degree of rotation.
- The nature of the over-refraction may be used as a guide with the toric prescription lens, although its absolute value is not very meaningful. If cylinder is present at the original axis or at

CD

Table 23.2 Residual refractive error induced by mislocation of toric lenses of various cylindrical powers (From Holden and Frauenhofer,[4] with permission)

Convention	(1) Axes in standard axis notation	
	(2) Anticlockwise is +ve, clockwise −ve	
Mislocation (degrees)	−1.00 D	−2.00 D (×2)
5	+0.08/−0.16 × 42.5	+0.17/−0.34 × 42.5
10	+0.17/−0.34 × 40	+0.35/−0.69 × 40
15	+0.26/−0.52 × 37.5	+0.52/−1.04 × 37.5
20	+0.34/−0.69 × 35	+0.68/−1.37 × 35
25	+0.43/−0.85 × 32.5	+0.85/−1.69 × 32.5
30	+0.50/−1.00 × 30	+1.00/−2.00 × 30
35	+0.57/−1.14 × 27.5	+1.14/−2.29 × 27.5
40	+0.64/−1.28 × 25	+1.29/−2.57 × 25
45	+0.71/−1.42 × 22.5	+1.41/−2.83 × 22.5
50	+0.76/−1.53 × 20	+1.53/−3.06 × 20
55	+0.82/−1.64 × 17.5	+1.64/−3.28 × 17.5
60	+0.87/−1.73 × 15	+1.73/−3.46 × 15
65	+0.90/−1.82 × 12.5	+1.81/−3.63 × 12.5
70	+0.94/−1.88 × 10	+1.88/−3.76 × 10
75	+0.96/−1.93 × 7.5	+1.93/−3.85 × 7 5
80	+0.98/−1.97 × 5	+1.97/−3.94 × 5
85	+0.99/−1.99 × 2.5	+1.99/−3.98 × 2.5
90	+1.00/−2.00 × 180	+2.00/−4.00 × 180

90° to this, under- or overcorrection is suggested. If it takes the form of a plus sphere with minus cylinder of approximately twice the power (e.g. +0.50/−1.00) at a different axis, it is because of cylinder axis mislocation. This may be due to lens rotation or inaccurate manufacture and may be assessed either from Table 23.2 or modern computer programs.

Practical advice

Depending on the type of axis markings, the position at which a lens settles on the cornea can be recorded as shown in Figure 23.4(a)–(c).

23.5 Fitting examples

FRONT SURFACE STOCK TORIC

Example:

Spectacle *Rx*: R.E.−3.00/−1.25 × 85

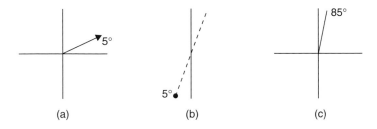

Figure 23.4 (a)–(c) Recording lens orientation

Keratometry: R.E. 7.85 mm (43.00 D) spherical

The astigmatism is entirely lenticular, so a front surface toric is required.

Best fitting: Ciba, WCE Toric: FL (flat): 14.60 −3.00

Over-refraction: Plano/−1.25 × 85

Trial lens: Locates with 5° nasal (anticlockwise) rotation.

The nearest options available for this stock design are:

Cylinders: −1.00 D or −1.75 D. It is nearly always better to under- rather than over-correct. Select −1.00 D.

Axes: 80° or 90°. Select 80° because of the 5° nasal orientation of the trial lens. The cylinder axis will therefore rotate to the required 85°.

Lens specification: FL:14.60 −3.00/−1.00 × 80

FRONT SURFACE TORIC WITH FULL RANGE OF PARAMETERS

Example:

Spectacle *Rx*: L.E. −2.50/−3.50 × 180

Keratometry: L.E. 8.23 mm along 180° (41.00 D)

7.72 mm along 90° (43.75 D)

The astigmatism is outside the range of a stock toric. Most is corneal but with 0.75 D lenticular. Select a front surface toric with a full range of parameters.

Best fitting: Hydron Z6 Toric   9.00:14.00   −3.00

Over-refraction: +0.50/−3.25 × 180

Lens specification: allowing for 5° nasal rotation (clockwise for left eye):

9.00:14.00 − 2.50/−3.25 × 5

Suppose this prescription lens proved too mobile and also settled consistently with 10° temporal rotation (anticlockwise for left eye). Re-order:

Final lens specification: 8.70:14.00   −2.50/−3.25 × 170

BACK SURFACE STOCK TORIC (e.g. Hydrocurve 3)

Spectacle   *Rx*:   R.E. −1.25 DS/−2.50 DC × 20

Keratometry: R.E. 7.96 mm along   20° (42.50 D)

                      7.50 mm along 110° (45.00 D)

The astigmatism is entirely corneal and possibly within the range of a stock toric.

Best fitting: 8.80:14.50   −1.50

Example A:

Over-refraction: +0.25/−2.25 × 20

Trial lens: Locates with 5° nasal rotation (anticlockwise for right eye).

Lens specification: 8.80:14.50   −1.25/−2.00 × 15

Example B:

Over-refraction: Plano/−2.75 × 25

Trial lens: Locates with 20° temporal rotation (clockwise for right eye).

With 0.75 D undercorrection of the cylinder and a required axis theoretically at an oblique 45°, this example is unlikely to give a successful result. Discontinue and try another variety of toric to give better orientation on the cornea.

BACK SURFACE TORIC FITTED BY CALCULATION

Example:

Spectacle *Rx*:   R. E. −0.75/−3.50 × 15

Keratometry: R.E.   8.23 mm along 15   (41.00 D)

7.63 mm along 105 (44.25 D)

The astigmatism is almost entirely corneal and outside the range of a stock toric. Suppose non-truncated designs give unstable and excessive rotation. Select a back surface toric with truncation.

Best fitting: Hydroflex TS   9.30:14.00   −3.00

Over-refraction: +2.50/−3.50 × 15

(N.B. This is required in minus cylinder form. There is also the typical +0.25 D difference in spherical power due to liquid lens and flexure effects − see Section 17.3)

Trial lens: Locates with 10° nasal rotation. Prescription lens therefore requires a compensated axis at 5° (designated T5)

Calculation of radii for principal meridians

The trial lens radius is taken as the flatter meridian and, using Table 23.1, converted to surface power (N.B. minus sign).

9.30 mm   →   −47.83 D   surface power

add   −3.50 D   correcting cylinder

8.70 mm   ←   −51.33 D

General advice

- A successful fitting usually returns consistently to the same orientation within one or two blinks or after rotational displacement of the eye.
- Where a lens mislocates on the eye, rather than attempt to change its orientation (e.g. by tightening the fit or adjusting the truncation), assume that the various stabilizing factors (*see* Section 23.2.1) will always act on the lens in a similar way. Compensate in the axis of the correcting cylinder for any lens rotation on the eye.
- Fitting is less reliable with oblique cylinders.
- Take particular care when fitting essentially monocular patients. They are much more disturbed by any instability of vision caused by temporary lens rotation on blinking.
- If no success is achieved after the second lens for a particular eye, try a different type of design.

The nearest value to 51.33 D in Table 23.1 is 51.13 D (8.70 mm) and is taken as the steeper meridian.

Final lens specification: 9.30/8.70:14.00 −0.50 T5

N.B. If the prescription lens overcorrects the astigmatism, this is possibly due to induced astigmatism, and a smaller toric difference is indicated.

References

1. Killpartrick, M.R. (1983) Apples, space-time and the watermelon seed. *Ophthalmic Optician*, **23**, 801–802
2. Grant, R. (1986) Mechanics of toric soft lens stabilisation. *Transactions of the British Contact Lens Association Annual Clinical Conference*, **3**, 44–47
4. Lindsay, R.G. and Westerhout, D. (1997) Toric contact lens fitting. In *Contact Lenses*, A.J. Phillips and L. Speedwell (eds), Butterworth-Heinemann, Oxford, pp. 464–493
5. Holden, B.A. and Frauenfelder, G. (1975) Principles and practice of correcting astigmatism with soft contact lenses. *Australian Journal of Optometry*, **58**, 279–299
6. Cooke, G., Green, T. and Young, G. (1996) Spreadsheet calculation of oblique cylinder power. *Optician*, **211** (5540), 28–30

Chapter 24

Bifocal lenses and presbyopia

24.1 Patient selection

24.1.1 New patients

INDICATIONS

- Patients who fulfil the normal criteria for successful contact lens wear.
- Fairly tolerant patients who can accept some compromise in their distance and near vision.
- Patients without exacting visual requirements.

CONTRAINDICATIONS

- Patients almost emmetropic for distance.
- Where there are basic contraindications to contact lens wear.
- Very critical patients.
- Patients who need good sustained close vision for work require particular care.
- Where the reason for fitting is obviously a spectacle dispensing problem.
- Poor handling.

Practical advice

To give prior assessment of adaptation, fit single vision distance first or try disposables if:
- The patient is uncertain about contact lenses.
- There are practitioner doubts about suitability.
- Handling may be a problem.

24.1.2 Existing lens wearers

- Early presbyopes often cope with +0.50 D added to the distance correction, usually in one eye.
- Many patients are happy to wear reading spectacles over their contact lenses to avoid both complications and expense.
- Some patients inadvertently using monovision because of refractive change are less happy when refitted with bifocals.
- If the patient is a successful hard lens wearer, soft bifocals should not be fitted.

INDICATIONS

- Long-term lens wearers who do not wish to resume wearing spectacles, even for reading.
- Physical problems with spectacles.
- Nuisance value of spectacles for one specific task.

CONTRAINDICATIONS

- Poor volume or quality of tears, common with presbyopes.
- Where tolerance is becoming marginal with single vision lenses.
- Patients taking systemic drugs (e.g. for arthritis or sometimes hormone replacement therapy).

24.2 Monovision

Monovision is a technique for correcting presbyopia in which reading power is incorporated into a single-vision contact lens worn usually on the non-dominant eye.

24.2.1 Advantages and disadvantages of monovision

ADVANTAGES

- The least complicated method of dealing with presbyopia.
- It is unnecessary to make any compromise in the fitting.
- Patient acceptability is high, provided that the concept has been explained.
- Stability of vision.

- Patients usually decide rapidly that they can or cannot accept the technique.
- Significantly less expensive than bifocals.

DISADVANTAGES

- Reduced stereopsis, but at optical infinity this is negligible and peripheral fusion is maintained.
- Some loss of contrast sensitivity, although this is also true of most bifocal contact lenses.
- Unacceptable blurring may reduce tolerance.
- Cannot be used with monocular patients.
- Requires fairly strong eye dominance.
- Care is required with driving, particularly at night.

24.2.2 Fitting for monovision

- Lenses, hard or soft, are fitted according to normal criteria.
- The non dominant eye is generally used for near vision.
- The left is more often the non-dominant eye; in the UK, this is more practicable for driving.
- The least minus or most plus is found for distance in the dominant eye.
- The minimum plus power for adequate near vision is included for the non-dominant eye.

Practical advice

- If right and left eyes are similar in prescription, the patient can experiment with which eye to use for near.
- If near vision is the main use, try changing the dominance and adapting the method to the patient's needs.
- For occasional optimum distance vision (e.g. prolonged driving), consider prescribing either a third distance lens for the non-dominant eye or spectacles to wear over the lenses.
- The easiest way of assessing eye dominance is to have the patient (1) point with the forefingers of both hands touching; or (2) fixate through a cardboard tube.

PARTIAL MONOVISION

A low add of +0.50 D or +0.75 D often gives sufficient convenience for intermittent near vision (e.g. price tags, menus, headlines) and patients are then happy to use reading spectacles for prolonged close work. This technique can sometimes be particularly effective with front surface aspherics.

24.3 Bifocal lens designs

24.3.1 Alternating designs (translating bifocals)

Alternating lenses contain two distinct sectors. These may be either fused or solid portions, or extend across the entire width of the lens (Figure 24.1). Segment lenses are more common, but the concept is equally valid with concentric designs. Distance and near portions can never be used in the same direction of gaze or at the same time. Lens stability and position are controlled by either prism or truncation.

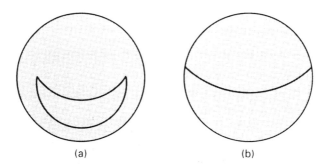

(a)   (b)

Figure 24.1 Bifocal lens design: (a) fused or solid portion; (b) solid portion extending across lens width

FACTORS FOR SUCCESSFUL FITTING

- The lens must move upwards on downward gaze to bring the near portion in front of the pupil area.
- A relatively taut lower lid is necessary; if it is too slack, the lens edge slides across the lower limbus.
- The bottom lid should be no lower than the inferior limbus in order to support the lens.

Rule of thumb

There must be sufficient movement to ensure that approximately three-quarters of the pupil area is covered by the correct section of the lens for both distance and near[1] (Figure 24.2).

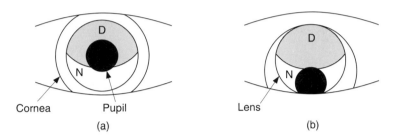

Cornea   Pupil   Lens

(a)   (b)

Figure 24.2 Bifocal lens movement: (a) primary gaze; (b) down gaze (D, distance portion; N, near portion)

- There should be minimal disturbance of the lens on blinking or the reading portion is drawn in front of the pupil for distance and the patient complains of variable vision.

24.3.2 Simultaneous designs (non-translating bifocals)

Simultaneous designs essentially provide distance and near vision together and do not rely on lens movement. They are commonly found with concentric or aspheric lenses where they are usually referred to as centre near (CN) and centre distance (CD), or with diffractive designs.

FACTORS FOR SUCCESSFUL FITTING

Stability of fit and the ability to discern between distance and near are important factors. Pupil size is also very significant in the performance of all simultaneous bifocals except diffractive lenses.

One of the main problems with simultaneous bifocals is a loss of contrast sensitivity of the superimposed retinal images. The problem is worse in low illumination and can give particular difficulties at near vision.

CENTRE NEAR LENSES

- Low illumination with CN concentric types favours distance vision because of the increase in pupil size.

- High illumination with CN concentric types favours near vision because of the decrease in pupil size; thus drivers should wear sunglasses.

- With CN aspherics, the larger the pupil the better the distance vision. Older patients with small pupils may not achieve good distance acuity.

CENTRE DISTANCE LENSES

- Low illumination with CD concentric types favours near vision.

- High illumination with CD concentric types favours distance vision; thus sunglasses should be worn to read on a beach.

- With CD aspherics, small pupils make available less reading addition; thus, the older the patient the less suitable for near.

24.4 Fitting hard bifocals

24.4.1 Alternating types

FUSED SEGMENTED BIFOCALS (E.G. FLUOROPERM ST)

PMMA lenses used to be ordered with fused upcurve segments of different refractive index,[1] whilst the modern ST bifocal has a straight-top, high refractive index segment encapsulated within the lens (Figure 24.3).[2] Optically, the two designs behave in a very similar fashion but the gas-permeable material of the ST bifocal gives a much better physiological performance during wear.

The anterior and posterior surfaces are smooth and the segment is monocentric, i.e. the optical centre of the segment is located at the segment top to give 'step-free' vision. Despite the use of prism for stabilization, the lens is thinner and lighter than the solid segment Tangent Streak version. Segment size and shape are fixed at 6 mm wide and 3 mm high but all other parameters are custom designed for the patient. The amount of prism can be varied from 1.25^Δ to 3.00^Δ and depends on the BVP. It is usually greater for more negative powers.

A fitting set is essential since trial lenses need to be truncated and have prism ballast to ensure accurate assessment. With min-

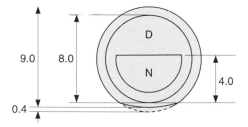

Figure 24.3 ST Bifocal lens drawn with measurements for ordering (D, distance portion; N, near portion)

imal astigmatism a lens is selected 0.05–0.15 mm flatter than 'K'. Over 1.00 DC, a steeper radius is used. The ideal fitting gives alignment or minimal apical touch with the truncation resting on the lower lid. Vertical movement should be about 1 mm with rapid recovery on blinking. There should be at least 2 mm between the top of the lens and the superior limbus in the primary position. On downwards gaze, the lens should be lifted by at least 2 mm and translate over the superior limbus.

The segment fluoresces and is easy to see with the Burton lamp. The segment top should be level with or slightly below the inferior pupillary margin in normal ambient lighting. With the slit lamp and a wide beam, the segment top should be 0.4–0.7 mm below the inferior pupillary margin. Excessive lens rotation can be controlled by changing the prism power and axis, or by altering the angle of the truncation.

Practical advice

- Additions below +1.50 D are not available.
- High-riding lenses can be improved by increasing the prism and centre thickness.
- Err on the high side for the segment top as this can subsequently be lowered by adjustment to the truncation.
- Increase the truncation if the segment is located too high.
- Avoid fitting patients with a very low lower lid as it may not be possible to control the lens position.

TYPICAL SPECIFICATION

7.80:8.00/9.40 × 9.00   –3.00   Add +2.00

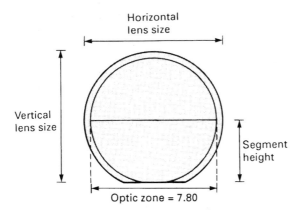

Figure 24.4 Design of Tangent Streak one-piece hard bifocal

Seg. height: 3.60 mm; 2.00$^\Delta$

ONE-PIECE HARD BIFOCAL (E.G. TANGENT STREAKS)

Consists of two wide segments meeting at a straight horizontal junction (Figure 24.4), similar to an executive-type spectacle bifocal.[3]

A trial set is necessary to assess movement of the lens and position of the segment line. A flat fitting is required so that the lens rides onto the lower lid between blinks. A low position is necessary to ensure sufficient clearance between the top of the lens and superior limbus for adequate translation, which is helped by truncation combined with 2$^\Delta$. The range of BOZRs is 7.42 mm (45.50 D) to 8.23 mm (41.00 D) and the initial lens is selected on the basis of Table 24.1.

The BOZD is a constant 7.80 mm, although there are two standard TDs of 9.90/9.40 mm and 9.40/9.00 mm. The position of the segment is observed with the ophthalmoscope or slit lamp. It is

Table 24.1 Tangent Streak

Corneal astigmatism (D)	Trial lens (BOZR)
0.00 D	'K' + 0.20 mm
0.50 D	'K' + 0.10 mm
>1.00 D	1/4 between flattest and steepest 'K'

ideally 1.50 mm below the centre of the pupil in distance gaze. In downward gaze, the lens should translate for the segment line to rise slightly above the pupil centre. If the lens is not pushed up by the bottom lid, then more prism or a flatter BOZR should be used. Where the lower lid is below the limbus, a lens should be used with larger TD, less truncation, and higher segment. Example:

HVID: 12.00 mm   Pupil size 4.00 mm   'K' 7.80 × 7.65
BOZR: 7.90 mm; TD 9.90/9.40; seg. height 5.20 mm

Practical advice

- Always use a trial set and take advantage of loan lenses where available.
- Use trial lenses as near as possible to the anticipated BVP because lenses of different power behave differently on the eye.
- Err on the flat side for the initial trial lens.
- The larger TD is used more frequently.
- If the fluorescein pattern is irregular and difficult to interpret, judge the fit according to movement and translation
- Lenses are supplied dry and require hydration for 24 hours before dispensing.

CONCENTRIC BIFOCALS (E.G. AVISION SYSTEM)

The Avision lens is a CD concentric construction with alternating design principles. The optic is monocentric, so rotation is not a problem and the average lens mass is less than with many other designs. Any material can be used.

Lens position is controlled by a range of anterior bevels (designated P or M, from 1 to 4) to ensure the correct degree of lid attachment. P lenses promote more and M lenses less lid grip. Prism ballast can also be incorporated if necessary to encourage a lower lens position. A diagnostic set is available with the eight different edge types and a diagnostic ring to demarcate the 4.00 mm distance portion. Trial lenses (with TD = 9.30 mm and AEL = 0.13 mm) allow assessment of centration, optic diameter and lens movement. The ideal lens has the size of the distance portion equal to that of the pupil diameter in ambient illumination.

The lens of first choice is selected on 'K' or 0.10 mm flatter than 'K' to give an alignment fitting with minimal mid-peripheral bearing and moderate edge clearance. The optimum edge type and fitting give a central position with 1 mm of rapid movement on blinking and a centre distance zone that provides full pupil coverage to avoid simultaneous vision effects. If the lens does not move by at least 2 mm to ensure translation for near vision, the TD should be reduced.

24.4.2 Simultaneous types

CONCENTRIC BIFOCALS

Concentric bifocals are especially suitable when good near vision is required above eye level, although some patients find the superimposed images difficult to ignore. The diameter of the distance portion is dependent on the pupil size and the lenses must be fitted to centre well with minimum movement. Back or front surface designs are possible (Figure 24.5), although the latter are more frequently fitted.[4]

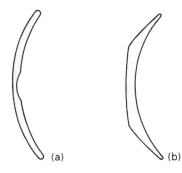

(a)   (b)

Figure 24.5 Concentric bifocals: (a) back surface design; (b) front surface design (from Phillips and Speedwell, *Contact Lenses*, 4th edn, Butterworth-Heinemann, Oxford, by permission)

Front surface

These are CD lenses made as lenticulars, with a central flatter curve giving a small optic area for distance surrounded by a steeper carrier, the radius of which is selected to give the correct power for near. The distance portion varies between 3.00 mm and 5.00 mm and should cover 50% of the pupil area. 4.00 mm is needed in 70% of cases. It is often useful to bias one eye for distance with a larger segment and the other for near with a smaller central area. A stable fit is achieved with large TDs between 9.60 mm and 9.90 mm, although some vertical movement is essential for satisfactory near vision. A low-riding lens works better than a high-riding one.

Typical specification

R and L: 7.80:7.50/8.40:8.60/10.50:9.80   –3.00   Add +2.00
Right seg. size 4.30 mm; Left seg. size 3.50 mm

Practical advice

The lenticular design means that it is possible to:
* Add negative power to the distance area.
* Add positive power to the near carrier.
* Increase to a small extent the size of the distance area.

Back surface

The de Carle lens is a CD design[5] with a very steep central back curve which relies on the partial neutralization effect of the tears. It has a typical radius of about 6.90 mm for an add of 12.50 D and a diameter between 2.00 mm and 4.00 mm. The surrounding annulus for near is used as a bearing surface (*see* Figure 24.5a and b).

'PROGRESSIONS' ASPHERIC MULTIFOCAL

Progressions is an aspheric varifocal rigid lens design which uses a variety of aspheric back surface geometries depending on corneal topography and spectacle prescription. The lens is designed on an individual basis to modify the spherical aberration of the combined optical system of lens, tears and cornea so as to provide a predictable varifocal effect. Although the lens can be prescribed using assumptions about the shape of the cornea, best results are obtained when the corneal topography has been measured by means of a videokeratoscope. The corneal data can be used in combination with the spectacle prescription to calculate an aspheric back surface geometry which will provide distance vision in the central zone with increasing positive power towards the edge of the optic zone. Some translation is necessary for the lens to function. Typically, the lens TD is 9.50 mm. The Progressions lens is more likely to be successful with low myopes and hyperopes than with high myopes needing large reading adds.

ASPHERIC (E.G. NISSEL AQUALINE MF200, CONTEX ASPHERIC LIFESTYLE)

The aspheric front surface is designed to produce a progressive power curve which increases from the centre outwards. The lens therefore gives centre distance with an intermediate to near addition of up to +2.00 D within the pupil area. Plus power is further enhanced in upwards or downwards gaze.

Control of spherical aberration within the power gradient gives a smooth transition from distance to near vision. Some designs (e.g. Contex) require a steep fitting to achieve the change in power gradient over the pupil area, whilst others (e.g. Nissel) can be fitted in alignment as a standard lens.

The design of the steep fittings depends on the front surface eccentricity which can range from 0.9 to 0.5. Lenses are fitted 1.25–3.50 D (0.2–0.7 mm) steeper than 'K' to give a range of additions from +1.25 D to +2.25 D. Lower eccentricities require lenses to be fitted steeper and vice versa. The TD ranges from 8.00 mm to 12.20 mm but the ideal diameter lies between 10.00 mm and 10.60 mm.

The reading addition cannot work effectively if the lens is fitted too steep or too flat. If a higher add is required, the non-dominant eye can be over-plussed by +0.50 D but care should be taken not to over-minus distance. For best near vision while reading, the patient should hold the chin up to use the intermediate zone.

The Lifestyle lens is fitted to the mid-periphery of the cornea rather than the centre. The base curve is therefore not critical and the second aspheric curve, the equivalent base curve (EQ), is aligned with the cornea to achieve the desired fit. No corneal positioning is required and although initially it was fitted as a high riding lens this is no longer necessary.

HARD GAS-PERMEABLE DIFFRACTIVE BIFOCALS (E.G. DIFFRAX)

These diffractive bifocals were designed with a circular phase plate incorporated into the lens optic so that light could be made to interfere constructively at two focal points and to interfere destructively at other points on the optic axis.[6] The design, which was pupil-independent, has been withdrawn from use with hard gas-permeable lenses.

24.5 Fitting soft bifocals

24.5.1 Alternating type

Alternating bifocals have not generally proved successful with soft lenses because of the difficulty of large lenses translating effectively. Lenses which have been produced consist of:

- Crescent segments stabilized by truncation and prism ballast.
- Concentric designs with a high minus edge to interact with the lower lid and translate.

24.5.2 Simultaneous types

CONCENTRIC BIFOCALS (SPHERICAL)

Both CD and CN designs have been available. CD designs, which are currently out of production, tended to be more beneficial for drivers, while CN are better for VDU operators. All designs are pupil-dependent, so a trial set is necessary for both fitting and power determination.

The optimum fitting should give minimal movement with good centration. The initial lens, however, should be the flattest choice that is reasonable because older, presbyopic eyes have a reduced volume of tears and less free lens movement over the conjunctiva.

The position of the central portion within the pupil area is more easily checked with either the retinoscope or ophthalmoscope than with the slit lamp. A decentred segment is unlikely to give good vision. It is often advantageous to use a different segment size in each eye, e.g. the smaller CN for the dominant distance eye and the larger CN as the reading lens.

Centre near (e.g. Simulvue)

- The diameters available for the CN portion are 2.35 mm and 2.55 mm.
- Different segment sizes should be used, choosing the smaller near diameter for the dominant eye. It may be necessary to fit very small or very large pupils respectively with the 2.35 mm or 2.55 mm segments in both eyes. Pupils that vary widely may encounter problems in extreme conditions of light or dark.
- The near add should be at least +0.50 D more than the spectacle reading addition, myopes requiring more plus for near than hyperopes.
- There is a choice of two base curves (8.70 mm and 9.00 mm); adequate but not excessive movement is required.
- The CN zone needs to cover only 50% of the pupil diameter and does not need to be exactly centred to achieve good results.

- Against-the-rule astigmatism may cause lateral decentration of the CN portion. Increasing the near zone diameter may well give better acuity.
- Monocular over-refraction should be carried out, but not using a phoropter.
- The distance over-refraction should be confirmed before checking the required reading add.

Typical specification

R. and L. 8.70:14.00 –3.00   Near add +2.50
Right segment 2.35 mm; Left segment 2.55 mm

Centre distance (e.g. Ciba Bisoft)

This CIBA Bisoft design had 'steep' and 'flat' fittings with TDs of 13.00 mm and 13.80 mm. Distance powers ranged from –10.00 D to +7.00, with adds from +1.50 D to +4.00 D, both in 0.25 D steps. The diameters of the central distance portion were either 3.2 mm or 3.8 mm.

Acuvue Bifocal

Unlike previous concentric and diffractive bifocals with a 'bulls-eye' construction, the Acuvue Bifocal is designed to provide the optimum correction needed under different lighting conditions. Using a series of concentric rings, the so-called 'pupil intelligent' lens gives different levels of near and distance correction depending on the size of the patient's pupil. The multiple ring configuration is intended to provide vision which is more specific to the available lighting conditions.

- The material is the same 58% Etafilcon A used for other Acuvue lenses.
- Power range is from +4.00 D to –6.00 D.
- There are four adds; +1.00 D, +1.50 D, +2.00 D and +2.50 D.

ASPHERIC BIFOCALS

Back surface aspheric (e.g. Occasions)

Progressive addition lenses of CD design with the periphery providing a near addition of up to +1.50 D. They are one-fit monthly disposables and are selected entirely on the basis of distance power. Optimum performance is achieved with good centration under conditions of average illumination and pupil size. Lenses work better for early presbyopes because of the limited reading add and can be made more successful with over-plussing in one eye or if fitted in combination with another lens type.

Front surface aspherics (e.g. Esstech PS, Unilens, Softline, PV2000/2500)

CN designs based on the overcorrection of spherical aberration. The power becomes relatively less positive towards the lens periphery. Distance vision is better with large pupils, whereas near is relatively unaffected by pupil size. Distance powers range from ±7.00 D and near powers of +1.00 D or +2.00 D are available depending on the manufacturer. Good centration is essential to give optimum vision. Where possible the lens of first choice is selected approximately 1.00 mm flatter than 'K'; some designs are one-fit. Lenses are essentially fitted for near vision and a full trial set is necessary to assess acuity using binocular refraction with lenses within 0.50 D of the anticipated result. Success is often increased by undercorrection in the dominant eye and over-plus in the other or by using lenses with different adds.

Example: Softline
Spectacle *Rx*:   +2.50/−1.50 × 90; near add +1.75
Best sphere: +1.75 plus +1.75 add = +3.50 combined power
Select trial lens: +1.50, add +2.00   = +3.50 combined power
   or: +1.25, add +2.00   = +3.25 combined power
   or: + 1.00, add +2.00   = + 3.00 combined power

Multi-aspherics (Variations, Polyvue)

CN simultaneous vision lenses offering a range of power profiles for near correction within a progressively corrected zone of spherical aberration. Variations is a front aspheric with three profiles equivalent to +1.25 D, +2.00 D and +2.75 D. The parameters are the same as those for the ES70.

Polyvue has a unique fitting factor which is the use of a white ring and black central dot on trial lenses to help easy assessment of centration. The near addition profiles are either LOW (up to +1.50 D) or HIGH (up to +3.00 D), with a choice of two base curves and central accommodation areas of either 1.50 mm or 1.90 mm.

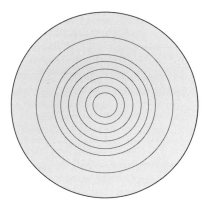

Figure 24.6 Diffractive soft bifocal (Echelon design)

DIFFRACTIVE BIFOCALS (E.G. ECHELON)

The optical principle is similar to that of the hard Diffrax bifocal and is based on Fresnel-type diffraction facets (Echelettes) less than 3 μm in depth (Figure 24.6). Chromatic aberration is reduced and there is virtually no pupil dependence. With distance vision, however, light scatter is observed around point sources and some patients have problems with sunlight and driving at night. At near, there is sometimes a ghosting or '3-D' effect.

The lens is a one-fit design in 38% HEMA. Distance powers range from +4.00 D to –6.00 D, with near adds of +1.50 D, +2.00 D and +2.50 D.

Typical specification

8.70:13.80   –3.00   Add +2.00

COMBINATIONS

A combination of one single vision lens and one bifocal, or two different designs of bifocal, increases the chance of success. The following combinations can be tried to give better distance vision to a dominant right eye:

Right eye	*Left eye*
Distance single vision	Centre near bifocal
Centre near bifocal (2.35)	Centre near bifocal (2.55)

General advice

- Have available a variety of soft bifocals in order to fit the majority of suitable patients.
- It is essential to use trial lenses to obtain any idea of potential success for any particular type of bifocal.
- Try different combinations of bifocals and single vision lenses according to eye dominance.
- Avoid fitting poor lens handlers because of the potential expense with breakages.
- Monovision has a higher success rate than bifocals.
- Do not fit patients with very small pupils of 3 mm or less. They are unable to use the area beyond the central power.

References

1. Stone, J. (1983) Fitting bifocal contact lenses. *Ophthalmic Optician*, **23**, 350–352
2. Ruston, D.M. and Meyler, J.G. (1995) How to fit alternating vision RGP bifocals, Part 2. The Fluoroperm ST bifocal contact lens. *Optometry Today*, Dec 4th, 34–40
3. Ruston, D.M. (1995) How to fit alternating vision RGP bifocals: the Tangent Streak bifocal – Part 1. *Optometry Today*, Oct 23rd, 24–30
4. de Carle, J.T. (1997) Bifocal and multifocal contact lenses. In *Contact Lenses*, 4th edn, A.J. Phillips and L. Speedwell (eds), Butterworth-Heinemann, Oxford, pp. 540–565
5. de Carle, J.T. (1959) The de Carle bifocal contact lens. *Contacto*, **3**, 5–9
6. Freeman, M.H. and Stone, J. (1987) A new diffractive bifocal contact lens. *Transactions of the British Contact Lens Association Annual Clinical Conference*, **4**, 15–22

Chapter 25

Special lens features and applications

25.1 Lens identification

25.1.1 Hard gas-permeable lenses

- A single dot engraved on the right lens is the British Standards recommendation.
- 'R' and 'L' engravings. Sometimes only the 'R' is used.
- Partial or complete lens specification is engraved by some manufacturers (e.g. CIBA Vision). This is intended for practitioner rather than patient information.
- Location of cylinder axis or prism base.
- Position of segment to assist bifocal fitting.
- Aphakics and hypermetropes, with poor unaided near vision, sometimes find it useful to have right and left lenses made in different tints. Usually the right is grey and left blue.
- A black dot is easier to see on high powered minus lenses than an engraving.

25.1.2 Soft lenses

Modern laser techniques have largely eliminated earlier problems with mechanical engravings which could either develop fractures or attract deposits. Information can also be imprinted onto the lens photographically and the same method has been used by the practitioner to mark 'R' and 'L'.

- 'R' and 'L' engravings.
- 'R' and 'L' photographic markings.
- A code, serial or lot number.
- Details of partial or complete lens specification.

- Location of cylinder axis or prism base.
- Position of segment to assist bifocal fitting.

25.2 Tinted, cosmetic and prosthetic lenses

Lenses are tinted for a variety of reasons:

- To reduce adaptive photophobia.
- To assist handling.
- To enhance or change the natural eye colour.
- To reduce photophobia in albinism and aphakia.
- For identification.
- To improve colour vision (*see* Section 25.2.4).

The potential disadvantages of tinted lenses are:

- Change in colour values.
- Difficulty with night vision, particularly driving.
- Possible toxicity of dyes.

Tinted lenses are sometimes referred to as *enhancer tints* where they accentuate rather than change the natural eye colour.

Cosmetic lenses, in this context, may be defined as those used to change the colour of the eyes, whereas prosthetic lenses are used to conceal unsightly scarring or abnormalities of the iris.

25.2.1 Hard gas-permeable lenses

Most modern lenses are available in a fairly restricted range of tints. Many materials are made only in pale blue and do not give the option of clear lenses. Grey (and sometimes brown) is usually possible. Green is not available in several widely used materials, and in addition the colour reproducibility tends to be unreliable. There is often poor consistency of colour between different batches of most tints and patients should be advised of the potential problem with replacement lenses.

Hand-painted cosmetic and prosthetic lenses are limited to stable, relatively low *Dk* materials such as XL20 (Nissel).

25.2.2 PMMA lenses

PMMA lenses, in contrast, have been available in a wide range of stable, consistently reproducible tints. The most common, standardly used colours are marked with an asterisk.

Grey		*Brown*	
911	very pale grey	2285-1*	light brown
912*	light grey (the most common)	2285-2	medium brown
512	medium grey/brown	2285	dark brown
999	dark grey		

Blue		*Green*	
1077-1*	light blue	2240-2*	light green
700	light/medium blue/violet	2240-3	medium green
1077-3	medium blue	600	bright green
1077-2	dark blue	2240-1	dark green

Other tints

Yellow	200
Amber	300
Red	2241-1, 400
Pink	2241-2
Lavender	2242-2
Violet	10910

Clinical quality (CQ) materials use inert carbon particles within the monomer to avoid any possible toxic effect of dyes in commercial grade PMMA:

Clear
Very light grey/brown   – 9042   (previously 911 CQ)
Light grey/brown   – 9043   (previously 912 CQ)

COSMETIC AND PROSTHETIC LENSES

Cosmetic and prosthetic corneal lenses are available with painted laminated inserts (e.g. Nissel). These are colour-matched from photographs or sets of sample iris buttons and are usually painted by hand with the appropriate clear or black pupil. Although they give excellent cosmetic results, there are several difficulties associated with the use of corrective lenses:

- They are necessarily thick with large total diameters (about 11.50 mm) to give good corneal coverage and appearance.
- Comfort is often poor, with limited wearing time.
- There is a high risk of corneal oedema.
- The artificial pupils often give visual disturbance on blinking.
- There is a tunnel vision effect, with restricted field of view.
- It is not possible to assess the fitting of opaque lenses with fluorescein.

Some of these problems are overcome with the use of scleral lenses (*see* Section 32.1).

General advice

- Order most hard gas-permeable lenses with a light tint to assist handling and reduce adaptive photophobia.
- Do not fit tinted soft lenses just for the sake of it. Unless a specific cosmetic effect is required or the lens type is made with a standard handling tint, the advantages may be outweighed by practical difficulties of colour matching, time delays, colour fading and the constraints of which solution systems can be used.
- Avoid tints where colour values are important (e.g. artists).
- Care is required with the choice of solutions for tinted and cosmetic soft lenses. Oxidizing systems, especially those based on chlorine, can cause colour fading or laminates to peel apart.
- It is difficult to persuade many patients, particularly emmetropes, that tinted and cosmetic lenses are more than just a fashion accessory. Careful explanation is necessary that they must be fitted with the same skill and accuracy as conventional lenses and that proper care and maintenance are essential to avoid the risk of infection.
- The effect of a tinted lens cannot be judged unless placed on the eye. The final result is a combination of lens tint, iris colour and ambient lighting.
- To enhance eye colour, do not use a tint that is too dark. The most pleasing cosmetic effect is usually achieved with a subtle colour change.
- Dark brown eyes are virtually unaffected by purely tinted lenses. Use opaque or dot matrix soft lenses to give a cosmetic colour change.
- Grey eyes respond well to blue and green tints.
- Light and medium brown eyes may sometimes respond to green tints.
- Brown eyes can sometimes be lightened with a yellow tint.
- Blue eyes may become brown with an orange tint.

25.2.3 Soft lenses

There is much less clinical need for tinted soft lenses because of the low incidence of adaptive photophobia. Numerous laboratories, however, offer a range of enhancer tints for mainly cosmetic reasons.[1] Opaque and semi-opaque lenses are also available for cosmetic and prosthetic fitting. The most common variations are shown in Figure 25.1:

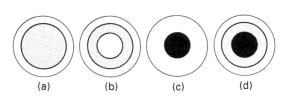

(a)   (b)   (c)   (d)

Figure 25.1 Variations possible with soft lens tints: (a) tinted iris with clear peripheral annulus; (b) tinted iris with clear peripheral annulus and clear pupil; (c) black (opaque) pupil on clear lens; (d) tinted iris with clear peripheral annulus and black (opaque) pupil

(a) Tinted iris with clear peripheral annulus. The iris diameter is usually standardized at 11.50 mm, with a clear periphery to give a natural appearance on the eye. Some laboratories (e.g. Hydron and Igel International) offer both a range of tints and colour densities. Very pale handling tints are also possible (e.g. Optima, Excelens, Durasoft 3 Lite Tint).

(b) Tinted iris with clear pupil and clear peripheral annulus. The clear pupil partially avoids problems with changed colour values and light reduction at night. The cosmetic appearance is not as satisfactory for many patients as a completely tinted iris

(c) Clear lens with black pupil. Used for occlusion or prosthetic reasons.

(d) Tinted iris with black pupil and clear peripheral annulus. Used for occlusion or prosthetic reasons.

Soft lenses are also produced with inhibitors, specifically to eliminate the ultraviolet part of the spectrum (e.g. Precision UV, Actifresh 400, Acuvue) and 'sun filters' (e.g. Lunelle).

OPAQUE PAINTED AND PRINTED LENSES

For cosmetic, prosthetic and theatrical purposes it is also possible to manufacture soft lenses with an opaque laminated backing or insert. This may be either painted or printed with clear or black pupils. Depending upon the laboratory, a limitless range of colours and cosmetic effects is possible, but the additional lens thickness of inserts can cause problems with comfort and oedema. Despite their greater stability on the eye compared with hard lenses, opaque corrective soft lenses with a clear pupil can also give visual disturbance on blinking and a reduced field of view.

Very large lenses with total diameter of up to 18.00 mm can be stabilized with prism ballast. By painting a decentred iris, they can be used cosmetically to correct squints.

DOT MATRIX LENSES

Another successful cosmetic approach is the manufacture of lenses with coloured dot matrix patterns (e.g. Wesley Jessen.PBH, Durasoft). These avoid most of the visual problems that occur with opaque lenses. A further refinement of design to overcome the restricted field of view is to have the patterns more widely spaced towards the pupil area.

25.2.4 Lenses to enhance colour vision

THE X-CHROM LENS

A specialized application of tinting is the monocular use of the dark red X-chrom lens. Its particular transmission characteristics are reported to enhance colour discrimination in patients with red-green deficiency.[2] Lenses are now available in soft lens form.

CHROMOGEN

The Chromogen system aims to achieve the same enhancement to colour vision and is available in a selection of tints as a soft lens.[3]

25.3 Fenestration

USES OF FENESTRATION

PMMA (and occasionally modern hard) lenses are ventilated to:

- Resolve corneal oedema.
- Improve comfort in hot, stuffy atmospheres.
- Lengthen wearing time.
- Reduce the risk of overwear syndrome (*see* Section 29.1).
- Improve tear flow beneath the lens.
- Reduce spectacle blur.
- Give faster adaptation.
- Improve frothing and dimpling.
- Prevent adhesion.

PROBLEMS WITH FENESTRATION

- Discomfort in some cases.
- Visual disturbance on blinking with about 20% of patients.

- Lenses are weakened mechanically with the risk of cracking.
- The holes can become blocked with secretions from the tears.

Practical advice

- Use single holes for lenses smaller than 9.00 mm; two or more for larger total diameters.
- The size is usually 0.25–0.4 mm, but can vary from 0.1 mm to as large as 1 mm.
- Position fenestrations 1–2 mm off-centre with a minus lens to reduce the risk of cracking and allow the holes to cover a greater area of the cornea as the lens rotates on blinking.
- Avoid placing a peripheral hole on a transitional bearing area.
- If there is some doubt as to how the patient will react to the fenestrations, modify one lens at a time.
- Err slightly on the small side, as the ventilation holes can subsequently be enlarged.
- Instruct the patient to maintain the patency of the holes with the careful use of a soft, boxwood cocktail stick.
- Despite the obvious, always instruct the laboratory 'countersunk and very well polished'.

25.4 Overseas prescriptions

Most soft lens specifications are international. Some differences may be found with hard gas-permeable lenses. Prescriptions from continental Europe may be written in the order of radius (R_o) power (D), diameter ($\emptyset$).

Example: 7.80 –3.00 9.40

US prescriptions often give the BOZR (base curve or BCR) derived from keratometry fitting in dioptres. This is converted to millimetres using $n = 1.3375$. Peripheral (intermediate or secondary) curves are usually followed by their width and the overall diameter (OAD) in millimetres. The final back peripheral curve is usually called a *bevel*. A convex, front peripheral curve to reduce the edge thickness of minus lenses is sometimes called a *CN bevel*.

Example:

BCR	45.00 D	OZ 7.80 mm	OAD 9.60 mm
SCR	39.25 D	(0.6 mm)
Bevel	32.12 D	(0.3 mm)

is equivalent to 7.50:7.80/8.60:9.00/10.50:9.60

25.5 Contact lenses and sport

25.5.1 Advantages and disadvantages

Contact lenses offer considerable advantages over spectacles for sport.

ADVANTAGES

- Larger field of view.
- Unaffected by bad weather.
- With contact sports, both player and opponents are safer with no spectacle frame.

DISADVANTAGES

Disadvantages relate mainly to hard lenses:

- Loss or displacement.
- Increased photophobia.
- Foreign bodies.

Because of these potential disadvantages, the governing bodies of certain sports may disallow the use of some types of contact lens (e.g. rally driving, horse racing).

25.5.2 Lens types

SOFT LENSES

Stability is the prime consideration with sport. The lens must give virtually no risk of loss from the eye, even with contact sports; must avoid the intrusion of foreign bodies; and must give consistent vision despite rapid eye movements. Soft lenses are therefore the first choice in most cases. For serious sporting use where optimum acuity is required (e.g. cricket), toric soft lenses are often preferable to hard, even to correct quite small degrees of astigmatism. The main disadvantage is lens dehydration (*see* Section 17.3). Hard gas-permeable lenses.

For less serious sport, hard lens wearers may well find that they can continue with existing lenses. Lenses can also be fitted deliberately larger and tighter than PMMA. They are specifically indicated where optimum acuity is required (e.g. pistol shooting), and in the case of flying the authorities may insist on their use to the exclusion of soft lenses.

SCLERAL LENSES

Scleral lenses (see Chapter 15) give maximum stability of vision with no risk of loss. Their disadvantages are difficulty of fitting and limited wearing time. They are therefore used only rarely, but have occasional application for aquatic sports such as water polo or canoeing where the head may be underwater for a relatively long period.

25.5.3 Specific applications

SWIMMING[4]

Contact lenses, on balance, are not recommended for swimming unless well-fitted goggles are worn. Hard lenses, unless large and tight with a small palpebral aperture, are usually contraindicated because of the high risk of loss. Soft lenses, if used carefully, have been worn fairly successfully. Some patients are very sensitive to chlorine absorbed by the lenses and may show conjunctival injection for several hours after exposure. This can even occur when lenses have been removed during swimming, but replaced before the chlorine has been eliminated from the eyes.

Another factor is the saline concentration of sea water, since soft lenses fit more loosely in hypertonic solution. This could be used to advantage by rinsing lenses with hypotonic solution to tighten the fitting prior to swimming.

Practical advice

It should also be remembered that swimming pools are a frequent source of ocular infection, and micro-organisms such as *Acanthamoeba* may be unaffected by chlorine disinfection.

DIVING

Good results have been obtained with various water content soft lenses when used for scuba diving, with little risk of displacement. Air bubbles tend to form beneath lenses at depths of about 150 ft (45 m), but less with soft than with hard lenses, which are generally contraindicated for this reason.[5]
    Water replacing air in front of the cornea reduces its refracting power by about 40.00 D. Scleral lenses have therefore been designed either with a flat-fronted air cell or with a high index glass anterior surface.[6]

SKIING

Most forms of contact lens prove very successful for skiing. It is essential to use either goggles or large sunglasses to give protection from wind and cold and prevent soft lens dehydration.

CLIMBING AT HIGH ALTITUDE

High Dk hard or high water content soft lenses should be used because of the reduced level of oxygen in the atmosphere at high altitude.[7] Extended wear may well be preferred to avoid cold weather difficulties with both handling and solutions.

SHOOTING

Competition shooting usually requires the precision and stability of hard lens acuity. The binocular balance is important. Depending upon the type of weapon, it is sometimes necessary either to fog the alternate eye or undercorrect the fixating eye to assist focusing on the front sight.

References

1. Davies, I. and Davies, G. (1994) Tinted soft contact lenses – a review. *Optician*, **208** (5476), 18–28
2. Zeltzer, H. (1982) *X Chrome Manual*, 2nd edn, The X-Chrom Corp., Waltham, USA
3. Harris, D. (1997) A study of CL fittings with colour-enhancing lenses. *Optician*, **213** (5604), 38–41
4. Hill, R.M. (1985) The swimming eye. *International Contact Lens Clinic*, **12**, 175–179
5. Molinari, J. and Socks, J. (1987) Effect of hyperbaric conditions on corneal physiology with hydrogel lenses. *Journal of the British Contact Lens Association.* (Scientific Meetings 1987). p. 17

6. Douthwaite, W.A. (1995) *Contact Lens Optics and Lens Design*, 2nd edn, Butterworth-Heinemann, Oxford
7. Clarke, C. (1976) Contact lenses at high altitude. *British Journal of Ophthalmology*, **60**, 470–480

Chapter 26

Care systems

26.1 Components of solutions

All contact lens solutions are produced according to general principles of formulation and good manufacturing practice.

BUFFERS

Buffers (e.g. sodium phosphate, borate or tromethamine) are included where there is a need to keep the pH within the narrow limits necessary for contact lens wear (pH 6–8). The Antimicrobial Buffer System (ABS) patented by CIBA Vision combines three borate buffers (boric acid, sodium borate and sodium perborate) in bottled saline. These constituents yield 0.006% hydrogen peroxide which acts as an antimicrobial agent.[1] Other unpreserved salines are buffered with borate or bicarbonate; phosphate is used in only a minority of preparations.

PRESERVATIVES

Preservatives restrict the growth of micro-organisms and maintain the sterility of the solution remaining in the bottle and in the contact lens case. Typical examples are given below.

Benzalkonium chloride (BAK)

Frequently used with PMMA lenses. It destabilizes the tear film in concentrations over 0.004%, so wetting solutions or rewetting drops do not exceed this concentration. The majority of soaking and cleaning solutions can use 0.004–0.01% because they do not come into contact with the eye. Its use with modern hard lenses has been questioned because of surface adsorption.[2]

Chlorhexidine digluconate (CHX)

Usually included with other preservative systems in a concentration of 0.006% for hard lens solutions. If it is used alone, the kill

Warning!

Benzalkonium chloride is never used with soft lenses because of its toxicity to the cornea in large or sustained doses.

time is slow and lenses must be stored for a minimum of 10 hours. Soft lens solutions employ a reduced concentration of 0.002–0.005%.

Thiomersal

A mercurial derivative used in concentrations of 0.001–0.002% with both hard and soft lens solutions, more often found with the latter. Thiomersal is effective against fungi, but toxic reactions are fairly common. It is slow acting as a preservative and so is usually incorporated with chlorhexidine or EDTA.

Dymed

Dymed is the proprietary name for polyhexanide (polyamino-propyl biguanide or polyhexamethylene biguanide).[3] It is one of the new generation of high molecular weight preservatives used in multifunction soft lens solutions that come under the umbrella title of *polyquats*. Dymed is found in concentrations of 0.00005–0.0001%. All polyquats bind to negatively charged phospholipids found in the bacterial plasma membrane. Their action results in cellular lysis rather than disrupting bacterial cell walls like other antimicrobials (e.g. ReNu, ReNu MultiPlus, Complete).

Polyquad

Polyquad (polyquaternium 1) is a new generation polyquat used as a high molecular weight preservative. The molecular weight is 14 times that of chlorhexidine, nearly 4 times that of Dymed and comes in a concentration of 0.001% (e.g. Opti-Free, Opti-1).

Water-soluble cationics

Water-soluble cationics such as polyxetonium chloride 0.006% have low toxicity and are used in hard lens solutions (e.g. Total Care).

Phenylmercuric nitrate and chlorbutol

Phenylmercuric nitrate is found in some multipurpose hard lens solutions in a concentration of 0.004%. Chlorbutol binds to CAB and is now uncommon due to its volatile nature. Used in concentrations of 0.4% (e.g. Sterisoak, Liquifilm Tears).

Quaternary ammonias

Used in soft lens soaking solutions in concentrations of 0.013–0.03%.

Sorbic acid

Used in surfactant cleaners with a concentration of 0.1% (e.g. Pliagel).

TONICITY AGENTS (invariably SODIUM CHLORIDE)

To adjust the salt concentration and ensure compatibility with the tears.

VISCOSITY AGENTS (E.G. HYDROXY ETHYL CELLULOSE)

To improve the wetting time and comfort of the solution.

WETTING AGENTS (E.G. POLYVINYL ALCOHOL, POLYSORBATE 80)

To help the solution spread across the lens surface. Also found in soft lens disinfection solutions (e.g. polyvinyl pyrrolidone).

CHELATING AGENTS (E.G. ETHYLENEDIAMINE TETRAACETIC ACID (EDTA) KNOWN AS SODIUM EDETATE)

Found in concentrations of 0.01–0.2%. Used to enhance the action of preservatives, especially benzalkonium chloride with which it has a synergistic action. The main exceptions are mercurial derivatives.

SURFACTANTS (E.G. POLOXAMINE, MIRANOL)

The most common surfactants used in multipurpose soft lens solutions for their cleaning action are poloxamine and tyloxapol. These are supplemented in recent products with non-ionic surfactants, e.g. Lubricare (Quattro) and protein removal agents, e.g.

Hydranate (Renu Multi Plus). Those solutions not containing a surfactant (e.g. Opti-Free) do require a supplementary cleaner. Other cleaners or hard lens multifunction solutions contain miranol (e.g. Total Care) and phospholipid (e.g. Boston Elite).

26.2 Solutions for hard gas-permeable lenses

The surface of a hard gas-permeable lens is more prone to deposits and interaction with some formulations compared to the more inert PMMA.[4]

26.2.1 Wetting solutions

Wetting solutions are used on insertion to act as a cushion between the lens and cornea. They also enhance the spread of tears across the lens surface, although the effect only lasts for a maximum of 15 minutes and sometimes for as little as 5 seconds.[5]

Formulation: tonicity agent; viscosity agent; wetting agent; preservatives; chelating agent.

26.2.2 Soaking solutions

Soaking solutions keep lenses hydrated during overnight storage in a sterile, bacteriocidal environment. They facilitate good surface wetting and assist the removal of deposits. Hydration is important to maintain the correct BOZR both for modern hard lens materials[6] and for PMMA over about –10.00 D.[7]

Formulation: tonicity agent; wetting agent; detergent; preservatives; chelating agent.

26.2.3 Cleaning solutions

Cleaning solutions remove surface debris including lipids and mucus (e.g. LC65) and enhance the disinfecting action of the soaking solution. With the advent of fluorosilicon acrylates, greasing of the lens surface has become a more frequent problem. Manufacturers have therefore developed alcohol-based solutions (e.g. Boston Advance, Bausch & Lomb Elite, Miraflow) or cleaners with emollient and foam stabilizers (e.g. Total Care). The inclusion of microscopic polymeric beads in suspension gives a light surface polishing effect useful for removing denatured proteins (e.g. Boston, Bausch & Lomb).

Formulation: detergent; preservatives; chelating agent.

Practical advice

- Advise patients to take care not to cause an inadvertent power change with the polishing action.
- Take care with cleaners containing only an organic solvent (e.g. isopropyl alcohol) to avoid upsetting the surface wetting properties of some hard lens materials, especially fluoropolymers.[6]

26.2.4 Multipurpose solutions

These combine all of the above functions, but usually with some loss of efficiency:

- Wetting, soaking and cleaning (e.g. Total)
- Soaking and cleaning (e.g. Clean-N-Soak).
- Wetting and soaking (e.g. Bausch & Lomb, Total Care).

Formulation: wetting agent; detergent; preservatives; chelating agent

26.2.5 Rewetting solutions (comfort drops)

Comfort drops are used to rewet lenses while they are worn, especially in dry environments (e.g. Clerz).
Formulation: wetting agent; preservatives; chelating agent. Some are now produced without preservative (e.g. Revive).

26.2.6 Enzyme tablets

Proteinaceous films require enzyme removal with some hard lens materials, particularly silicon acrylates.
Formulation: (see Section 26.4.4).

Practical advice

- Depending upon the active ingredient, patients find it much more convenient to leave lenses soaking overnight.
- Enzymes may not be required with fluoropolymers and rarely with CAB.
- Advise hay fever sufferers to use them more frequently in the spring and early summer.

26.3 Solutions for soft lenses

The general principles for soft lens solutions are similar to those for hard lens solutions, but there are potentially more difficulties because of the possibility of interaction with the material. Viscosity agents are not generally employed and the pattern of use is often different, since many solutions must be partnered to ensure their complete antimicrobial efficacy.

26.4 Disinfection

Disinfection may be by means of either *chemicals* (cold) or *heat*.

26.4.1 Chemical disinfection

Cold disinfection uses either preserved chemicals or unpreserved oxidative systems.

PRESERVED SOAKING SOLUTIONS

Used for overnight storage (e.g. Prymesoak, Sterisal 2, Optifree).
   Formulation: tonicity agent; wetting agent; preservative; buffer; detergent.

MULTIPURPOSE SOLUTIONS

Combine disinfection and cleaning. Ideal for disposable lenses (e.g. Renu Multi Plus, Quattro, Optil, Solocare).
   Formulation: high molecular weight preservative; surfactant; chelating agent; buffer.

SALINE

A solution of 0.9% saline is referred to as *isotonic*, having an overall sodium chloride concentration equivalent to that of human tears. A solution with higher salt concentration is *hypertonic* and one with a lower concentration *hypotonic*.
   Normal (0.9%) saline may be either buffered or unbuffered and is available in the following formats:

* Preserved in multi-dose bottles (e.g. CIBA Vision).
* Unpreserved in unit dose form (e.g. Amidose).

- Unpreserved in aerosol form (e.g. Solusal, Lens Plus).
- Drip-feed bags with one-way valve (not obtainable in the UK except in some hospital departments).

N.B. Home-made saline, using purified water, ceased in the UK in 1988 with the withdrawal of salt tablets. *Acanthamoeba* infection in the USA has been linked to home-made saline.[8]

TAP WATER

In the past, the OptimEyes tablet, containing 0.004% chlorhexidine, was dissolved in *rising mains water* to create a simple and inexpensive disinfection solution. This system is no longer available.

Tap water must not be used for soft lens storage and insertion, or for cleaning the lens case, because of:

- Serious risk of microbial contamination (e.g. *Acanthamoeba*).
- Trace metals and salts.
- Lens adhesion as a result of hypotonicity.

Rising mains water can be used to flush hard gas-permeable lenses after cleaning and prior to overnight storage in a disinfecting solution. Boiled water or saline is safer for cleaning the lens case, which should then be air dried.

OXIDATIVE SYSTEMS

Oxidative systems are generally unpreserved and use hydrogen peroxide or chlorine-based compounds as the disinfecting agent.

Hydrogen peroxide (H_2O_2)

Most peroxide systems use a 3% concentration. They include a sodium or phosphate stabilizer to prevent the rapid decompensation of the otherwise unstable H_2O_2.[3]

A tablet of enzyme cleaner can be included with the peroxide solution (e.g. Ultrazyme).

Advantages of hydrogen peroxide

- No reaction to preservatives.
- Efficient method of disinfecting.
- Enhances cleaning.
- An enzyme cleaner can sometimes be avoided.

- Prolongs lens life.
- Less risk of red eye reaction with extended wear.

Disadvantages of hydrogen peroxide

- The peroxide must be neutralized.
- The neutralizing time is sometimes lengthy.
- Complicated to use and understand.
- High water content materials may deteriorate with prolonged storage in peroxide.
- Occasional allergies.
- The peroxide may lose its efficacy if kept too long (e.g. extended wear).
- Bulky for travel.
- Expensive.
- Possibility of patient error.

Three types of neutralization are available:

1. *Catalytic.* (a) Using catalase, a naturally occurring bovine catalyst which is highly specific for the speedy decomposition of hydrogen peroxide, either in solution (e.g. Oxysept) or with a time release tablet coated in hydroxypropylmethylcellulose (e.g. OxySept One Step). (b) Using a platinum coated disc (e.g. AOsept, EasySept), this is much slower than catalase because the molecules have to migrate through the buffered saline to the disc surface instead of being evenly distributed throughout the solution. The disc needs replacing every 3 months (sooner with some patients). If the neutralizing solution is buffered to a high pH (e.g. AOSept), the kill time is slower. The neutralization does not depend on the concentration of the catalyst and no byproducts are formed except water and oxygen.
2. *Reactive.* Chemicals such as sodium pyruvate (e.g. 10:10, MiraSept) or sodium thiosulphate (Perform) initiate an oxidation–reduction reaction which causes the hydrogen peroxide to decompose. The speed and degree of neutralization depend upon concentration and temperature. By products are formed such as sodium acetate, carbon dioxide and water (10:10); or sodium tetrathionate and sodium hydroxide (Perform).
   A further method uses a 22 mg sodium perborate tablet (e.g. FreeSept) which produces 0.1% hydrogen peroxide when dissolved in unpreserved saline. A soaking time of 6 hours is

needed for effective disinfection and it is necessary to give lenses a saline rinse in the case before insertion.

3. *Dilution.* By rinsing and soaking in saline (e.g. the now discontinued Quik-Sept).

Chlorine systems

Chlorine-based systems contain active ingredients such as sodium dichloroisocyanurate (e.g. Softab) or *para*-dichlorosulphamoyl benzoic acid (e.g. Aerotab).

Advantages of chlorine

* One-step systems which help compliance.
* Neutralization unnecessary.
* Unpreserved saline is the only solution used, either to dissolve the tablet or rinse the lens before use.
* Less irritation with patient error.
* Easy to understand.
* Minimum bulk and good for travel.
* Less expensive than peroxide
* Useful for disinfecting trial lenses.

Disadvantages of chlorine

* Residual traces of the disinfecting agent may be present on lens insertion.
* Slow kill time so overnight disinfection required.
* An effective surfactant cleaner is essential.
* May be confused with enzyme tablets.
* Patient may forget to add the tablet.
* Lenses have shorter life span than with H_2O_2
* Ineffective against *Acanthamoeba*, protozoa and some fungi.
* Tinted soft lenses may fade.

26.4.2 Heat disinfection

Heat disinfection is generally carried out using unpreserved normal saline at a pasteurization temperature of 70–80°C. The addition of sodium edetate gives calcium-removing properties. Lenses must always be allowed to cool before insertion.

ADVANTAGES OF HEAT DISINFECTION

- Easy to use.
- Economical.
- Efficient at killing micro-organisms.
- Suitable for some disposable lenses.

DISADVANTAGES OF HEAT DISINFECTION

- Difficult for travel.
- Denatures protein onto the lens surface.
- Accelerates lens ageing.
- Routine surfactant and enzyme cleaning essential.

METHODS

- Heating unit, preferably thermostatic and time-controlled.
- Vacuum flask or saucepan. The lens case is placed in boiling water for 10 minutes, after which the lenses are allowed to cool.

MICROWAVE

Non-pressurized microwave disinfection can be carried out with the Micro Clens system. This uses a saline solution which, following microwave action and cooling, is formulated to reduce to isotonicity for immediate lens insertion. The system consists of the disinfector unit containing Micro Clens saline into which the contact lens case, filled with the same solution, is placed. The unit is microwaved for 1–2 minutes and a visible change in the solution levels of the unit and case confirms that the microwave system has operated successfully. As with all moist matter, disinfection is achieved by microwave irradiation producing high-frequency oscillations within the molecules. These oscillations rapidly raise the temperature and can destroy vegetative micro-organisms within 2 minutes. Turbulence of the irradiated solution also cleans the lens surface by the emulsification of lipids.[9]

Practical advice

- Patients must not use 0.9% saline instead of Micro Clens solution, or the final pH will be incorrect.
- Lens vials with metal caps cannot be used in a microwave.

26.4.3 Cleaning solutions

Formulation: surface-active agents; preservatives.
In addition to cleaners specifically formulated for soft lenses
(e.g. Pliagel), hard lens cleaners which do not contain benzalkonium chloride can be used (e.g. LC65). Alcohol-based cleaners are
effective against lipids (e.g. Miraflow). For denatured protein, a
surfactant-polymeric bead cleaner (e.g. Opti-Clean) combines a
cleaning agent with microscopic, polystyrene-like beads.[10]
Daily surface cleaning is important to:

* Remove lipids, inorganic deposits, some proteins and insolu-
ble contaminants by manual action.
* Overcome the hydrophobicity of oily deposits with surface-
active agents.
* Assist chemical disinfection by removing deposits that could
interfere with antibacterial activity.
* Remove contaminants that supply nutrients to bacteria.

OTHER CLEANING METHODS

* Ultrasonic units.
ı Ultraviolet units.
* Spinning devices.

26.4.4 Periodic cleaners

ENZYME TABLETS

Enzyme tablets are used for the removal of protein from the lens
surface. Weekly cleaning is suggested, but patients on peroxide
are able to use them less frequently. Tablets are dissolved in
either saline or distilled water.

Practical advice

* Where papain causes an adverse reaction, especially with high
water content lenses, reduce the soaking time to 15 minutes.
* Hydrogen peroxide breaks down residual papain and should be
used after the enzyme cleaner.
* Advise hay fever sufferers to use them more frequently in the
spring and early summer

Formulation: papain (Hydrocare or Bausch & Lomb); subtilisin A (Ultrazyme); pancreatin (Clenzyme); lipase, pronase, protease, sodium edetate (Amiclair).

26.4.5 Professional cleaners

Strong oxidizing agents (e.g. sodium perborate) have been used by the practitioner for intensive cleaning and rejuvenation. Their action is enhanced by means of tonicity changes and should not be used more than once on a lens because of dimensional changes. High water content lenses are more susceptible and should be treated at a lower temperature for a shorter period of time (*see* Section 4.4.1).

Practical advice

A very small number of patients can give an extreme sensitivity reaction to professional cleaners, however thoroughly lenses are rinsed and boiled out in saline after use.

References

1. Franklin, V. and Tighe, B. (1995) Disclosure – the true story of multi-purpose solutions. *Optician,* **209** (5500), 25–28
2. Hoffman, W.C. (1987) Ending the BAK–RGP controversy. *Optican,* **193** (5095), 31–32
3. Christie, C.L. and Meyler, J.G. (1997) Contemporary contact lens care products. *Contact Lens and Anterior Eye,* **20** (Suppl), S11–S17
4. Walker, J. (1997) New developments in RGP lens care. *Optician,* **213** (5583), 16–19
5. Doane, M.G. (1988) In vivo measurement of contact lens wetting. *Transactions of the British Contact Lens Association Annual Clinical Conference,* **5**, 110–111
6. Lowther, G.E. (1987) Effect of some solutions on HGP contact lens parameters. *Journal of American Optometric Association,* **58**, 188–192
7. Phillips, A.J. (1969) Alterations in curvature of the finished corneal lens. *Ophthalmic Optician,* **9**, 980–1110
8. Stehr-Green, J. (1989) The epidemiology of Acanthamoeba keratitis in the United States. *American Journal of Ophthalmology,* **107**, 331
9. Hirji, N.K. (1997) A new device for disinfecting hydrogel contact lenses. *Optician,* **214** (5617), 38–39
10. Fowler, S.A. and Allansmith, M.R. (1984) Removal of soft lens deposits with surfactant – polymeric bead cleaner. *Contact Lens Association of Ophthalmologists Journal,* **10**, 229–231

Chapter 27

Lens collection and patient instruction

27.1 Lens collection

INSERTION OF LENSES

The lenses are inserted after verification and given time to settle before assessing acuities and fitting. An existing wearer needs only a few minutes, whereas a new patient requires 10–20 minutes depending upon lens type.

ASSESSMENT OF VISION

The visual assessment should confirm that acuities are the same as or better than those achieved during initial fitting.

ASSESSMENT OF FITTING

This should confirm:

- That the fitting appears as originally intended.
- The lenses have been accurately made. Apart from the main parameters, the practitioner should consider other factors such as blending, lenticulation, thickness and edge shape.
- The fitting appears satisfactory, even if the previous two criteria are met.
- Whether any discomfort is normal or excessive.

27.2 Insertion and removal

Patients often need to realize that handling is a hurdle to overcome, but has little to do with comfort, vision or eventual wearing time. Insertion should always be done over a flat surface or closed sink, while removal can be into the cupped hand for hard lenses. Patients should be taught initially with a mirror, but it is ultimately better for them to manage without. Soft and hard lens insertion follow the same pattern, but removal is different.

27.2.1 Hard lenses

INSERTION

The lens is cleaned, rinsed and wetted. The lids are held firmly apart while the patient looks at the reflection of the eye in a mirror. The head may be either vertical or horizontal and the lens is placed onto the cornea with the first or second finger of the dominant hand.

Practical advice

- The alternate eye must be kept open to prevent Bell's phenomenon.
- The lids should be held from underneath the base of the lashes to prevent reflex blinking.
- Reassure the patient that the lens does no harm on the sclera and cannot get lost 'behind the eye'.
- Show the patient how to recentre the lens with indirect finger pressure on the lid margins or by massaging through the closed lids.

REMOVAL

The eye must be held open wide enough for the taut lids to eject the lens from behind by means of blinking and:

- One finger pulling slightly upwards from the outer canthus.
- Two fingers from the same hand pulling from the lid margins.
- Two fingers, one from each hand, pulling with a sideways scissors motion.
- Two fingers, one from each hand, positioned vertically and pushing the lid margins against the globe of the eye and towards each other. This method, although more difficult to learn, is more consistently reliable.
- Holding the lids firmly and turning the eye nasally.

If all of these methods fail, a moistened suction holder can be applied perpendicular to the centre of the lens.

Practical advice

The patient should not be allowed to leave before being competent at lens removal (insertion can be safely practised at home).

27.2.2 Soft lenses

INSERTION

The general principles are the same as for hard lenses. The key difference is that as lenses are self-centring patients need not be concerned if they are inserted out of position. Where near fixation is uncontrollable, especially with hypermetropes, lenses can be inserted onto the inferior sclera while looking upwards at a distant fixation target.

Practical advice

- To stop lens ejection at the moment of insertion because of an air bubble, advise the patient to take both hands away and look down slowly. The eyes should be gently closed and the lids squeezed together to remove the bubble.
- A dry finger helps stop the lens reversing.
- Allow ultrathin lenses to dry on the finger for about 20 seconds to help insertion.
- With ultrathins, it may be necessary to pull the upper lid over the lens to prevent the lens rolling out of the eye on lid closure.
- If the lens is uncomfortable on insertion, it should be slid onto the temporal sclera and allowed to recentre. This usually dislodges a foreign body, make-up or very small air bubble; the lens should be removed, rinsed and reinserted if discomfort persists.

REMOVAL

Hard lens pulling methods do not generally work with soft lenses. They are removed by:

- Sliding onto the temporal or inferior sclera and pinching out.
- Pinching directly off the cornea (this is a less satisfactory method because of the risk of scratching the cornea).
- Squeezing at the edge of the lens with the upper and lower lid margins to create an air bubble and eject the lens.

27.3 Suggested wearing schedules

The aim is to achieve a wearing time with hard gas-permeable lenses of 8–10 hours by the time of the first aftercare check-up at about 2 weeks. This interval may be longer with soft lenses, although all-day wear is often achieved more rapidly. The recommended schedule can be recorded as the starting time, increment and maximum.

Examples:
Hard gas-permeable lenses: 3 + 1   →   8 h
Previous failure: 1 + 1/2   →   8 h
PMMA: 2 + 1/2   →   8 h
Low water content soft: 3 + 1   →   12 h
High water content soft: 4 + 2   →   all day
Refits of hard with soft: 6 + 2   →   all day

All-day wear is then achieved with hourly build-up if there are no contraindications at the first aftercare visit.

Practical advice

- The wearing schedules must be easy to understand and to follow.
- Advise the patient that, to avoid the risk of over-wear, the wearing schedule is a maximum and not a target.
- The total wearing time can be divided into two periods at different times of day, usually separated by a 4-hour gap.
- Lenses should be removed and advice sought in the event of persistent discomfort, redness or other unusual symptoms.

27.4 General patient advice

New patients should not be allowed to wear lenses home because of the risk of early loss or damage. Before leaving, they should be given further clear instructions both verbally and in writing to cover the following points.

- Lens identification.
- Wearing schedule.
- That lens comfort should be no worse than that already experienced on a tolerance trial and that the eyes should not become unduly red or sore.
- To bring to the first aftercare examination both their lens case and their spectacles.
- That unless there is a serious problem with comfort or vision they should come to the aftercare visit having worn lenses for as long as possible that particular day.
- The lens case, containing solution, should be carried at all times.
- To handle lenses in a well-lit area with spectacles nearby.
- To follow a routine, always dealing with the same lens first and to handle only one lens at a time to avoid mixing them up.

- Method of lens storage (hard) or disinfection (soft).
- Not to change the brand or type of solution without first consulting the practitioner.
- Names of solutions equivalent to the original recommendations.
- Some solutions are sold overseas with the same brand name but have a different formulation.
- The distinction between cleaning and disinfection.
- Lenses should be cleaned daily, immediately after removal from the eye.
- Never to use hard lens solutions with soft lenses and *vice versa*.
- That soft lenses are very fragile if they dry out but are not necessarily spoiled since they recover after rehydration.
- To avoid placing two soft lenses in the same compartment of the case since they may stick together and prove impossible to separate.

- The lens case should be changed at regular intervals.

- Sudden acute discomfort is probably caused by foreign bodies.
- Spectacle blur should not be experienced (except with PMMA).
- Difficulty with near vision may be noticed during the first few days.
- Some degree of adaptive photophobia is normal.
- Extreme environments in terms of temperature or humidity may affect both comfort and vision.
- Anything that makes the eyes feel dry may make the lenses temporarily uncomfortable. Factors include: air conditioning, central heating; using VDU screens; and some drugs (e.g. antihistamines, HRT and alcohol).
- Falling asleep with the lenses in or entering extreme environments may give temporary lens adhesion, which may be released by the application of normal saline and gentle lid pressure.

PRECAUTIONS

- What to do and where to go in case of an emergency.
- Soft lenses should not be worn while eye drops or ointment are used for any reason (wait 1 hour for drops and 4 hours for ointment).
- Hard lenses could be worn with drops but not with ointment.
- Environments containing fumes, chemicals or sprays should be avoided.
- Traces of noxious chemicals must be very carefully removed from the hands before touching the lenses.
- If soft lenses have been left in their case without being worn for more than a few days, they should be disinfected again before use.
- Not to lick lenses prior to insertion.
- Not to use detergents like washing-up liquid with hard gas-permeable lenses because they may damage the surface.
- To use goggles or photochromatic glasses for activities such as

cycling or skiing to protect the eyes from wind, dust and dehydration.

- To take care with driving because of altered spatial judgement, and flare at night.
- When travelling or sunbathing, to be careful not to fall asleep with lenses in unless they are for extended wear.
- To avoid wearing lenses where possible on long flights because of the dry atmosphere on aircraft and the possibility of eye infection.
- Swimming is unwise with hard lenses because of the risk of loss. Soft lenses are often better but may still be lost; they might also cause stinging and red eyes if chlorine is absorbed into the material. There is also the risk of infection if lenses are not subsequently cleaned and disinfected. Overall, it is better to use a well-fitted pair of prescription swimming goggles.

Chapter 28

Aftercare

28.1 First aftercare visit

The first aftercare examination should ideally take place after 2–3 weeks. If good progress has not been made by this time, success with the initial lenses is unlikely and significant changes may well need to be made. If the timing is too soon, nearly all patients complain of a multitude of genuinely adaptive symptoms; if too long after fitting, disturbing signs may have arisen or patients may have discontinued because of problems which are not adaptive.

The timing of aftercare appointments is important. Daily wear patients should be examined during the afternoon following several hours of contact lens use, whereas extended wear patients should be seen in the morning so that any overnight effects can be observed.

The results of this and subsequent visits should be recorded according to one of the grading scales outlined in Section 3.3.

28.1.1 Initial discussion

Initial discussion should cover the following points which may require further assessment during the course of the examination:

- What progress the patient feels has been made.
- Are there any particular problems?
- Has the patient come in wearing the lenses – if not, why not?
- Maximum wearing time.
- Wearing time on the day of examination.
- Is handling satisfactory?
- Have all instructions been understood?
- Are instructions being followed?

- Are solutions being used correctly?
- Is the wearing schedule being followed?
- Are lenses being worn in the correct eye?
- Are soft lenses inside out?
- Is the patient in a happy and positive frame of mind?

Practical advice

- Carefully distinguish between visual and physical symptoms. Patients often complain of discomfort which really relates to vision.

28.1.2 Visual acuity and over-refraction

Snellen acuities are recorded monocularly and binocularly in the normal way. The quality of retinoscopy reflex is particularly important during assessment of vision and over-refraction (*see* Section 28.2).

28.1.3 Assessment of fitting with white light

White light examination either with low magnification or unaided gives a preliminary assessment of:

- Lens centration in primary position.
- Lens movement on blinking.
- Lens position with lateral and vertical eye movements.
- Blink rate.
- Completeness of blink.
- Conjunctival injection.
- Head position.
- Eye movements.
- Palpebral aperture.

Some of these factors may well be different during slit lamp examination where the head position is unnatural and light intensity much greater.

Practical advice

- Some conditions such as swelling of the bulbar conjunctiva or eyelids are seen more easily without magnification or with diffuse illumination on the slit lamp.
- With a soft lens, movement is best seen by directing the beam from a hand-held pen torch, not necessarily from in front but from the side or below, so that the junction of the lenticular portion of the lens casts an easily observed annular light pattern and shadow onto the iris background. The movement of this is more easily discernible than that of the lens itself.

28.1.4 Assessment of fitting with fluorescein

Examination with fluorescein is mainly directed at hard lens fittings, although it can also be used with other specialized lenses such as silicon. Ultraviolet light does not give a useful assessment of fitting with hard lenses containing UV blockers (e.g. Boston 7). High molecular weight fluorescein can be used with soft lenses, but generally adds little to white light observation. Fluorescein examination should reveal:

- The central fitting in respect of touch and clearance.
- Peripheral fitting and edge clearance.
- The speed of fluorescein mixing as an indicator of tear flow.
- 3 and 9 o'clock staining.
- Other areas of gross corneal staining or desiccation.

28.1.5 Slit lamp examination with lenses in situ

The slit lamp is the major diagnostic instrument both at initial fitting and at all aftercare examinations. With lenses *in situ* it is used with varying degrees of magnification to check:

- Lens fit (centration and movement).
- Tear lens with slit beam.
- Signs of gross corneal oedema.
- The bulbar conjuctiva for signs of vessel irritation.
- The condition of lenses.
- Any air bubbles trapped under the lenses.
- Any debris trapped under the lenses.

- Wettability of lens surface

28.1.6. Supplementary procedures with lenses *in situ*

Supplementary procedures at this stage, with lenses still *in situ*, may include:

- Photography or computerized image capture.
- Contrast sensitivity.
- Keratometry over front surface of lens (with soft lenses).
- Placido disc or Klein keratoscope (with soft lenses).

28.1.7 Slit lamp examination with lenses removed

Lenses are removed and ideally stored in the patient's own case. Fluorescein is then instilled and the eyes examined for:

- Any signs of corneal staining, noting both extent and depth.
- Any signs of corneal oedema (e.g. central clouding, microcysts, striae), with both sclerotic scatter and direct observation.
- Corneal indentation (from hard lens adhesion).
- Scleral indentation (from tight soft lenses).
- Foreign bodies.
- Corneal desiccation.
- Qualitative assessment of tear film.
- Conjunctival injection or desiccation.
- Engorgement of limbal vessels.
- Irritation of lid margins.
- Lid oedema.
- Changes to tarsal plate (seen with lid eversion).

28.1.8 Supplementary tests with lenses removed

Examination may indicate that supplementary procedures are advisable:

- Keratometry.
- Quantitative assessment of tear flow (*see* Section 5.6).
- Staining with rose bengal.
- Photography or computerized image capture.

- Pachometry.
- Aesthesiometry.

28.1.9 Clinical adjustments or changes

The practitioner is now able to decide whether any symptoms are purely adaptive and can be temporarily ignored or whether some action is needed. There are several possible changes which may be necessary:

- Alteration to power or fitting. Hard gas-permeable and PMMA lenses may be either modified or exchanged, depending upon the laboratory policy. Soft lenses require replacement.
- Refitting with the same general type of lens. For example, a hard gas-permeable lens with a higher Dk material; a soft lens with a different water content.
- Refitting with a totally different type of lens. For example: hard gas-permeable with soft; soft with hard gas-permeable; or spherical with toric.
- Different solutions, e.g. completely changing the regimen because of allergy, adding saline as an extra rinsing solution, or using a more efficient cleaner.
- Adjustment to the wearing schedule. Adaptation can often be helped with a change of wearing schedule, either slower or occasionally faster (e.g. to span a working day as soon as possible). A single period can be divided into two or *vice versa*.

28.1.10 Further discussion with the patient

The aftercare examination should conclude with further discussion, particularly to maintain patient enthusiasm. It should include:

- Reassurance concerning any subjective symptoms.
- Any lens changes with reasons.
- Any changes to solutions regimen.
- Recommended date of next visit.

28.2 Visual problems

28.2.1 General factors

First look for spherical errors and, if this improves acuity to a satisfactory level, small cylinders can be ignored.

- Distance acuity should be assessed separately from near and intermediate vision, since different and independent problems can arise.
- Snellen acuity is recorded in the usual way. Binocular acuity is often significantly better than that expected from monocular results. Contrast sensitivity measurements may explain visual problems where recorded acuities appear to be satisfactory.
- Retinoscopy reflex is an important diagnostic aid. It can show optical aberrations in a lens because of poor manufacture which may not be apparent with verification.
- A retinoscopy reflex improving after a blink with a soft lens indicates a tight fitting (see Chapter 18).
- The ophthalmoscope can also reveal lens aberrations as well as special features such as the position of a bifocal segment.
- Spectacle blur should not be present with hard gas-permeable and soft lenses. It is almost to be expected with PMMA.

DISTANCE VISION

Adaptive problems

- Variable vision. Most patients are affected to some degree during the early stages of adaptation.
- 'Foggy' vision due to greasy lenses. Usually worse in the afternoon and associated with poor blinking.
- Asthenopia, because of minor refractive changes or while the patient gets used to a different type of vision.
- Distorted vision. Myopes and hypermetropes notice, respectively, larger and smaller retinal image sizes.
- An apparently unequal change in over-refraction, with one eye requiring more minus and the other less, is a frequent indication that right and left lenses have been reversed.

Non-adaptive problems

- Blurred vision because of refractive changes. When tear flow has returned to normal, changes in refraction of 0.50 D can sometimes occur. An increase in minus may also indicate corneal oedema, so keratometry and slit lamp findings should also be assessed.

- Blurred vision because of residual astigmatism. This should be predictable at initial fitting, but is sometimes not observed until lenses have fully settled. Patients typically complain of ghosting. Consider a front surface toric.
- 'Foggy' vision because of greasy lenses. Tends to be worse immediately on insertion because of poor wetting or late in the day because of surface drying. Look for CLIPC by everting the lids; this can sometimes occur within a few days of lens wear. Ensure solutions are being used correctly and possibly change to a different system. Hard lenses may need to be repolished and re-edged (sometimes necessary even with new lenses) or require an entirely different edge shape. Alternatively, consider a different lens material.
- Blurred vision because of oedema. Patients typically complain of 'foggy' or 'cloudy' vision. It can be differentiated from greasy deposits because if the lenses are cleaned and reinserted there is no temporary improvement in vision. It is much more common with PMMA, which should be fenestrated or refitted. Modern hard and soft lenses can be refitted with higher *Dk* materials.
- Asthenopia may be due to residual astigmatism, over-correction, binocular imbalance or change in eye dominance (e.g. because of residual astigmatism in the dominant eye).

NEAR VISION

Near vision problems are frequently encountered in the early stages of adaptation with all types of lens (*see* Section 5.4).

INTERMEDIATE VISION

Music reading is a common problem because of the working distance, poor lighting conditions and instability of vision during adaptation. VDUs and painting can cause similar difficulties.

28.2.2 Hard gas-permeable and PMMA lenses

- Flare is worse with small PMMA lenses and flat peripheries. Possible modifications are thinning the mid-periphery or edges to improve centration. Otherwise fit a lens with a larger BOZD and total diameter; use less edge lift, especially in aspheric form; or change to a soft lens.

- Variable vision on blinking because of excessively mobile lenses.
- Blurred vision because of flexure. More common with hard gas-permeable than PMMA lenses. Consider a flatter fitting, greater centre thickness or a more rigid material.

28.2.3 Soft lenses

- Flare is uncommon with soft lenses, but can occur with some designs of toric and with a displaced pupil. Where the patient cannot adapt, the lens should be remade with a larger FOZD or refitted with a different design.
- Blurred vision except after a blink suggests a tight fitting. This may be confirmed by the retinoscopy reflex.
- Variable vision, worse after a blink, suggests a loose fitting.
- Deterioration of vision during the course of the day may be due to lens dehydration.

28.3 Wearing problems

28.3.1 General factors

The practitioner must decide whether the fitting:

- Still looks as intended at the initial fitting. It is possible for either the eyes or the lenses to have altered.
- Is satisfactory in terms of position, movement, central fit, peripheral fit and centration.
- Is responsible for any subjective symptoms. Problems can arise, however satisfactory the fitting and quality of lens manufacture.
- Is causing any asymptomatic problems (e.g. oedema with an immobile lens).

28.3.2 Cornea

OEDEMA

Oedema is common with PMMA and quite feasible with hard gas-permeable and soft lenses where they are low-riding, sticking, or the cornea has high oxygen requirements. Sclerotic scatter in a darkened room shows central oedema most clearly. This technique is not so successful with soft lenses, where the oedema tends to extend from limbus to limbus and may give rise to striae. Microcysts and bullae are other signs of corneal swelling. Subjectively, patients may complain of photophobia, cloudy vision or spectacle blur.

STAINING

Several types of staining are observed in practice.

Arcuate staining

Arcuate staining with hard lenses is usually found in the superior mid-periphery of the cornea (Figure 28.1). It is often asymptomatic and can be caused by:

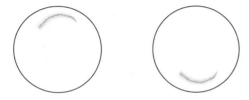

Figure 28.1 Arcuate staining

- Sharp or poorly blended transitions
- Sharp or poorly finished edges.
- Insufficient edge lift.
- Lens adhesion
- Overall tight fitting.
- Tight lids giving excessive force during blinking.
- Badly finished or blocked fenestrations.
- Deposits on posterior lens surface.

Pseudo-arcuate staining is sometimes observed with narrow edge lift. The lens periphery gives an arcuate pressure effect which does not actually take up fluorescein stain. It is sometimes sufficient to reveal the Fischer–Schweitzer corneal mosaic. Remedies to arcuate staining include:

- Fully blending all transitions.

- Re-edging.
- Greater edge lift.
- Smaller BOZD.
- Flatter BOZR.
- Changing to a different total diameter.

Arcuate staining is also observed with both daily and extended wear soft lenses. Although it can occur in most regions of the cornea, it is more commonly found towards the superior limbus with thicker and higher water content lenses. It has been referred to as superior epithelial arcuate lesions (SEALS)[1] and usually causes discomfort with reduced wearing time, particularly when associated with corneal drying. In severe cases there is gradually advancing superior vascularization. It is usually resolved by changing the design or water content, but may occasionally necessitate refitting with hard lenses.

Arcuate staining in the lower third of the cornea is sometimes referred to as a *smile stain*. It is usually caused by lens dehydration and is often associated with poor or incomplete blinking. It may be asymptomatic but more frequently causes a gritty or burning sensation. A looser fitting lens or one with different dehydration characteristics is required.

3 and 9 o'clock staining

3 and 9 o'clock staining is created by drying in the nasal and temporal areas of the cornea (Figure 28.2). It is a more frequent

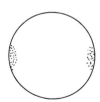

Figure 28.2 3 and 9 o'clock staining

problem with hard gas-permeable lenses than with PMMA, with several possible causes. These must be recognized before the correct remedial action can be taken:

- Poor blinking.
- Inadequate tear film.

- Wide palpebral apertures.
- Periphery too flat or edges too thick (lid held away from the corneal surface – *lid gap*).
- Periphery too tight (physical disruption of tear film).
- Total diameter too large (physical disruption of tear film).
- Total diameter too small (disincentive to proper blinking).
- The lens material (tear film disrupted by poor surface wetting properties).

3 and 9 o'clock staining may be resolved by:

- Correct blinking.
- A thinner lens.
- Refitting with a lid attachment design.
- A different total diameter.
- A different lens periphery.
- Refitting with a better wetting material.
- Refitting with soft lenses.

Central staining

Central staining is caused by the breakdown of the corneal epithelium as a result of corneal oedema (Figure 28.3). It is possible with any type of lens, but is usually associated with PMMA.

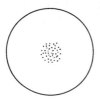

Figure 28.3 Central staining

Punctate staining (corneal stippling)

Punctate staining may be either intense or diffuse and has a variety of causes:

- Corneal desiccation between the lower periphery of a hard lens and the limbus due to exposure of the epithelium where it is not lubricated by the lids on blinking (Figure 28.4). It may be regarded as a more superficial and more diffuse type of 3

Figure 28.4 Inferior punctate staining

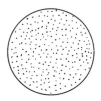

Figure 28.5 Diffuse punctate staining

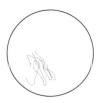

Figure 28.6 Foreign body tracks

and 9 o'clock staining and responds to the same remedial actions.

- Solutions. Punctates vary from extremely fine and diffuse over the entire corneal surface with no apparent symptoms (Figure 28.5), to large coalescent areas with gross hyperaemia, lacrimation and discomfort.
- Material allergies.
- Toxic reactions (e.g. to contaminated soft lenses or unreacted monomers).

Foreign body

Staining is typically superficial and linear with a curved or zig-zag shape (Figure 28.6), although sometimes a foreign body may be trapped by the lens deep into the cornea. The sudden sharp pain associated with foreign bodies is a constant minor hazard with hard gas-permeable lenses and, because the corneal sensitivity is not depressed to the same extent as PMMA, often causes greater problems.

Irregular staining

Irregular staining may have a variety of possible causes:

- A poor fitting lens.
- Damaged lens.
- Deposits on posterior lens surface.
- Badly finished or blocked fenestration.
- Fingernail scratch from poor insertion or removal.

Air bubbles (dimpling)

Dimpling occurs mainly with hard lenses, but is also possible with soft. The small air bubbles trapped in a pool of tears beneath a contact lens act as foreign bodies. They give a fairly dramatic appearance with fluorescein, but do not give true staining (Figure 28.7). If the lens is removed and the eye rinsed with saline, irregular depressions can be seen in the corneal surface, but the apparent staining disappears with no actual uptake of fluorescein by the epithelium. Dimpling causes no discomfort, but gives blurred vision if it occurs within the pupil area where it is easily detected with both the retinoscope and ophthalmoscope. As the bubbles coalesce, they can either froth or occasionally form a single large bubble which may lead to corneal desiccation. Dimpling is found:

- Centrally, with a steep fitting.
- Superiorly, under a flat periphery in a stable high-riding lens.
- With highly astigmatic corneas.
- With keratoconus and other irregular corneas.

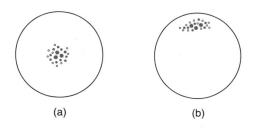

(a)   (b)

Figure 28.7 (a) Central dimpling; (b) superior dimpling.

It can be helped by:

- Loosening the fit to promote better tear flow.
- Changing the BOZD or total diameter.
- Fenestration, although this could make it worse.

Practical advice

Small, discrete areas of staining (grade I) and isolated punctates can often be safely ignored with hard lenses. Much more careful assessment is necessary with soft lenses to ensure that they are not a precursor to more serious corneal complication.

28.3.3 Limbus

BLOOD VESSELS

It is always important to examine carefully the superior corneoscleral junction, since the limbal blood vessels dilate in response to any adverse stimulus such as physical irritation, insufficient oxygen or solutions reaction. It is also possible for 'ghost' vessels from previous contact lens wear to refill within a few days if stimulated by these same factors.

STAINING

Staining at the limbus can occur for various reasons:

- Solutions reaction.
- Abrasions from lens edges.
- Desiccation (3 and 9 o'clock).
- Inferior, because of exposure.
- Hypoxia beneath the upper lid.
- Nasal or temporal decentration of a soft lens.

With soft lenses, an accumulation of fluorescein rather than staining may sometimes occur around the limbus where the lens has created a pressure effect.

DELLEN

The long-term consequence of severe 3 and 9 o'clock desiccation with hard gas-permeable and PMMA lenses is dellen formation.

This shows as marked corneal thinning at the limbus associated with severe conjunctival injection. Recovery, however, can occur within a few days on ceasing contact lens wear.

LIMBAL OPACIFICATION

Although limbal opacification is usually a long-term response to PMMA, it can occur more rapidly with modern hard lenses. It is observed together with an advancing area of corneal drying, and on rare occasions it is observed by the time of the first aftercare examination.

PINGUECULA

Pingueculae may become injected during contact lens wear, particularly where associated with poor blinking and dry eyes. Patients often notice them for the first time when beginning to use contact lenses and may require reassurance that they are benign and are not actually caused by the lenses.

28.3.4 Bulbar conjunctiva

INJECTION

Some minor degree of redness is frequently adaptive and there may be staining with either fluorescein or rose bengal. More severe conjunctival injection can be due to:

- Solutions reaction.
- Other allergies.
- Poor blinking.
- 3 and 9 o'clock staining.
- Other desiccation.
- Infections.
- Physical irritation.

28.3.5 Lids

CONTACT LENS-INDUCED PAPILLARY CONJUNCTIVITIS

CLIPC is an inflammation of the papillary conjunctiva of, usually, the upper lids, characterized by the presence of irregularly shaped papillae. These may appear similar to those found with vernal catarrh, but are histologically different and progress in four distinct stages:[2]

1. Preclinical stage with mild increase in mucus production.
2. Conjunctival hyperaemia and thickening with slight elevation of normal papillae. Vascular tufts can be seen in the papillae.
3. Formation of larger papillae from coalescent smaller papillae, often starting from the inner and outer canthi.
4. Formation of elevated, giant papillae with flattened heads which can stain with fluorescein.

Contact lens wearers are usually seen at stages 1 or 2. The symptoms are quite distinctive:

- Itching on lens removal.
- Discharge in the morning, typically yellow in colour.
- Severe lens deposits causing blurred vision.
- Excessive movement of the lens which is pulled by the rough inner surface of the upper lid.
- Gradually deteriorating comfort.

The condition can be either unilateral or bilateral and, although more typically a problem of soft lens wear, can be found with all lens types.[3] There are several causative factors, working either on their own or in conjunction:

- Allergic response to the lens material.
- Autoimmune allergic response to protein deposits on the lens surface.
- Solutions sensitivity.
- Mechanical irritation.
- Environmental irritation.
- Predisposition with atopic patients (e.g. hay fever sufferers).

Resolving CLIPC may require several courses of action:

- Consider referral for medical treatment with either sodium cromoglycate 2% (e.g. Opticrom) or steroids such as Predsol-n.
- Discontinue extended wear, at least until condition is resolved.
- Fit new soft lenses or repolish hard lenses.
- Fit new soft lenses before the hay fever season.
- Ensure regular lens replacement or fit disposables.
- Eliminate all preserved solutions

- Change to a peroxide system.
- Ensure regular use of enzyme tablets.
- With soft lenses, consider a different material or refitting with hard gas-permeable lenses.
- With hard lenses, avoid silicon acrylates and consider CAB or fluoropolymers.

PTOSIS

Ptosis is observed in long-term wearers of both hard gas-permeable and PMMA lenses and may be either unilateral or bilateral.[4] It appears unrelated to any particular fitting philosophy or oxygen permeability and is not usually improved by altering the fit. As long as any neurological factors have been eliminated, there may be no need to take any action but merely keep the condition under observation. If ptosis is interfering with vision or cosmetic appearance, the following may be tried:

- Change to soft lenses, which may sometimes prove effective.
- Discontinue contact lens wear.
- Surgical intervention, but this is not always successful.

MISCELLANEOUS LID PROBLEMS

There are several minor lid problems. The majority are unconnected with contact lenses, although patients may require reassurance of this point.

- Concretions.
- Make-up trapped on palpebral conjunctiva.
- Blocked meibomian glands and frothing at lid margin.
- Styes and cysts.
- Blepharitis exacerbated by contact lens wear.
- Vesicles on lid margins.
- Skin allergies, often caused by make-up but sometimes by solutions.
- Lid spasms and twitching.

28.3.6 Lens adhesion

Adhesion has been regarded as a hard lens extended wear problem (*see* Section 21.5). It is not uncommon, however, with daily wear towards the end of the day where the impression of the lens can be seen on the cornea after removal. Patients are often asymptomatic, but the possible problems are:

- Arcuate staining.
- Redness.
- Trapped debris.
- Corneal distortion.
- Infection.

Lens adhesion can be caused by a variety of factors:

- Dry eyes.
- Tight lids.
- Periphery too narrow.
- Lens material (more common with greater flexibility).
- Lens design (more common with aspheric lenses).

Lens adhesion can be an intractable problem but may sometimes be helped by:

- Flattening the periphery or adding an extra edge curve with a radius of 15.00 mm or 18.00 mm.
- Steepening the central fit.
- Changing the lens design to increase the width of the periphery.
- Increasing the thickness.
- Changing to a more rigid material.
- Improved blinking.
- Lubricating drops.

28.3.7 Environmental and general factors

Some of the most difficult problems in contact lens practice are not caused by the lenses but by the environment or external factors over which the practitioner has no control:

- Central heating.
- Air conditioning.
- Low humidity.
- High altitude.

- Staring at VDU screens.
- Polluted atmospheres.
- Poor lighting.

Symptoms of discomfort are exacerbated by other factors:

- Alcohol.
- Diet.
- Systemic drugs (*see* Section 29.3).
- Oral contraceptives.
- HRT
- Tiredness.
- Poor general health.
- Pregnancy.
- Psychological effects of tension.

28.3.8 Blinking

Infrequent or incomplete blinking is a particular difficulty with hard gas-permeable and PMMA lenses. It causes several problems:

- Oedema because of insufficient tear pump.
- 3 and 9 o'clock staining.
- Other corneal and conjunctival desiccation.
- Conjunctival injection.
- General discomfort.
- Lens deposits and blurred vision.

Incomplete blinking with soft lenses also causes problems because of dehydration. This in turn can lead to inferior or lower mid-peripheral staining (smile stain) and lens deposits.

Practical advice

Hard lenses act as a strong disincentive to correct blinking, so retraining is rarely successful. Refitting with soft lenses is often the best solution.

28.4 Aftercare at yearly intervals or longer

Examination after 12 months or a longer period is particularly concerned with the possible long-term consequences of contact lens wear and the condition of the lenses. It includes the same stages as the first aftercare routine (*see* Sections 28.1.1 to 28.1.10) with the key additions of:

* Reassessment of contact lens refraction and refitting with trial lenses.
* Spectacle refraction (*see* Section 29.4).
* Ophthalmoscopy – this may be the only opportunity for fundus and ophthalmic examination.
* Assessment of contact lens condition.

28.4.1 Ocular examination

* Vascularization or neovascularization.
* Oedematous responses (microcysts, bullae, striae).
* Signs of infection (nummular or other infiltrates).
* Corneal thinning.
* Endothelial polymegathism.
* Chronic staining.

CONJUNCTIVA

* Desiccation.
* Injection.
* Pingueculae.

LIDS

* Position, including ptosis.
* CLIPC.
* Concretions.
* Patency of meibomian glands.

TEARS

* Qualitative assessment.
* Break-up time.

OVER-REFRACTION

- Comparison with previously recorded acuities.
- Change in myopia or hypermetropia.
- Change in astigmatism.

28.4.2 Other factors

REASSESSING CONTACT LENS REFRACTION AND FITTING

Old and deposited lenses frequently give reduced acuity. Hard lenses may have distorted with repeated handling and soft lenses become less flexible with age. Spurious refractive changes of up to 1.00 D can be found, so it is essential to reassess both refractive result and fit with fresh trial lenses (preferably those used at the original fitting) in order to obtain a reliable result.

ASSESSING CONTACT LENS CONDITION

It is also important to examine the lens condition both on the eye with the slit lamp and off the eye with a projection microscope. These instruments allow easy demonstration to the patient of surface and edge defects or signs of ageing (*see* Section 29.5).

SOLUTIONS

It is important to establish that the patient is using solutions correctly. Common errors are:

- Changing brands without consulting the practitioner.
- Omitting to use a daily cleaner.
- Insufficient rinsing of cleaning solution.
- Forgetting to use enzyme tablets.
- Using preserved instead of unpreserved saline.
- Thinking saline is a storage and disinfection solution.
- Forgetting to add the disinfection tablet with chlorine systems.

References

1. Hine, N., Back, A. and Holden, B.A. (1987) Aetiology of arcuate epithelial lesions induced by hydrogels. *Transactions of the British Contact Lens Association Annual Clinical Conference*, 4, 48–50
2. Allansmith, M.R., Korb, D.R., Freiner, J.V., Henriquez, A.S., Simon, M.A. and

Finnemore, V.M. (1977) Giant papillary conjunctivitis in contact lens wearers. *American Journal of Ophthalmology*, **83**, 697–708

3. Efron, N. (1997) Contact lens-induced papillary conjunctivitis. *Optician*, **213** (5583), 20–27
4. Epstein, G. and Potterman, A.M. (1981) Acquired blepharoptosis secondary to contact lens wear. *American Journal of Ophthalmology*, **91**, 634–639

Chapter 29

Supplementary aftercare

29.1 Emergencies and infections

Emergencies, either perceived or real, are a fairly routine occurrence in contact lens practice. It is a common assumption by patients that the lenses are the invariable cause of any ocular problem and it may require all of the practitioner's skill to differentiate between contact lens and non-contact lens emergencies.

29.1.1 Infections

Infections may be either connected or unconnected with contact lens wear. In serious cases, immediate medical treatment is required to minimize any risk of permanent visual loss.

MICROBIAL KERATITIS (SUPPURATIVE KERATITIS)[1,2]

Microbial keratitis is a potentially sight-threatening condition and requires urgent diagnosis and referral. It is caused by bacteria such as the Gram-negative *Pseudomonas aeruginosa* or the Gram-positive *Staphylococcus aureus* or *Streptococcus pyogenes*. Patients typically present with:

- Severe pain.
- An epithelial defect.
- A central lesion over 1 mm in diameter.
- Corneal suppuration (ulceration) which can be rapidly progressive.
- Uveitis.
- Lid oedema.

If patients are observed early, before ulceration occurs, epithelial disturbance or superficial punctate keratitis may be the only signs. Corneal ulcers associated with Gram-positive bacteria are usually smaller and less purulent. The Gram-negative *Pseudomonas*, in particular, is highly virulent and characteristically produces large epithelial defects with dense anterior stromal infiltrates. Treatment usually commences with a broad-spectrum antibiotic until the specific micro-organism has been identified.

Microbial keratitis in contact lens wearers is associated with soft extended wear,[3] poor patient hygiene, poor compliance and contaminated lens cases.[4]

Practical advice

- Corneal ulceration can progress with great rapidity so that serious visual loss can occur within 12–24 hours. Immediate referral direct to an ophthalmologist is absolutely essential.
- Chloramphenical which is currently the only antibiotic available to optometrists as a first aid treatment is ineffective against Gram-negative micro-organisms such as *Pseudomonas aeruginosa*.

STERILE KERATITIS

Some cases of keratitis are described as *sterile*, where no micro-organism can be cultured and identified. Compared with microbial keratitis, patients usually present with:

- Mild pain.
- Small peripheral lesions, less than 1 mm in diameter.
- Non-progressive corneal suppuration.
- No uveitis.

Sterile keratitis should be treated as possibly microbial in origin until proved otherwise. The condition responds to topical steroids.

ACANTHAMOEBA KERATITIS[6]

Acanthamoeba keratititis is an uncommon but devastating ocular condition. There are several reports that associate it with the use of contact lenses[5,6] so that the practitioner should always be open to its possibility in a patient presenting as a painful emergency.

Acanthamoeba is a non-flagellate protozoon occurring in trophozoite and cyst forms. The double-walled nature of the cyst accounts for its strong resistance to treatment. The organism is widely distributed in air and water so that tap water should never be recommended for rinsing contact lenses or their cases. Patients should also be advised to be particularly careful with cleaning and disinfection after swimming with lenses. Miraflow is specifically effective against *Acanthamoeba*.

The later, characteristic feature of *Acanthamoeba* is an extensive ring infiltrate in the cornea. There is often hypopyon and secondary glaucoma. The condition produces a high incidence of corneal scarring requiring keratoplasty and immediate referral is therefore essential. The earlier the diagnosis, the more successful the treatment, and a referral note should include the practitioner's suspicions.

Early features of *Acanthamoeba* infection are:

- Severe ocular pain or aching, out of all proportion to any initial signs of infection or inflammation.
- Red eye.
- Reduced acuity.
- Central punctate epithelialopathy which often breaks down to an erosion. The lesion may well be dendritiform and therefore mistaken for ocular herpes simplex.
- Perineural infiltration of corneal nerves, extending from the centre to periphery.
- Superficial nummular keratitis.

Treatment is still being developed but Brolene drops (propamidine) and ointment (dibromopropamidine) both have some efficacy. Steroids are usually contraindicated.

Viral keratitis

The contact lens practitioner may encounter two main types of viral keratitis, although there is no particular association with contact lenses. Viral infections typically produce a profuse serous discharge.

- Herpes simplex. Very painful and typically showing dendritic lesions or disciform keratitis. There is generally scarring with the risk of recurrence. Acyclovir is used in treatment.
- Adenovirus. Mildly painful, showing multiple subepithelial infiltrates which may fade very slowly. The condition is extremely infectious but self-limiting with only a small chance of visual loss.

29.1.2 Acute red eye syndrome (contact lens-induced acute red eye (CLARE); red eye)[7]

The red eye reaction is an inflammatory response sometimes occurring with soft extended wear lenses (*see* Section 21.4.2.). There is gross unilateral hyperaemia, associated with varying degrees of pain, photophobia, lacrimation and limbal infiltrates.

29.1.3 Overwear syndrome (acute epithelial necrosis; 3 am syndrome)

This is commonly associated with PMMA, although not unknown with either hard gas-permeable or soft lenses. The patient is typically awakened in the middle of the night with extreme pain ('red-hot needles' is the usual description), photophobia and lacrimation. It is an extreme response to gross corneal oedema as a result of excessive contact lens wear. Typical causes are:

*   Too fast an initial wearing schedule.
*   Patient forgetting to remove lenses at a specified time.
*   All-day use after a gap in lens wear because of loss.
*   Falling asleep with lenses in.
*   Chronic oedema with longer than normal wear in a hot and stuffy atmosphere.

Examination, where feasible, shows large areas of corneal staining. Treatment may well require local anaesthetic and antibiotics to minimize the risk of secondary infection. In extreme cases, medical treatment is necessary with 'pad and bandaging' in a darkened room for 24 hours. The epithelium usually recovers within 2–3 days, although contact lens wear should not be resumed for at least a week and not until the practitioner has confirmed that the cornea is clear. A very slow wearing schedule is then indicated. Patients require considerable reassurance that they will not suffer permanent damage to their eyes.

Practical advice

Local anaesthetics tend to retard epithelial healing and should only be used in cases of extreme pain. The preferred analgesic is aspirin with whisky

---

29.1.4 Foreign bodies

These are much more common with hard gas-permeable and PMMA lenses. The damage to the corneal epithelium, however, can sometimes be greater with soft lenses because the foreign body remains trapped behind the lens for a longer period of time. Patients complain of sudden, acute pain during the wearing day. The lens must be removed and fluorescein instilled to assess the depth of staining with slit lamp optic section. Treatment consists of antibiotics, with 'pad and bandaging' in severe cases.

29.1.5 Corneal abrasions

Severe abrasions cause symptoms similar to those resulting from foreign bodies. They may be caused by poor lens handling, typically by fingernails, inserting or wearing damaged lenses, lenses breaking in the eye, and fitting problems.

29.1.6 Solutions problems

A high proportion of soft lens emergencies relate to solutions reactions. Careful questioning is sometimes necessary to reveal either patient error or the offending solution. Typical problems are:

- Genuine allergic response.

- Thimerosal keratopathy, also known as contact lens-induced superior limbic keratoconjunctivitis (CLSLK).
- Using hard lens solutions with soft lenses.
- Not neutralizing lenses stored in hydrogen peroxide.

- Confusing soaking and cleaning solutions.
- Reaction to enzyme tablets.
- Using enzyme tablets in conjunction with an incorrect solution.
- Adverse reaction after intensive cleaning.
- Using preserved comfort drops in an otherwise non-preserved regime.
- Using preserved therapeutic drops.
- Patients changing to a brand different from that originally recommended by the practitioner.
- Patients being sold an incorrect solution.

29.1.7 Contaminated lenses

This problem mainly applies to soft lenses contaminated by products like paint, varnish, hairspray and make-up, either by direct contact or indirectly via the hands. Hard lenses are occasionally affected.

29.2 Grief cases

Not all patients adapt well to contact lenses, however carefully they are fitted. This may be due to the practitioner, the patient or limitations in available lens designs.[8]

29.2.1 Causes

The main reasons for grief cases wishing to consult another practitioner are:

- Poor vision or comfort because of fitting or refitting with the wrong type of lens.
- Wearing the correct type of lens but an unsatisfactory fitting.
- Poor vision or comfort because of badly manufactured lenses.
- Using inappropriate solutions.
- Recurrent deposits or greasy lenses.
- Persistent red eyes or 3 and 9 o'clock staining because of poor blinking.
- Dry eyes.
- Spectacle blur.
- Allergic response to materials or solutions.
- The patient does not understand or follow instructions.
- The presence of an eye infection, either connected or unconnected with the contact lenses.
- The patient may no longer be suitable for contact lens wear because of corneal exhaustion, dry eyes or environmental factors.
- The patient has never really been suitable for contact lenses.
- The patient may have lost confidence in the previous practitioner, although the lenses are perfectly satisfactory.

29.2.2 Courses of action

The new practitioner must decide on the main reason for previous dissatisfaction and whether successful contact lens wear is feasible. The following are the most common courses of action:

- Modify existing lenses. This applies mainly to PMMA and hard gas-permeable lenses.
- Refit lenses of the same general type (e.g soft with soft or hard gas-permeable with hard gas-permeable), but use a different material, *Dk* or design.
- Refit with lenses of an altogether different type (e.g. soft with hard gas-permeable or hard gas-permeable with soft).
- Change the solutions or disinfection system. This is often advisable, even where refitting is also carried out.
- Give advice on correct blinking.
- Give clear instructions in the correct use of solutions, even where there is no sensitivity problem.
- Give correct instructions in lens handling and maintenance.
- Refer for medical opinion.
- Advise patients that they are now unsuitable for lenses. They will be disappointed, but at the same time should accept the fact that they have at last been given unequivocal advice.

Practical advice

- Grief cases have generally been disillusioned with contact lenses and are seeking a swift and positive resolution to their problems.
- Where refitting is necessary, dispense lenses from stock where possible.
- Give a safe but rapid wearing schedule.
- Put a time limit of 2–3 weeks on any course of action to prevent an unsuccessful case dragging on interminably.
- Where only partial success is possible, advise patients to be realistic, accept a restricted wearing time or discontinue.

29.2.3 Avoiding grief cases

- Do not refit lenses just for the sake of it. If a patient is entirely happy with existing lenses and examination reveals no serious, asymptomatic problems (e.g. corneal oedema or vascularization), then leave well alone. This often applies to old-fashioned low *Dk* lenses, either hard or soft.

- Explain, nevertheless, any relevant new developments and clarify misconceptions (e.g. disposables are not appropriate for toric hard lens wearers).
- Do not refit PMMA wearers with soft lenses (see Section 13.6.3).
- If a patient has been refitted with theoretically better lenses (e.g. PMMA with hard gas-permeable or low water content soft with high) and they do not settle rapidly, then return to the previous type without delay.
- If a replacement lens does not settle rapidly with an experienced lens wearer, change it or refit.
- Use only the best possible quality lenses. Poorly made examples can waste more in practitioner time than the cost of the lenses.
- Adopt a flexible and open-minded approach to contact lens fitting and be prepared to change from one type to another if problems arise.

29.3 Side effects of systemic drugs

Many systemic drugs have side effects which give rise to symptoms of discomfort, blurred vision, dryness and lens discolouration (Table 29.1).

Practical advice

- Pathologies of the cornea due to side effects are serious and tend to be progressive as the dosage continues.
- Use the yellow card system to report any adverse response to either contact lens products or systemic drugs.

29.4 Prescribing spectacles for contact lens wearers

The factors to consider include:

- Establishing the correct *Rx*.
- Providing a correction that is visually comfortable.
- Time of examination.

Table 29.1 Systemic drugs and their side effects

Drug	Side effect
CENTRAL NERVOUS SYSTEM	
Carbamazepine (Tegretol)	Conjunctivitis and photophobia
Maprotiline (Ludiomil)	Intolerance to contact lenses and loss of tear fluid
Diazepam (Valium)	Lowered visual acuity and reduced tear production
Dothiepin (Prothiaden)	Reduced tear flow
Amitriptyline (Tryptizol)	Reduced tear flow
Lorazepam (Atavan)	Dry eye
BLOOD PRESSURE AND HEART CONDITION	
Atenolol (Tenormin) ⎤	Smarting eyes and diffuse conjunctival
Isosorbide (Binitrat) ⎦	injection with very dry eyes
Amiodarone (Cordarone)	Faint striae in both corneas and yellow brown deposits
Oxprenolol (Trasidrex)	Dry eye/conjunctivitis
Cyclopenthiazide	Dry eye/conjunctivitis
Methyldopa (Aldomet)	Keratoconjunctivitis sicca
MUSCULOSKELETAL DISORDERS (ANTI-INFLAMMATORY)	
Penicillamine (Distamine)	Dry eye and reduced vision
URINARY ANTI-INFECTIVES	
Trimethoprim ⎤	
Sulphamethoxazole (Septrin) ⎦	Dryness and irritation
Nitrofurantoin (Furadantin)	Marked irritation with profuse lacrimation
ANTI-OBESITY	
Diethylpropion (Tenuate Dospan)	Reduced tear production and over-wear syndrome
ANTI-ALLERGIC	
Sodium cromoglycate (Opticrom)	Reduced tear production
ANTIBIOTICS	
Doxycycline (Vibramycin)	Marked photophobia and contact lens sensitivity
RESPIRATORY SYSTEM	
Beclomethasone (Becotide) ⎤	Increased sensitivity to contact lenses and
Salbutamol (Ventolin) ⎦	solutions
Rifampicin (for TB)	Discolours soft lenses yellow
ORAL CONTRACEPTIVE AND OESTROGEN	
Levonorgestrel (Microval)	Increase in astigmatism
Ovranette	Reduced tolerance to contact lenses
HRT	Dryness and irritation
ALIMENTARY SYSTEM	
Sulphasalazine (for Crohn's disease)	Discolours soft lenses
NASAL DECONGESTANTS	
Brompheniramine ⎤	Reduced tolerance to soft contact lens
Phenylephrine ⎦	wear
Adrenaline (epinephrine)	Discolours soft lenses
ANTIHISTAMINES	
Piriton ⎤	
Triludan ⎦	Dehydration

- When the spectacles are likely to be worn.
- Type of contact lens worn.

Non-tolerances are a frequent problem because, irrespective of contact lens type, many patients find great difficulty in adapting to the different nature of a spectacle correction worn in front of rather than on the eye. Typical problems are:

- Visual distortion (e.g. sloping floors and bowed door frames).
- Different spatial perspective.
- Different image size.
- Restricted field of view.
- Reflections, especially at night.
- Intolerance to full correction.
- Intolerance to cylinders.

Typical causes are:

- No spectacle refraction for several years and a correction showing a very marked increase in myopia.
- Astigmatism very different in axis and power compared with any previous correction.
- Patients may literally have worn no spectacles for decades because with PMMA it was not feasible to obtain a satisfactory result.
- Contact lens monovision (deliberate or accidental) may give difficulty with either bifocals or separate distance and near spectacles.

29.4.1 PMMA

Long-term PMMA wearers are the most difficult for prescribing spectacles because:

- There is almost invariably some degree of corneal distortion or moulding.
- There is frequently some level of corneal oedema.
- Refraction often gives a poor and unreliable end-point.
- Acuity may be depressed.

The main problem, however, is that after PMMA lenses have been removed, the refraction continuously changes for several weeks while the corneal curvature is undergoing an equivalent

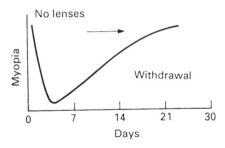

Figure 29.1 Myopia after PMMA lens removal (Rengstorff, 1967)

cycle of change. Although there are wide individual differences, there is an average decrease in myopia of 1.32 D over the first 3 days, followed by an increase in myopia up to 21 days (Figure 29.1).[9] At the same time, there is a strong trend towards increased with-the-rule astigmatism.

In practical terms, therefore, there is no merit whatever in leaving out lenses for periods of several days. Not only is it extremely inconvenient for the patients, especially if they are highly myopic with no current spectacles, but it is also liable to give a wildly inaccurate result. The once common advice of removing lenses for two or three days before refraction, in fact gives an examination time at the point of maximum change.

There are two realistic times for examination, the choice of which should be discussed with the patient according to when the correction is to be used:

1. Afternoon, immediately on removal of lenses, gives the closest approximation to a correction for use in the evenings when lenses have been removed for the day.
2. Morning, prior to insertion of lenses, simulates the occasion when contact lenses will not be worn for a day.

The morning result is usually 0.50–0.75 D less. Undercorrecting the evening refraction can often give a satisfactory compromise.

29.4.2 Hard gas-permeable lenses

Most modern hard lenses cause few problems compared with PMMA, but some degree of corneal moulding may be encountered, particularly with astigmatic eyes and where aspheric designs are used. Pronounced distortion occurs in cases of lens adhesion, and refraction should be postponed

Satisfactory refraction is usually achieved immediately on removal of lenses. If the result does not correlate with the contact lenses, keratometry and any previous spectacles, it should be repeated as a morning refraction.

Where PMMA has been refitted with hard gas-permeable lenses, wait about 2 months before refracting for spectacles, by which time most corneal changes will have resolved. This is confirmed by monitoring 'K' readings.

29.4.3 Soft lenses

Corneal curvature and refractive changes are far less common with soft lenses, although some steepening of the vertical meridian may occur. There is little mechanical moulding, and where oedema is present it generally extends from limbus to limbus without localized changes in curvature or physical distortion. Refraction on removal of soft lenses generally gives a good result, but where there is any doubt it should be repeated in the morning.

Practical advice

- Explain the potential problems to the patient.
- Take notice of any pre-contact lens spectacles, however old.
- Give maximum possible binocular addition.
- Consider undercorrecting spheres by 0.25–0.50 D.
- Consider undercorrecting or omitting cylinders, especially if oblique.
- Be careful not to change eye dominance.
- Repeat refraction on another occasion if it does not correlate with the contact lenses, keratometry and previous correction.

29.5 Lens ageing

29.5.1 Soft lenses

Soft lenses stored in sealed vials remain in good condition for several years, but once they are worn regularly lens deterioration occurs in a variety of ways. Unlike hard lenses, ageing is a common cause of lens replacement influenced by a variety of factors:

- Lens material. High water content ionic lenses deteriorate more rapidly than low water content and non-ionic because of deposits and discolouration (*see* Section 6.3).

- Wearing schedule. Extended wear lenses are more badly affected by deposits than those used daily.

- Tear chemistry. Some patients' lenses last only a few weeks, whereas others can remain in acceptable condition for several years. Dry eyes cause particular problems.

- Method of disinfection. Lenses have a shorter life span when sterilized by heat compared with solutions. Hydrogen peroxide is particularly good at keeping lenses in optimum condition (*see* Section 26.4.1).

- Regularity and method of cleaning.

- Patient care.

- The environment in which lenses are worn. Dry atmospheres enhance lens deposits.

PROTEIN FILM

All lenses suffer protein deposits to some extent. With HEMA in particular, there is a chemical bonding between tear protein and the polymer's hydroxyl groups.[10] Heat disinfection exacerbates the problem by denaturing any surface protein that has not been removed by proper cleaning. It is observed as a blue-grey film by oblique illumination against a dark background (dark-field illumination). It can also be seen during slit lamp examination if the patient stares and the lens surface is allowed to dry.

DISCOLOURATION

Most high water content lenses suffer from brown discolouration to some extent. HEMA can also be affected and heat aggravates the problem. Adrenaline compounds in the tears, nicotine and make-up have been suggested as other causes. Some lenses fluoresce with ultraviolet light. This effect may be due either to the material (with new lenses) or chlorhexidine bound to surface deposits. Acuity may be reduced and significant reductions in light transmission occur.[11] Hormonal problems and systemic drugs have also been implicated (*see* Section 29.3).

WHITE SPOTS

White spots almost invariably occur on the front surface of the lens. In the early stages they appear as fine punctate dots and gradually develop into discrete, elevated deposits scattered irregularly within the area of the exposed palpebral aperture. High water content lenses and those for extended wear are much more affected, particularly with dry-eyed patients and poor blinkers. In severe cases, white spots can be over 1 mm across and extremely uncomfortable. These larger deposits have also been referred to as *mulberries* and *jelly-bumps*. The composition of white spots has been variously described as a combination of mucoprotein and lipids, mucopolysaccharides, and calcium phosphate and calcium carbonate.[12]

RUST SPOTS

Rust spots are mainly due to atmospheric pollution and are more often observed in patients from industrial areas or who travel by train. They are a form of benign ferrous contamination affecting all types of soft lens and are occasionally found as a manufacturing fault.

SURFACE AND EDGE DETERIORATION

As lenses become older and less flexible, they become uncomfortable because of surface scratches and edge chips. Engravings can either crack or become encrusted with deposits. Uneven drying of protein film at the lens periphery can cause crenellated edges.

FITTING CHANGES

Lenses with deposits are more influenced by the upper lid and significant changes in fitting characteristics can occur. Usually they become looser and corneal diameter lenses may become badly decentred. High-riding lenses are frequently associated with CLIPC where the irregular tarsal plate pulls the deposited lens out of position.

REFRACTIVE CHANGES

Old and less flexible lenses frequently give reduced acuity as well as spurious changes in over-refraction of as much as 1.00 D. The lens power, therefore, should always be rechecked with a fresh trial lens when refitting is necessary.

Practical advice

- Before undertaking professional cleaning, advise patients that it will be carried out 'at their own risk'. Unpredictable and irreversible changes can occur to lens dimensions.
- A small minority of highly allergic patients can produce a severe reaction to professionally cleaned lenses.
- Use a shorter cleaning time and lower temperature with high water content lenses.
- Protein film and discolouration can usually be removed or improved by professional cleaning.
- White spots do not respond well and lenses may fail to survive intensive cleaning.
- It is sometimes beneficial to leave lenses in hydrogen peroxide for up to a week, changing the solution every 2 or 3 days, before intensive cleaning with a product like Liprofin.
- Lenses with cracks and chips harbour micro-organisms and should be replaced.
- Patients should be encouraged to replace lenses on a regular basis, rather than expect an unrealistically long life span.

29.5.2 Hard gas-permeable lenses

Hard lenses do not deteriorate in the same way as soft lenses. Their life span is approximately 2–4 years but, depending upon the material, they do deteriorate in various ways.

DEPOSITS

Silicon acrylate materials (see Section 6.1) attract protein from the tears and most patients benefit from the use of enzyme tablets. Monthly soaking is usually sufficient, although some patients require more frequent treatment.

Fluorosilicon acrylates present less of a problem with protein and many of the materials do not require enzyme tablets.

CAB lenses do not contain silicon. Protein deposits are rarely a problem and enzyme tablets are almost always unnecessary. Lenses do attract lipids, however, so greasing is sometimes a problem.

DISCOLOURATION

Discolouration is rarely a problem with most materials. However, some (even when new) show haziness and lack of optical transparency. CAB lenses may also become hazy after 12–18 months.

SURFACE AND EDGE DETERIORATION

Some of the fluorosilicon acrylates have proved quite brittle, and edge damage or complete breakage are not uncommon. Certain of the high Dk silicon acrylates suffer from surface crazing. CAB lenses are more prone to surface scratching.

29.5.3 PMMA

PMMA is still the most stable and inert material. It attracts little in the way of permanent deposits, although some patients are troubled by greasing with older or scratched lenses. It can readily be repolished and frequently gives a life span in excess of 5 years.

29.6 Lens modification

Modifications may be found necessary either during initial adaptation or at annual aftercare examinations. Adjustments are usually better left to the laboratory, especially with the less stable modern hard lenses. There are some occasions, however, when it is essential for lenses to be modified on the spot, and the following minimum equipment should be available:

- Drum with motorized spindle.
- Velveteen pad.
- Reversible suction holder or chuck.
- Selection of convex radius tools with polishing tape.
- Polishing medium.

29.6.1 Hard gas-permeable and PMMA lenses

It is possible to make the following modifications:

- Blend and flatten peripheral radii.
- Reduce TD.
- Minor changes to BVP.
- Repolish or reshape edges.
- Repolish front surfaces.
- Fenestration.
- Truncation.

BLENDING AND FLATTENING OF PERIPHERAL CURVES

- The lens is held centrally by the convex surface with a suction holder or negative chuck.
- A tape-covered convex tool of the required radius is selected.
- The lens is rotated against the tool in the opposite direction of motion to the spindle.

Practical advice

- Ensure the pad or tool is wet at all times.
- All modifications tend to make the fit looser.
- It is not feasible to tighten the fit by modification.
- Do not attempt to modify surface-treated lenses.
- Modern hard lens materials require greater care to avoid distortion and far less pressure than PMMA.

CHANGING THE BVP

It is easier to add minus than plus power without upsetting the image quality. The limits for successful modification are about −0.75 D and +0.50 D for hard gas-permeable lenses; −1.00 D and +0.75 D for PMMA.

PLUS POWER

The lens is mounted centrally by the concave surface with a suction holder or long-stemmed chuck. It is held against the centre of a velveteen pad moistened with polish and gently rocked, working from periphery to centre.

NEGATIVE POWER

The lens is pressed with one finger against a stationary pad, well oiled with polish. It is rotated in small circles about 10 times clockwise and then anticlockwise, working from centre to periphery. This adds about −0.25 D and is repeated for more minus.

POLISHING THE EDGES

The lens is attached to a strong suction holder or chuck and the edge rocked and rotated against a well-oiled, spinning pad.

POLISHING THE SURFACE

The lens is mounted as if for adding positive power, but also drawn across the pad. This adds minus to neutralize any power change. After two passes, both the surface and the focimeter image are checked.

29.6.2 Scleral lenses

Possible modifications:

- Back optic grind-out.
- Transitional grind-out.
- Fenestration.
- Channelling.
- BVP.
- Back scleral size reduction.

References

1. Bull, J.K.G., Stapleton, F. and Minassian. D. (1991) Contact lenses and other risk factors in microbial keratitis. *Lancet*, **338**, 650–653
2. Efron, N. (1997) Contact lens-induced microbial infiltrative keratitis. *Optician*, **214** (5617), 24–32
3. Schein, O.D., Buehler, P.O., Stamler, J.F. *et al.* (1994) Impact of overnight wear on the risks of contact lens-associated ulcerative keratitis. *Archives of Ophthalmology*, **112**, 186–190
4. Gray. T., Cursons, R., Sherwan, J. and Rose, P. (1995) Acanthamoeba, bacterial and fungal contamination of contact lens storage cases. *British Journal of Ophthalmology*, **79**, 601–605
5. McCully, J.P., Alizadeh, H. and Niederkorn, J.Y. (1995) Acanthamoeba keratitis. *Journal of the Contact Lens Association of Ophthalmologists*, **21** (1), 73–76
6. Illingworth, C.D., Cook, S.D., Karabatsas, C.H. and Easty, D.L. (1995) Acanthamoeba keratitis: risk factors and outcome. *British Journal of Ophthalmology*, **79** (12), 1078–1082
7. Efron, N. (1997) Contact lens-induced sterile infiltrative keratitis. *Optician*, **214** (5606), 16–22
8. Gasson, A.P. (1984) Aftercare – the good, the bad and the ugly. *Transactions of the British Contact Lens Association Annual Clinical Conference*, **7**, 143–145
9. Rengstorff, R.H. (1967) Variations in myopia measurements: an after-effect observed with habitual wearers of contact lenses. *American Journal of Optometry*, **44**, 149–161
10. Cummings, J.S. (1973) The future of soft contact lenses. *Manufacturing Optics International*, **26**, 309–312
11. Gasson, A.P. (1975) Visual considerations with hydrophilic lenses. *Ophthalmic Optician*, **15**, 439–448
12. Ruben, M., Triparthi, R.C. and Winder, A.F. (1975) Calcium deposition as a cause of spoilation of hydrophilic soft contact lenses. *British Journal of Ophthalmology*, **59**, 141–148

Chapter 30

Contact lenses and children

30.1 Management

30.1.1 Parent management

Sympathetic management is essential, because parents are naturally concerned about eye problems which become evident within a few weeks of birth, whether the treatment is surgery or simply optical correction. Ametropic children as young as 4 or 5 years may be brought in for contact lenses because the parents cannot accept the idea of spectacles. A contact lens trial may help appreciation of vision where children have reacted against spectacles.

30.1.2 Child management

Babies are easy to manage as no communication is necessary, whereas infants need the stimulation of toys to help with attention. Children of 5 years and older need a great deal of patience and kindness at the initial fitting, for the essential building up of confidence. Apart from fear of the unknown, they are disturbed by the manipulation necessary for insertion and removal and can be frightened of the optical equipment. Keratometry and slit lamp examination can be performed from an early age with a cooperative child, who can be held by the parent, kneel on a stool or stand at the instrument.

Table 30.1 Approximate corneal dimensions for children*

	Keratometry (mm)	*Corneal diameter* (mm)
Baby (2 months old)	6.90	10.0
Infant (4 years old)	7.60	11.0

*Adult dimensions are reachd at approximately 10 years of age.

30.2 Refractive applications

30.2.1 Myopia

The correction of high myopia may improve both acuity and the field of view. Near vision develops without any optical correction. The first choice is often soft, but the thick edge of a high minus lens may lead to vascularization in the long term.

Hard materials of medium Dk are usually the most suitable, except where PMMA is necessary to provide a robust lens for handling. Myopia control is achieved with PMMA[1] and to a lesser extent with modern hard lenses,[2] which are physiologically superior. Hard lenses may prove more acceptable after previous soft lens wear.

30.2.2 Hypermetropia

Strabismic children, especially those with accommodative esotropia, derive greatest benefit. Normal hypermetropes may find vision better with spectacles, but comments at school may initiate contact lens wear.

Soft lenses are the first choice for infants under 6 years and for most older children, depending on the degree of astigmatism, the acceptance of a hard lens, and sporting and other school activities.

30.2.3 Anisometropia

Unilateral myopes or hypermetropes, whether axial or refractive, may benefit from a combination of contact lens wear and part-time occlusion. Success is often greater than with spectacles, although in some cases they merely keep an amblyopic eye straight.[3] If extended wear is necessary with dense amblyopia, the risks outweigh the visual benefits and contact lenses are contra-indicated.

30.3 Therapeutic applications

30.3.1 Aphakia

Early treatment and optical correction are essential for bilateral aphakic infants, so that contact lenses give significant long-term visual benefits.[4] Extended wear soft lenses may be used initially, but only as a prelude to daily wear because of the risk of infection. Hard lenses can be fitted with confidence for children over

5 years but can also be attempted at an earlier age. Silicon can be used with success where soft lens loss is a major problem.

TYPICAL SPECIFICATION

Baby (1–6 months)   75% water content   7.00/12.00 + 32.00 D
Infant (1–4 years)   60% water content   7.60/13.50 + 25.00 D
Child (5–10 years)   60% water content   7.80/14.00 + 15.00 D

Practical advice

- Overcorrect babies for arm's-length vision, which is the range of their visual world.
- Prescribe bifocal spectacles over the lenses for close work at school.

30.3.2 Albinism

Albinism is associated with nystagmus, ametropia (often with high astigmatism) and photophobia. A tinted hard lens is best, but often there is no visual improvement over spectacles.[5] Tinted soft lenses are more comfortable and may well help infants.

Practical advice

- Carefully observe any nystagmus with hard lenses because it may increase with the stress of adaptation.
- 'K' readings are more easily obtained using an autokeratometer because of speed of measurement.

30.3.3 Aniridia and iris coloboma

These conditions require an opaque iris lens to occlude the light (*see* Section 25.2). Colour matching of the good eye is important at school, for psychological reasons.

30.3.4 Microphthalmos

Microphthalmic eyes are usually fitted for cosmetic rather than visual reasons. They tend to have steep corneal radii (e.g.

6.80 mm) with high hypermetropia (e.g. +10.00 D), so that aphakic design can be used with an arbitrary power of about +10.00 D.
Unilateral cases can be fitted with a tinted soft lens where the plus
power makes the eye look larger. This is easier to fit and more
comfortable than a scleral shell.

Practical advice

- A cosmetic lens for one disfigured eye is more often the parent's
  idea rather than the child's.
- Carefully consider the long-term effects, since a child often refus-
  es to go out without the lens.

30.4 Non-therapeutic fitting

If a child is happy wearing spectacles, the parents are best dis-
suaded from the idea of contact lenses. However, lenses can
sometimes be very successful as young as 7 years old, although
10–12 years is a more usual age to consider fitting.[6] The following
criteria apply:

- Visual correction is required all the time.
- The child wants lenses.
- The parents want the child to have lenses.
- The child is old enough to understand handling and main-
  tenance.

Keratometry readings are in the same range as those for adults
and the fitting technique is therefore the same. Aftercare is im-
perative because of the potential number of years lenses may be
worn, and the material with the best physiological characteristics
should be used.

   The advantages and disadvantages of the various lens types
are mainly as given in Section 5.3, but hard lenses are the probable first choice for myopes and high water content soft lenses for
hypermetropes. Torics should initially be avoided because of the
expense and risk of loss.

References

1.   Stone, J. (1976) The possible influence of contact lenses on myopia. *British
     Journal of Physiological Optics*, **31**, 89–114

2. Perrigan, J., Perrigan, D., Quintero, S. and Grosvenor, T. (1990) Silicone-acrylate contact lenses for myopia control: 3 year results. *Optometry & Vision Science*, **67**, 764–769
3. Morris, J. (1979) Contact lenses in infancy and childhood. *Contact Lens Journal*, **8**, 15–18
4. Taylor, D., Morris, J., Rogers, J.E. and Warland, J. (1979) Amblyopia in bilateral infantile and juvenile cataract. *Transactions of the Ophthalmological Society of the United Kingdom*, **99**, 170–176
5. Speedwell, L. (1997) Contact lens fitting in infants and pre-school children. In *Contact Lenses*, 4th edn, A.J. Phillips and L. Speedwell (eds), Butterworth-Heinemann, Oxford, pp. 731–742
6. Morris, J. (1996) Paediatric contact lens practice. In *Paediatric Eye Care*, S. Barnard and D. Edgar (eds), Blackwell Science Limited, Oxford, pp. 312–323

Chapter 31

Therapeutic fitting with hard and soft lenses

Contact lenses are used for therapeutic reasons to:

- Correct vision in eyes with existing pathology.
- Correct irregular corneal astigmatism by providing a smooth optical surface.
- Promote healing by protecting denuded cornea and new epithelium from the lids.
- Prevent epithelial breakdown. Relieve pain or foreign body sensation.
- Protect the cornea and, when used in conjunction with lubricating solutions, provide a moist environment.

31.1 Aphakia

Unilateral aphakics derive considerable visual benefit from lenses because the reduced image size and lack of distortion allow some degree of both fusion and binocular vision to be established. The field of view is also considerably improved. Visual acuity, however, is often reduced by about one line because of the absence of spectacle magnification.

The key problems with aphakic contact lens wearers are:

- Different retinal image sizes.
- Handling difficulties.
- Centration problems.
- Pupil shape and flare.

Particular care is now required with aphakia as the most straightforward cases will have received intraocular implants.

31.1.1 Hard lenses

Hard gas-permeable and PMMA lenses give excellent visual results and are therefore the ideal optical correction for those able to handle lenses.

CORNEAL LENS FITTING

* The BOZR is often fitted between mean and steepest 'K' to help stability and centration and give the preferred fluorescein pattern of apical clearance.
* The BOZD is chosen between 7.00 mm and 8.50 mm, depending on pupil size and position.
* The TD is generally larger than with the equivalent low-powered lens to help centration; it varies between 8.80 mm and 10.50 mm.
* The peripheral curves are usually spherical. The axial edge lift is greater than normal, of the order of 0.15 mm.
* Lenses are lenticular in form to reduce weight and thickness. The FOZD is often 0.50 mm larger than the BOZD. 8.00 mm to 8.50 mm is fairly standard, depending on pupil shape and position and where the lens sits. The reduced optic varies inversely with power.
* The front peripheral curve is often in the form of a negative carrier, although parallel and even positive shapes are used.

Practical advice

* Some high plus lenses always assume a decentred, superior temporal position because the corneal apex has been drawn in this direction during surgery. Choose the TD and BOZD to give sufficient pupil coverage for adequate vision.
* If lenses decentre down because of gravity and lens mass, fit larger ones.
* Use a negative carrier to give a 'hitch-up' lens.
* Avoid a back surface toric unless centration is a problem. Toric peripheries are sometimes necessary with high degrees of astigmatism.
* Tints reduce photophobia and assist handling; a different density or colour between right and left lenses helps identification.
* If exposed corneal sutures cause peripheral staining or are rubbed by the lens, they should be removed to enable comfortable wear. This may be necessary up to several months later.

- A typical centre thickness is 0.35–0.45 mm because of the high powers required.
- Peripheral fenestrations are often used with PMMA to help tears exchange. Central fenestrations can cause flare and visual disturbance.
- Edge thickness should be at least 0.16 mm to avoid a fragile 'knife edge' and make removal easier.

APEX (CORNEOSCLERAL) LENS

The Apex is a very large, modified corneal lens with a scleral rim of about 2.00 mm and reduced optic to minimize mass[1,2]. It is a bicurve construction, with the peripheral curve at least 0.70 mm flatter than the BOZD. The lens is used where the corneal curvature is very flat in one meridian, grossly irregular or where an eccentric pupil requires a very large optic. The lenses give stable acuity because of their limited movement on the cornea and are especially useful for uniocular senile aphakics and also for grafted aphakic eyes. The wearing times can be reasonably long because of reduced corneal sensitivity.

- The BOZR is chosen approximately 0.50 mm flatter than 'K' to give apical touch.
- The BOZD varies from 8.00 mm to 9.50 mm to allow corneal alignment over a fairly large central area.
- The TD varies between 11.50 mm and 13.00 mm, depending on the corneal diameter. The large size assists handling.
- The lens periphery usually has up to six fenestrations.

Typical specification: 8.20:8.50/10.50:12.00 BVP +17.00 Tint 912 Reduced Optic

---

Practical advice

- Expect some degree of corneal staining because of the fitting technique.
- The wearing time may be limited, but even a few hours of good vision is appreciated if nothing else has worked.

It is important to ensure that the patient can handle the lens before ordering. Elderly aphakics often have loose lids, so removal is difficult. A suction holder is more useful if it incorporates a light source, but should only be used by patients who are aware of the lens position and can aim correctly. Bilateral aphakics can use a spectacle frame glazed on one side only. The help of a friend or relative is invaluable.

The success rate is greater with binocular cases, whereas young unilateral aphakics often find tolerance difficult with a hard lens. The cause is often traumatic and they find it difficult to appreciate the potential consequences of lost binocular vision, amblyopia and divergence. A comfortable hydrophilic lens often achieves greater success.

31.1.2 Soft lenses

Most major companies produce lenses in a range of water content, in powers of +10.00 D to +20.00 D. Fitting criteria are mainly as given in Chapter 18.

Low water content lenses

Lenses may vary in size from 12.50 mm to 14.50 mm, with BOZRs from 8.10 mm to 9.50 mm. The design is usually a bicurve construction, with FOZDs between 10.00 mm and 13.00 mm. A front surface aspheric (e.g. Hydron) minimizes centre thickness but makes handling more difficult.

The BOZR is chosen to be approximately 0.50 mm flatter than 'K' for corneal diameter lenses and from 0.70 mm to 1.30 mm flatter than 'K' for semi-scleral lenses.

Lens size must always be chosen to avoid the limbus and give good centration. Irregularities at the limbus such as sutures or drainage blebs influence the choice of diameter. Exposed sutures should be removed, while deformities at the limbus may need to be vaulted with a diameter as large as 16.00 mm.

Medium water content lenses

Lenses have TDs between 13.00 mm and 14.50 mm. BOZRs range from 7.80 mm to 9.30 mm and are chosen 0.50–1.00 mm flatter than 'K' for semi-scleral designs.

High water content lenses

Lenses are mainly semi-scleral bicurves, with BOZDs from 7.00 mm to 8.00 mm and TDs between 13.50 mm and 14.50 mm.

16.00 mm diameters are available from some small manufacturers. BOZRs range from 7.80 mm to 9.00 mm and are selected only about 0.3 mm flatter than 'K' for diameters up to 14.00 mm. The range is steeper than with lower water content lenses because the softer materials require fitting closer to 'K' to ensure stability.

Practical advice

- Try more than one lens design, because different makes can give very different acuities.
- Always over-refract with the type of lens to be used, since the BVP may vary by at least 1.00 D between different designs.
- Centration also varies with design and lenticulation.

CONTINUOUS WEAR (see also Chapter 21)

Elderly aphakics who are unable to handle lenses may leave them in continuously. Careful practitioner management and regular aftercare visits are extremely important, since most documented infections associated with extended wear have been with this type of patient [3.]

Lens movement is especially important because of overnight dehydration and the need to ensure the removal of debris. A saline eyewash in the morning and evening can be recommended, ideally using minims. Deposits are a major problem and some patients need a new lens every 3–6 months.

31.2 Keratoconus

Keratoconus is the classic case in which a hard contact lens provides a new refracting surface for an irregular cornea and gives good acuity where spectacles are unable to manage adequate improvement. Corneal lenses are the preferred form of correction in the early stages of the condition.

The apex of the cone is usually displaced inferior and nasal relative to the pupil. The common problem in all keratoconus fitting is to make the BOZD of the lens, which tends to centre at the apex of the cone, sufficiently large to cover the pupil area without the formation of either dimples or a stagnant pool of tears.

Keratometry readings are typically steep, astigmatic and irregular, except in the early stages. As the cone advances, readings eventually fall outside the range of the instrument, although this can be extended with a supplementary plus lens (*see* Section 2.2.4). Modern autokeratometers have a much greater range and despite corneal distortion can sometimes gives readings as steep as 4–5 mm.

The main problems with keratoconus fitting are:

- Decentration on the irregular cornea.
- Discomfort because of increased lid and corneal sensitivity.
- Photophobia (helped by a tint).
- Lens thickness because of the high negative power
- Dimpling, which may necessitate fenestrations or a change in peripheral design.
- Oedema, often due to lack of lens mobility and reduced tears exchange.

31.2.1 Hard lenses

The three major techniques[4] for fitting hard lenses in keratoconus are:

1. Flat, or *two-point touch*, with primary lens support on the apex of the cornea, where the central optic zone of the lens touches or bears on the corneal apex.
2. Divided support, or *three-point touch*, with lens support and bearing shared between the corneal apex and the paracentral cornea.
3. Steep, with lens support and bearing directed off the apex and onto the paracentral cornea, with clearance or vaulting of the corneal apex.

SPHERICAL LENSES TO GIVE TWO-POINT TOUCH

- Use the apex of the cone as a fulcrum.
- Allow the lens to be held by the top lid to achieve a high-riding fitting.
- Need to be fitted sufficiently flat to allow for lid attachment.
- Possibly change the non-affected part of the cornea by mechanical pressure.

SPHERICAL LENSES TO GIVE THREE-POINT TOUCH

- The BOZR is chosen on or near the flattest 'K'.

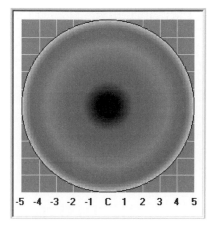

-5 -4 -3 -2 -1   C   1   2   3   4   5

Figure 31.1 Typical 'bull's-eye' fluorescein pattern (dark shading represents the fluorescein)

- The BOZD is between 5.00 mm and 7.00 mm.
- The TD ranges from 8.50 mm to 9.50 mm.
- The peripheral curves are designed to flatten off rapidly to follow the topography of the cornea.
- When the patient is using the cone area, the BVP is usually much higher minus than expected because of the steep BOZR. In advanced cases, the patient may use the periconal area and require less power.

The optimum three-point touch fluorescein fit (Figure 31.1) gives the overall effect of a 'bulls-eye' pattern. There is touch on the cone surrounded by a ring of fluorescein which is in turn surrounded by an annulus of mid-peripheral bearing with peripheral edge clearance. If the central touch is too heavy, it may allow rocking of the lens and cause corneal abrasion. This can be improved either by changing the BOZR or by altering the degree of peripheral bearing.

Typical trial lenses:[5]

5.50:5.60/6.50:7.60/8.50:8.60   –11.00
6.50:6.00/7.50:8.00/9.50:9.00   –5.50
7.00:6.00/8.00:8.20/10.00:9.20   –3.00

Rule of thumb

A change in radius of 0.05 mm ≡ 0.50 D with lenses steeper than 6.90 mm

---

Rule of thumb

Select the initial BOZD to be approximately equal to the BOZR + 0.20 mm (e.g. 7.40 mm with 7.20 mm radius; 6.20 mm with 6.00 mm radius).

The rule that a radius change of 0.05 mm $\equiv$ 0.25 D breaks down because of the very steep curves.

APICAL CLEARANCE LENSES

- A spherical central zone is chosen to vault the apex of the cone with minimum clearance.
- A spherical or non-conic peripheral zone is designed to slide over the flatter superior corneal surface.
- In some cases a junctionless transitional zone is used, broad enough to allow adequate edge clearance.
- Careful selection of the peripheral curves achieves best fitting results.

SPHERICAL LENSES TO FIT THE CORNEAL PERIPHERY

In fairly early keratoconus, especially with large corneas, lenses can be fitted on the basis of matching the relatively unchanged corneal periphery[6] but with the addition of a much steeper BOZR. The actual peripheral curves are very similar to those found in a lens designed for a normal cornea, but to allow for the steep centre a tricurve becomes a four- or possibly five-curve lens.

Examples:

'K' 6.60 mm along 170°   × 6.10 mm along 65°
    central fitting   peripheral fitting
    6.75:7.00/   7.80:7.70/8.60:8.50/10.50:9.50

'K' 6.60 mm along 50°   other meridian off the scale
    central fitting   peripheral fitting
    6.90:7.10/7.70:7.60/   8.50:8.20/9.30:9.00/10.50:10.00

'K' 6.25 mm along 65°   other meridian off the scale
    central fitting   peripheral fitting
    6.50:6.80/7.20:7.40/   8.20:8.20/9.00:9.00/10.50:9.60/
                      12.25:10.00

OFFSET AND ASPHERIC LENSES

These designs have the advantage that, if the conical zone of the cornea lies in front of the visual axis, a small-diameter lens can be fitted.

- The BOZR is chosen on flattest 'K' to give an area of central touch.
- The BOZD varies from 2.00 mm for a true conoid to 7.70 mm for some offsets.
- The TD is typically 8.00 mm, but may be as small as 7.00 mm.
- Axial edge lift is the standard 0.10–0.15 mm and assessed by fluorescein.
- Fenestrations may be used to improve tears exchange and reduce frothing.
- A parabolic curve with edge flattening of 0.7 mm (e.g. Zeiss) is sometimes useful when it is no longer feasible to fit spherical or aspheric lenses.
- Typical offset trial lens[7]: 6.00:5.50/AEL (ff) 0.1 at 8.50.

ELLIPTICAL 'K' (PERSECON E)

The design has a bi-elliptical back surface and works well for early keratoconus, especially where patients have large pupils.[8]

- The BOZR is chosen on flattest 'K'.
- The optic zone is 8.00–8.50 mm, allowing an even pressure distribution over the lens centre.
- The TD is either 9.30 mm or 9.80 mm.
- The eccentricity of 0.39 is the same as that of the standard Persecon E (see Section 11.2).
- The peripheral zone flattening has an elliptical curve of the same eccentricity but flatter vertex radius.[9]

The design is predetermined by the laboratory, so that if the fluorescein pattern is unsatisfactory another type of fitting should be used.

ASPHERIC PERIPHERY LENSES

Designed with a spherical back surface and either a flatter edge curve with an aspheric edge (e.g. Conflex/KE) or a spherical back surface with an aspheric-type peripheral bevel for greater edge lift (Aspheri-KD).

SHEPHARD ACUITY LENSES

Fitted from a trial set with a combined aspheric and multicurve design. Each lens is categorized according to a cone radius. A trial lens is selected on the basis of flattest 'K'.

Parameters available:

Radii	4.60 mm to 8.00 mm (0.20 mm steps)
Cone diameter	6.20 mm
Lens diameter	9.60 mm
Material	High *Dk* fluorocarbon

The Shephard design is useful for cases of advanced keratoconus more usually found in hospital contact lens practice.[10]

ROSE K LENS

A multicurve lens with spherical radii clearing the flat mid-peripheral and peripheral cornea. The radii are blended to form a controlled 'aspheric' peripheral lens geometry. These curves can be adjusted to give a looser or tighter peripheral fit.

- TD: 7.90 mm to 10.20 mm. Usually 8.70 mm is used; if not, then as the TD is increased or decreased the BOZD and secondary curve widths are also increased or decreased in a fixed ratio.
- Base curves: 4.75 mm to 8.00 mm.
- To keep pooling at the base of the cone to a minimum, the back optic zone must decrease as the base curve steepens. It will vary with diameter.
- The secondary curve width will vary with diameter.
- AELs: standard, flat and steep, increasing as the base curve is steepened.
- Choose a trial lens 0.20 mm steeper than average K.
- ª Initially obtain a light touch at the cone apex. A low riding lens means the radius is too steep or the optic zone too large.
- Consider the peripheral fit and order increased or decreased edge lift as needed. It is acceptable to have lower edge stand-off and it may be needed to ensure adequate superior alignment.
- Smaller TDs work well on steep corneas (8.10 to 8.30 mm). A large TD will tend to make the lens sit higher.

General advice on keratoconus

- Do not fit too steep as this may result in a large air bubble.
- The steeper the radius, the higher the minus power.
- Small changes in BOZR can give larger than expected changes in refraction.
- Modifying peripheral curves can affect the lens position and the required BVP.
- Even if the first trial lens is not ideal, over-refract to get an idea of the likely acuity. It is always better to assess the vision with at least two trial lenses.
- Lens design may depend on visual improvement.
- Expect to use at least two lenses per eye.
- The first lens can be made in PMMA and the final lens in a modern material.
- Sometimes a high Dk material is less comfortable than a low Dk material.
- Sometimes PMMA is the most comfortable of all.
- PMMA is more stable and can be made thinner.

31.2.2 Soft lenses

Soft lenses can sometimes be used for keratoconus, depending upon the degree of corneal distortion. Centre thickness is deliberately increased or a conical back surface used.

SPHERICAL SOFT LENSES

The minimum centre thickness should be 0.35 mm, but 0.60 mm is advisable. The edge is reduced to 0.18 mm by means of lenticulation. A relatively rigid +5.00 D HEMA lens masks a considerable degree of corneal distortion and reasonable acuity may be obtained with the additional use of spectacles.

TRAPEZOID LENSES

The trapezoid lens is designed to vault the conical area of the cornea.[11] The back surface has a central portion between 11.00 mm and 15.00 mm in radius, with a steeper peripheral curve of 8.50 mm. The TD is 15.00 mm, and a third curve of radius 9.50 mm is introduced if the edge is too tight.

The lenses are made in HEMA for rigidity, with a centre thickness of 0.60 mm and low plus power. Some degree of corneal moulding occurs, but it is less than with a conventional lens. The fitting depends on the size and steepness of the cone and should be assessed with a trial lens.

Example:

HEMA trapezoid trial lens:
12.00:8.50/8.00:14.00/9.00:15.00   +5.00 D t_c 0.60 mm

SCLERAL SOFT LENSES

A multicurve soft scleral lens with a diameter of 23.00 mm can be designed from a mould of the eye using a shadowgraph.

31.3 Corneal grafts (keratoplasty)

31.3.1 Hard lenses

The main considerations are:

- The size of the graft. It is better to keep the TD within the limits of the graft tissue.
- The tilt of the graft, which may cause a problem in position and stability. Lens decentration often occurs but is acceptable if the graft is not compromised.
- Stability. Sometimes a very large lens (> 12.00 mm) is necessary even to stay on the cornea with blinking.
- Staining of the grafted tissue is less acceptable than with a normal cornea and requires careful observation. Any coalescent areas are unacceptable.

Examples:
Offset 1   7.60:6.50/AEL (ff) 0.10 at 8.50
Apex   7.80:8.00/10.50:12.50

REVERSE GEOMETRY LENSES

It is sometimes beneficial to fit reverse geometry lenses consisting of :

- A spherical back optic zone.
- An aspheric intermediate curve,1.00 D flatter than the equivalent intermediate curve for standard reverse geometry lenses (*see* Section 8.6).

- An aspheric peripheral curve, wider than that used for a standard reverse geometry design.

31.3.2 Soft lenses

A soft bandage lens can compress or mould a low rigidity graft or realign a partially everted graft and is often used as a protective membrane immediately the sutures have been inserted. Soft lenses are also used to treat graft rejection. The soft 'splint' is often kept in place for several weeks.

31.4 Corneal irregularity

31.4.1 Hard gas permeable lenses

The initial lens is chosen on the basis of the best keratometry readings obtainable. The lens is fitted in the normal way, but the fluorescein pattern nearly always shows the irregularity of the corneal surface. The fitting is decided according to visual improvement. In some cases a small amount of apical clearance gives stability and good vision, whereas in others alignment or touch is necessary. The TD may need to be larger than normal for lens stability.

Bubbles over an irregular area can cause long-term corneal desiccation and may ultimately require a scleral lens.

31.4.2 Soft lenses

Soft lenses usually conform too closely to the cornea to give any great optical benefit. Some improvement is occasionally achieved with a thick lens or rigid material (e.g. CSI).

31.5 High myopia and hypermetropia

31.5.1 Hard gas permeable lenses

The main problem with powers over +10.00 D is the lens mass. Stability and position may be improved by fitting:

- A TD about 0.50 mm larger than usual.
- On mean 'K' to show apical clearance with the fluorescein pattern.
- Lid attachment (hitch-up) lenses (*see* Section 7.5).

- A reduced optic and ordering the optimum design of carrier (e.g. parallel for a high minus with tight lids; negative for high plus).

31.5.2 Soft lenses

The main difficulty with myopes is the mass of material at the limbus. Even with a reduced optic, long-term problems such as oedema and vascularization can arise. The size of the optic is important: HO3 and HO4 lenses (Bausch & Lomb) have a large optic and greater average thickness, whereas CSI (Pilkington) have a small optic and more satisfactory thickness. The highest power normally available is −22.00 D, which is equivalent to −35.00 D in spectacle form.

Hypermetropes, on the other hand, have all the lens mass centrally. This can cause central oedema even with high water content materials. A normal cornea is under greater stress than an aphakic eye because it has higher oxygen demands.

Radii are chosen in the normal way, but larger overall sizes are necessary to aid stability.

Practical advice

- Use a trial lens close to the anticipated power to give an accurate assessment of both BVP and fitting.
- Ensure that the back and front surface designs are consistent when replacing a lens to avoid visual and fitting difficulties.

31.6 Albinos

Hard lenses do not always give visual improvement despite frequently heavy and restrictive spectacles for bilateral hypermetropic astigmatism. Magnification is lost by fitting a contact lens and the cylinder gives unstable vision. The main benefit of contact lenses is to help photophobia by means of a tint, and occasionally soft lenses may also be used (*see* Section 25.2). Adaptation is a stressful period and any nystagmus can increase initially, although it tends to stabilize once the lenses have settled down. Nystagmus sometimes reduces where vision is improved.

31.7 Radial keratotomy and photo-refractive keratectomy

Radial keratotomy (RK) is a surgical technique to reduce myopia by flattening the cornea with radial incisions.

Photo-refractive keratectomy (PRK) is a laser technique to sculpt the central corneal surface producing a reduction in myopia, hypermetropia or astigmatism. Following PRK in myopes, the peripheral cornea retains its normal contour but the central, ablated zone is much flatter.

Hard lens fitting with conventional designs for both RK and PRK results in central fluorescein pooling, although an acceptable fit may sometimes be achieved using aspherics (e.g. Quantum, Persecon E). Reverse geometry lenses can often give much better corneal alignment and improved comfort (*see* Section 31.3.1). Lenses are best designed from topographical maps of the cornea (*see* Section 8.5 to avoid the use of numerous trial lenses.

Soft lens designs can work with RK and PRK, but trial and error is often necessary to find a lens that fits adequately, achieves good centration and avoids bubble formation.

References

1. Fraser, J.P. and Gordon, S.P. (1967) The 'apex' lens for uniocular aphakia. *Ophthalmic Optician*, **7**, 1190–1253
2. Bagshaw, J., Gordon, S.A.P. and Stanworth, A. (1966) A modified corneal contact lens: binocular single vision in unilateral aphakia. *British Orthoptic Journal*, **23**, 19–30
3. Carpel, E. and Parker, P. (1985) Extended wear aphakic contact lens fitting in high risk patients. *Contact Lens Association of Ophthalmologists Journal*, **11**, 231–233
4. Korb, D.R., Finnemore, V.M. and Herman, J.P. (1982) Apical changes and scarring in keratoconus related to contact lens fitting techniques. *Journal of the American Optometric Association*, **53**, 199–205
5. Woodward, E.G. (1997) Contact lenses in abnormal ocular conditions – keratoconus. In *Contact Lenses*, A.J. Phillips and L. Speedwell (eds), Butterworth-Heinemann, Oxford, pp. 693–706
6. Shephard, A.W. (1989) Keratoconus contact lens fitting. *Journal of the British Contact Lens Association* (Scientific Meetings 1989), pp. 21–25
7. Ruben, M. (1975) *Contact Lens Practice*, Baillière-Tindall, London, pp. 283–284
8. Astin, C. (1987) Fitting of keratoconus patients with bi-elliptical contact lenses. *The Journal of the British Contact Lens Association*, **10**, 24–28
9. Achatz, M., Eschmann, R., Rockert, H., Wilken, B. and Grant, R. (1985) Keratoconus – a new approach using bi-elliptical contact lenses. *Optometry Today*, **25**, 581–586
10. Hood, A. (1997) Advanced contact lens fitting part three: hospital contact lens practice. *Optician*, **214** (5612), 16–22
11. Ruben, M. (1978) *Soft Contact Lenses*. Baillière-Tindall, London, pp. 256–260

Chapter 32

Other lenses for therapeutic fitting

32.1 Scleral lenses

VISUAL INDICATIONS

- Ocular topography makes corneal lens fitting difficult.
- Eccentric pupils.
- Where a high-powered corneal or soft lens fails to centre.

PROTECTIVE INDICATIONS

- Tears retention in some dry-eye conditions (e.g. Stevens–Johnson syndrome, Sjögren's syndrome).
- Corneal exposure (e.g. inadequate lid closure, exophthalmic precorneal tear film failure).
- Fornix support (e.g. following reconstruction surgery, alkali burn).
- Entropion and trichiasis.
- Protection for anaesthetic cornea.
- Occlusion.
- Ptosis.

FITTING INDICATIONS

- Poor centration with other designs.
- Poor stability with a corneal lens.

Impression fitting is the preferred method because it can deal with virtually any eye. Subsequent lens modifications are made according to the specific condition.

A ptosis prop is made by using a shelf-type support by cutting through the full thickness of a 2–3 mm thick shell.[1]

In symblepharon, a hard scleral ring can be used. This is usually 4 mm wide and is effectively the scleral portion without the optic.

32.2 Combination lenses

32.2.1 'Piggy-back' lenses

The combination of a hard lens on top of a soft lens is used with keratoconus and graft cases to achieve good vision with improved comfort where all else has failed.[2]

The foundation soft lens has a large diameter for stability and a typical front surface radius of about 7.60 mm. This is achieved by altering the power of the best fitting, so that a minus lens is necessary for 'K' readings between 6.00 mm and 7.00 mm. A low plus lens is required if the cornea is flatter than 8.00 mm.

The hard lens has a TD of 9.50 mm or larger to give good centration. The BOZR is based on the front surface curvature of the soft lens, measured with the keratometer.

The problems with combination lenses are:

- An extensive trial set of large steep soft lenses is required to find a satisfactory fitting.
- Stabilizing the hard lens on the soft lens takes practice.
- Different solutions are needed for each part of the combination.
- Lenses are removed separately. In some cases, the soft part is used for extended wear with the hard lens put in place to help vision during the day.

The reverse combination of a corneal hard lens covered by a thin soft lens is used for sporting purposes.

32.2.2 Hard centre with soft periphery

This combination (e.g. Softperm) is designed to give the acuity of hard lenses with the comfort of soft.

The hard central portion has a diameter of 8.00 mm and is made from synergicon A material. The soft peripheral flange has a diameter of 14.30 mm. The basic fittings consist of radii from 7.10 mm to 8.10 mm in 0.1 mm steps and the first choice of lens is near to flattest 'K'. Fitting characteristics of movement and centration are based on soft lens criteria.[3] Large molecular weight fluorescein can be used.

Problems prior to Softperm were:

- The soft skirt detaching from the hard centre.
- Bubbles often forming at the hard–soft transition not eliminated by a change in fitting.
- Lenses fitting tightly to the eye, making removal difficult.
- The solutions must be compatible with both hard and soft lenses. Peroxide is now recommended.
- The low *Dk* of current materials.

32.2.3 Flexible lenses (e.g. Epicon)

The Epicon (Ultravision/Igel) is a flexible lens, in carbosilfocon material, mainly designed to be used for keratoconus and after keratoplasty, PRK and RK. The lens has a TD of 13.5 mm to vault over the limbal area. The BOZRs range from 6.4 mm to 7.6 mm and the aspheric peripheries come in four 'lifts', progressively flattening from A to D. The fit is checked with fluorescein in the normal way. Lenses are maintained with soft lens multifunction solutions and non-abrasive cleaners.[4]

Epicon K, specifically designed for for keratoconus, is fitted with light apical touch. The sagittal depth and degree of touch are adjusted by choosing flatter or steeper base curves while maintaining peripheral alignment. Lens movement and tears exchange are essential to avoid adhesion to the cornea.

32.3 Silicone lenses

Silicone lenses (*see* Section 6.5) have the following therapeutic uses:[5]

- Aphakia.
- Dry eyes, especially following therapy.
- Exposure problems following lid reconstruction.
- Corneal perforations.
- Corneal ulceration.

Trial sets consist of radii from 7.40 mm to 8.40 mm, with diameters from 11.70 mm to 13.20 mm in 0.50 mm steps (Zeiss) and 10.80 mm (Danker). A wide range of powers is available, including plano and aphakic.

ADVANTAGES

- Very high *Dk* permits continuous wear.
- Good vision.
- They do not dehydrate and are ideal for dry eyes or tear film problems.
- Low risk of loss or damage.
- Good for corneal reconstruction. The radius can be refitted as the cornea reforms under the lens.
- Resistance to bacterial colonization and therefore ideal for eyes open to infection.
- They do not absorb foreign substances, so medication can be used without fear of contamination.
- Fluorescein can be used to ensure the optimum fitting.

DISADVANTAGES

- Difficult to fit.
- Surfaces deposits. Six-monthly replacements are advisable.
- Lenses can be difficult to remove.
- Adhesion can occur with lenses fitted either too steep or too flat.
- Expensive.

32.4 Bandage lenses

Soft bandage lenses are used on an extended wear basis to relieve pain and allow denuded epithelium to regain its normal structure. They are available in high or low water contents and are usually of plano power, since they are not primarily intended for visual improvement.[6] Lenses are not generally handled by the patient and may require replacing every 4–8 weeks because of deposits. They are ideally fitted from stock and are used in cases of:

- Chronic keratitis.
- Post-keratoplasty.
- Bullous keratopathy.
- Exposure keratitis.

- Recurrent erosions.
- Corneal perforation.

32.4.1 General considerations

- Low water content is better where there is a tear film problem because it dehydrates less (e.g. exposure keratitis).
- High water content is better where a painful eye needs several weeks of continuous wear (e.g. bullous keratopathy).
- 'K' readings are not usually possible. A good starting point with a high water content lens is 8.50:14.50.
- Radii range from 7.80 mm to 9.50 mm, the flatter lenses often being made in the higher water content materials.
- Diameters vary between 13.50 mm and 16.50 mm, the larger lenses being made in the higher water content materials.
- Centre thickness varies between 0.10 mm and 0.25 mm, the lower water content lenses being thinner.
- Some lenses such as the Plano T (Bausch & Lomb) are one-fit.

32.5 Additional therapeutic uses

DRUG-RELEASE LENSES

Soft lenses or shields of a collagen material are used as a drug release mechanism.[7]

LOW-VISION AID

A Galilean telescope can be of benefit to the low-vision patient, but its cosmetic appearance is improved by using a high minus contact lens as the eyepiece. The powers required to achieve a minimum ×1.5 magnification are at least −25.00 D for the contact lens and +20.00 D for the spectacle lens. The problems are that the field of view reduces as the powers increase, and movement of the contact lens causes apparent movement of the visual field. However, the technique has been used with occasional success.[8,9]

VETERINARY BANDAGE LENSES

Veterinary bandage lenses (e.g. i-protex/Cantor & Silver) represent a good alternative to tarsorraphy to promote corneal healing.

They can be used on the eyes of cats, dogs, horses and lions for a wide variety of conditions including symblepharon, bullous keratopathy, adnexal problems, indolent ulcers and following superficial keratectomy. Lenses usually have a 74% water content and TDs of up to 25 mm. They are marked with a coloured dot for ease of viewing on the eye.

References

1. Trodd, T.C. (1971) Ptosis props in ocular myopathy. *Contact Lens*, **3**, 3–5
2. Westerhout, D.I. (1973) The combination lens and therapeutic uses of soft lenses. *The Contact Lens Journal*, **4**, 3–22
3. Astin, C. (1985) Saturn II lenses and penetrating keratoplasty. *Transactions of the British Contact Lens Association Annual Clinical Conference*, **2**, 2–5
4. Sturm, B. (1994) Development of the Ultracon and Epicon. *Optical Prism*, January, 25–28
5. Woodward, E.G. (1984) Therapeutic silicone rubber lenses. *Journal of the British Contact Lens Association*, **7**, 39–40
6. Astin, C.L.K. (1991) Therapeutic contact lenses – an overview of some lens types. *Journal of the British Contact Lens Association*, **14** (3), 129–133
7. Weissman, B. and Lee, D. (1988) Oxygen transmissibility, thickness and water content of three types of collagen shields. *Archives of Ophthalmology*, **106**, 1706
8. Silver, J.H. and Woodward, E.G. (1978) Driving with a visual disability – case report. *Ophthalmic Optician*, **18**, 794–795
9. Speedwell, L. (1986) 'Yet it does move' A successful and inadvertent Galilean telescopic system. *Optometry Today*, **26**, 109

Glossary of contact lens-related terms

*Denotes separate entry.

ANOXIA: The complete absence of oxygen.

APICAL CLEARANCE (apical pooling): A contact lens fitting, usually steep, in which there is a pool of tears between the back surface of a hard lens and the anterior surface of the corneal apex. Generally observed with *fluorescein.

APICAL TOUCH: A contact lens fitting, usually flat, in which the back surface of the lens rests on the apex of the cornea. Generally observed with *fluorescein.

ASEPTICIZATION: *See* pasteurization.

ASPHERIC (aspherical) LENS: Lens design where one or both surfaces are of non-spherical construction. Aspherics usually take the form of a parabola, ellipse or hyperbola, and are defined by *eccentricity.

AUTOCLAVE: Instrument for heat sterilization of contact lenses under pressure, usually at a temperature of 121°C for a minimum of 15 minutes.

AXIAL EDGE LIFT (AEL): Distance between a point on the back surface of a lens at a specified diameter and the continuation of the back central optic zone, measured parallel to the lens axis.

BACK OPTIC ZONE DIAMETER (BOZD): Diameter of the central, optic zone of a contact lens. Previously known as the optic diameter.

BACK OPTIC ZONE RADIUS (BOZR): Radius of curvature of the central, optic zone of a hard contact lens; previously known as back central optic radius (BCOR).

BACK PERIPHERAL RADIUS (BPR): Radius of curvature of a peripheral curve of a contact lens.

BACK SURFACE TORIC: Lens design where part or all of the back surface is of toric construction. The front surface may be either spherical, or toroidal in which case it is a *bitoric.

BANDAGE LENS: Soft contact lens used to protect the cornea, reduce pain and assist healing in conditions such as bullous keratopathy, ulcers and burns.

BASE CURVE: Term used to specify the back optic radius of a soft contact lens. For hard lenses, see back optic zone radius.

BI-ASPHERIC: Lens design having a back surface consisting of two different aspheric curves.

BICURVE: Lens design consisting of the central radius and one peripheral curve.

BIOCOMPATIBILITY: The ability of a material to interface with a natural substance without provoking a biological response.

BIOMIMESIS: Where the principles of the complex structure and chemistry of nature are emulated by much simpler scientific means which nevertheless achieve the same results.

BITORIC: Lens design with both front and back surfaces of toric construction.

BLENDING: The smoothing of a lens *transition with a curve intermediate between the two radii. Blending may be light, medium or heavy.

BREAK-UP TIME (BUT): The time in seconds for the break up of the precorneal tears film in a non-blinking eye. Generally observed with fluorescein and the slit lamp. A normal eye has a BUT of 15 seconds or greater. An important diagnostic test in assessing dry eyes (see non-invasive break-up time).

BULLOUS KERATOPATHY: A degeneration of the cornea, often following trauma, resulting in vesicles or bullae which cause severe pain on bursting. Frequently assisted by the use of a *bandage lens.

BURTON LAMP: A source of ultraviolet (blue) light of approximate wavelength 400 nm used to excite *fluorescein and for observation.

CARRIER (BS): That part of a lenticulated lens surrounding the front optic zone.

CAST MOULDING: Method of soft lens manufacture employing heat and closed moulds.

COMPRESSION MOULDING: Method of hard lens manufacture employing granules of polymer, heat and pressure.

CONDITIONING SOLUTION: A storage solution used to enhance the biocompatibility of lens surfaces.

CONOID: Design of fenestrated PMMA lens introduced in the 1960s fitted 0.3 mm steeper than 'K'. Noted cause of corneal moulding.

CONSTANT AXIAL EDGE LIFT (CAEL): A lens design in which the axial edge lift of the peripheral curves is calculated to remain constant for all BOZRs in a series.

CONTACT ANGLE: Angle formed by a tangent to a sessile drop of fluid at the point where the drop meets a surface. A more wettable material has a smaller angle of contact. The angle is 0° for a completely hydrophilic material.

CONTACT LENS-INDUCED PAPILLARY CONJUNCTIVITIS (CLIPC); giant papillary conjunctivitis: Condition of the palpebral conjunctiva characterized by the presence of large papillae. Suggested causes with contact lens wearers are allergic, mechanical and chemical.

CONTINUOUS WEAR: The use of contact lenses without removal for periods in excess of 1 week. *See* *extended wear and *flexible wear.

CONVENTIONAL LENS: Soft lens intended for repeated, non-disposable use.

CORNEAL EXHAUSTION: Loss of tolerance to contact lenses from long-term hypoxia resulting in chronic oedema.

CORNEAL LENS: A hard gas-permeable lens fitted within the area of the cornea. Typical overall sizes are 8.50–10.00 mm.

CORNEAL MOULDING: Change in corneal curvature caused by the presence of a contact lens. Predominantly associated with PMMA-induced oedema but also found with hard gas-permeable lenses, especially aspherics, and occasionally with soft lenses.

DIMPLING: The formation of trapped air bubbles beneath a contact lens. Usually associated with hard lenses but can also occur with soft lenses.

DISINFECTION: The process of reducing the number of viable micro-organisms to a level which is harmful neither to ocular health nor to the quality of contact lenses and accessories.

DISPOSABLE LENS: Soft lens designed for frequent replacement, usually on a daily, weekly or monthly basis.

Dk and *Dk/t*: *See* oxygen permeability and oxygen transmissibility.

ECCENTRICITY: Defines mathematically the departure of an aspheric curve from a circle. Used to describe both a lens form or the curvature of the cornea which has a typical eccentricity of 0.5.

EDGE LIFT: *See* Axial edge lift and radial edge lift.

EXPIRY DATE: The date, designated by the manufacturer, beyond which a product should not be first used.

EXTENDED WEAR: The regular use of contact lenses without removal, overnight or during sleep, for periods of up to 1 week. *See* flexible wear and continuous wear.

FENESTRATED LENS FOR OPTIC MEASUREMENT (FLOM): A diagnostic hard lens with typical overall size of 13.50–14.50 mm, used to assess the optic fitting and power of a scleral lens.

FENESTRATION: A ventilation hole drilled in a contact lens. Provides additional oxygen to the cornea and may assist the dispersal of air bubbles or dimples.

FLEXIBLE WEAR: The intermittent use of contact lenses overnight or during sleep.

FLEXURE: The bending of a soft contact lens fitted flatter or steeper than 'K' to conform to the corneal curvature. Usually applied to soft lenses where negative power is induced, but also applicable to steep-fitting hard lenses where visual distortion may occur.

FLUORESCEIN (sodium fluorescein): A dye which stains live tissue, used in 1% solution or by applicator strips to (1) reveal lesions in the corneal or conjunctival epithelium; (2) assess hard lens fitting characteristics; and (3) evaluate tears film (see break-up time). The dye is orange under white light but fluoresces bright green when excited by ultraviolet light. Molecular weight 330.

FLUOROSILICON ACRYLATES: Hard lens copolymers composed of fluoromonomers and siloxy acrylate monomers. Sometimes loosely called fluorocarbons.

FOOD AND DRUGS ADMINISTRATION (FDA): The regulatory authority in the USA that licenses the manufacture and supply of contact lenses, solutions and ancillary products.

FREQUENT REPLACEMENT: The regular replacement of soft lenses at predetermined intervals, usually at 1, 3 or 6 months. *See* disposable lenses.

FRONT SURFACE TORIC: Lens with a spherical back surface and toroidal front surface, used for the correction of *residual astigmatism. Stabilization is necessary to control axis orientation.

GHOST VESSELS: Vessels in the cornea caused by vascularization and which have emptied of blood after the removal of the stimulus (e.g. hypoxic or chemical).

GIANT PAPILLARY CONJUNCTIVITIS (GPC): also called *contact lens-induced papillary conjunctivitis. Condition of the palpebral conjunctiva characterized by the presence of large papillae. Suggested contact lens causes are allergic, mechanical and chemical.

HARD GAS-PERMEABLES: Hard lenses made from materials such as *silicon acrylates and *fluorosilicon acrylates which permit the flow through their structure of gases, particularly oxygen and carbon dioxide.

HYDRATION: The uptake of water by a hydrogel material.

HYDROGEL: A material made from a hydrogel polymer which absorbs and binds water into its molecular structure. Describes those lenses which have a percentage water content, although not all hydrogels are necessarily soft.

HYDROPHILIC (water loving): Frequently used as a synonym for soft lenses but more properly applied to define the surface characteristic of a material in relation to its wetting angle.

HYDROPHOBIC (water hating): A surface characteristic of a material which causes the surface to repel water.

HYPERCAPNIA. The accumulation of carbon dioxide within the ocular tissues.

HYPOXIA: Reduced supply of oxygen to the ocular tissues.

IMPRESSION LENS: *Scleral lens fitted by taking a mould of the eye.

INDUCED ASTIGMATISM: Astigmatism created optically when a toric lens is fitted on the cornea because of the difference in the refractive index between tears and contact lens material.

INFILTRATES: Inflammatory cells within the cornea occurring as a response to viral or other infection, toxic or chemical stimulus. Typically seen as greyish disciform patches near the limbus.

ISOTONIC SOLUTION: A solution having the same tonicity as 0.9% sodium chloride.

KERATOMETER: *See* ophthalmometer.

LID-ATTACHMENT: Hard lens fitting technique to ensure that the lens periphery is held in a superior 'hitch-up' position by the upper lid and moves with it on blinking. Reduces lid sensation and can avoid 3 and 9 o'clock staining.

MICROCYSTS: Small vesicles in the corneal epithelium containing fluid and cellular debris. Occur as a typical response to corneal stress, particularly extended wear.

MICRON; micrometre (µm): Unit of length (1/1000th of a mm or 10^{-6} m) used, for example, in defining *tear layer thickness.

MONOVISION: Technique for correcting presbyopia in which reading addition is incorporated into the contact lens for the non-dominant eye.

MULTICURVE: Lens design consisting of the central radius and multiple peripheral curves.

NEOVASCULARIZATION: Growth of blood vessels within the corneal stroma towards the pupil area (see vascularization).

NEUTRALIZATION: The process by which active ingredients in contact lens care products are rendered inactive and non-toxic to ocular tissues. Usually applied to systems containing hydrogen peroxide.

NON-INVASIVE BREAK-UP TIME (NIBUT): Methods used to measure the stability of the tears film without a staining agent, employing a cold diffuse light source or grid pattern for observation (see Break-up time).

OPHTHALMOMETER (keratometer): Instrument used for measuring the curvature of the anterior surface of the cornea. Can also be used to measure the radius of curvature of a contact lens.

OPTIC ZONE DIAMETER: Diameter of a specified optic zone, measured to the surrounding junction. If the latter is not circular, the major and minor diameters define the size. N.B. The term may be qualified, for example, 'back central optic zone diameter'.

ORTHOKERATOLOGY: The reduction, modification or elimination of a visual defect by the programmed application of contact lenses. The technique for reducing myopia consists of changing the shape of the cornea by fitting a series of hard lenses progressively flatter than 'K'.

OVER-REFRACTION: Refraction carried out with a contact lens on the eye.

OVERWEAR SYNDROME (acute epithelial necrosis; 3 am syndrome): Extreme, painful response to gross corneal oedema as a result of excessive contact lens wear. Usually found with PMMA and typically occurring in the middle of the night.

OXYGEN PERMEABILITY (*Dk*): The rate of oxygen flow under specified conditions through the unit area of contact lens material of unit thickness when subjected to unit pressure difference.

OXYGEN TRANSMISSIBILITY (*Dk/t*): The value for oxygen permeability divided by the thickness of the measured sample under specified conditions.

PACHOMETER (pachymeter): Instrument for measuring the thickness of the cornea using optical alignment.

PASTEURIZATION: Method of lens disinfection employing heat which reduces micro-organisms to a safe level. Falls short of the absolute efficacy of *sterilization.

PERMEABILITY. See oxygen permeability.

PHOTO-REFRACTIVE KERATECTOMY: Surgical technique employing a laser beam to sculpt the central corneal surface. Reduces myopia, hypermetropia or astigmatism.

PLACIDO DISC: Instrument to assess qualitatively the regularity of the cornea or a contact lens surface using concentric circles and a magnifying lens. An illuminated version is known as a Klein keratoscope and when combined with a camera as a photokeratoscope.

PMMA (polymethyl methacrylate): The plastics material from which nearly all rigid lenses were made prior to the introduction of *hard gas-permeables. Also known as perspex or plexiglas

POLYMEGATHISM: Irregularity in the size of cells of the corneal endothelium. Observed in extended wear and in long-standing PMMA wearers.

PREFORMED LENS: Scleral lens fitted from trial sets without taking a mould of the eye.

PRESERVATIVE: Agent intended to prevent the growth of micro-organisms in a care product.

PRISM BALLAST: The use in a contact lens of base down prism as a weighting or stabilizing device to assist with correct orientation on the eye in toric or bifocal fitting. The amount of prism is usually between $1^\triangle$ and $2^\triangle$. $3^\triangle$ is about the maximum available.

RADIAL EDGE LIFT (REL; 'Z' factor): Distance between a point on the back surface of a lens at a specified diameter and the continuation of the back central optic zone, measured along a radius of curvature of the latter.

RADIAL KERATOTOMY (RK): Surgical technique to reduce myopia by flattening the cornea with radial incisions.

RADIUSCOPE: Instrument used to measure the radius of curvature of a contact lens by means of Drysdale's method.

RESIDUAL ASTIGMATISM: Uncorrected astigmatism found by refraction when a spherical contact lens is placed on the cornea. Derives from the crystalline lens and is usually against-the-rule.

ROSE BENGAL: A deep red dye used to stain devitalized (dead) epithelial cells in the cornea and bulbar conjunctiva.

SCHIRMER TEST: Diagnostic test to assess quantitatively the volume of tear flow using strip of absorptive filter paper placed in the outer temporal part of the lower fornix. Normal tears flow wets at least 15 mm in 5 minutes. A frequently quoted but unreliable procedure.

SCLERAL LENS: A contact lens which fits over both the cornea and bulbar conjunctiva. Typical overall sizes are 22–24 mm.

SEMI-SCLERAL (mini-scleral): A soft lens which extends beyond the limbus onto the bulbar conjunctiva. Typical overall sizes are 14.00–15.00 mm.

SILICON ACRYLATES (siloxanes): Hard lens copolymers with varying proportions of acrylate and silicon.

SOAKING SOLUTION: A solution designed to keep a contact lens in its functional condition when not in the eye.

SPECTACLE BLUR: Blurred vision with spectacles after wearing contact lenses because of oedema and corneal moulding. Mainly caused by PMMA but also encountered with hard gas-permeable and soft lenses.

SPIN CASTING: Method of soft lens manufacture employing liquid polymer spun to the required shape in rotating open moulds.

STABILIZATION: Used to ensure the correct orientation of a contact lens. Important in the fitting of torics and bifocals (*see* truncation and prism ballast).

STAINING: Usually refers to the uptake of *fluorescein by lesions in the corneal epithelium but applies to any of the commonly used tissue stains (*see* rose bengal).

STERILIZATION: The killing of all micro-organisms (*see* disinfection).

STRIAE: Vertical stress lines observed as folds in the corneal stroma, caused by hypoxia. Vogt striae of different origin are observed in keratoconus.

SURFACTANT: Agent that modifies the surface energy of a contact lens solution.

TEAR LAYER THICKNESS: The thickness of the layer of tears between the back surface of a contact lens and the front surface of the cornea. Usually expressed in microns.

THREE AND NINE O'CLOCK STAINING: Staining of the nasal and temporal areas of the peripheral cornea. Frequently associated with conjunctival injection in the horizontal meridian. Influenced by dry eyes, poor blinking, lens design and lens material.

TORIC LENS: Lens with all or part of at least one surface of toroidal construction (*see* back surface toric, front surface toric, bitoric, toric periphery).

TORIC PERIPHERY: Lens with one or more peripheral curves of toric construction.

TRANSITION: The junction between two adjacent curves on the surface of a contact lens; usually applied to the central radius (BOZR) and first peripheral radius. Transitions may be sharp or blended.

TRANSMISSIBILITY: *See* oxygen transmissibility.

TRICURVE: Lens design consisting of the central radius and two peripheral curves.

TRUNCATION: The shaping of a lens, normally with a straight edge, to assist with correct orientation on the eye in toric or bifocal fitting. Truncation may be single, usually at the base, or double, at top and bottom of the lens.

VASCULARIZATION: Superficial extension of blood vessels from the limbal arcades into the cornea.

WATER CONTENT: Volume of water (0.9% saline) absorbed by a hydrophilic lens, expressed as a percentage of the total weight of the fully hydrated lens.

WATER UPTAKE: Volume of water (0.9% saline) absorbed by a hydrophilic lens, expressed as a percentage of the weight of the lens prior to hydration.

WETTABILITY: A property of the contact lens surface as defined by the contact angle and measured under specified conditions.

WETTING SOLUTION: A solution used with hard lenses to improve the wettability of the lens surface.

XEROGEL: Hydrogel lens prior to hydration.

Appendix

Vertex conversion table

Spectacle lens power	Vertex distance (mm)							
	Plus lenses				Minus lenses			
	8	10	12	14	8	10	12	14
4.00	4.12	4.12	4.25	4.25	3.87	3.87	3.87	3.75
4.50	4.62	4.75	4.75	4.75	4.37	4.25	4.25	4.25
5.00	5.25	5.25	5.25	5.37	4.75	4.75	4.75	4.62
5.50	5.75	5.75	5.87	6.00	5.25	5.25	5.12	5.12
6.00	6.25	6.37	6.50	6.50	5.75	5.62	5.62	5.50
6.50	6.87	7.00	7.00	7.12	6.12	6.12	6.00	6.00
7.00	7.37	7.50	7.62	7.75	6.62	6.50	6.50	6.50
7.50	8.00	8.12	8.25	8.37	7.12	7.00	6.87	6.75
8.00	8.50	8.75	8.87	9.00	7.50	7.37	7.25	7.35
8.50	9.12	9.25	9.50	9.62	8.00	7.87	7.75	7.62
9.00	9.75	9.87	10.12	10.37	8.37	8.25	8.12	8.00
9.50	10.25	10.50	10.75	11.00	8.87	8.62	8.50	8.37
10.00	10.87	11.12	11.37	11.62	9.25	9.12	8.87	8.75
10.50	11.50	11.75	12.00	12.25	9.62	9.50	9.37	9.12
11.00	12.00	12.37	12.75	13.00	10.12	9.87	9.75	9.50
11.50	12.62	13.00	13.37	13.75	10.50	10.37	10.12	9.87
12.00	13.25	13.62	14.00	14.50	11.00	10.75	10.50	10.25
12.50	13.87	14.25	14.75	15.25	11.37	11.12	10.87	10.62
13.00	14.50	15.00	15.50	16.00	11.75	11.50	11.25	11.00
13.50	15.12	15.62	16.12	16.62	12.25	11.87	11.62	11.37
14.00	15.75	16.25	16.75	17.50	12.62	12.25	12.00	11.75
14.50	16.50	17.00	17.50	18.25	13.00	12.62	12.37	12.00
15.00	17.00	17.75	18.25	19.00	13.37	13.00	12.75	12.37
15.50	17.75	18.25	19.00	19.75	13.75	13.50	13.00	12.75
16.00	18.25	19.01	19.75	20.50	14.25	13.75	13.50	13.00
16.50	19.00	19.75	20.50	21.50	14.50	14.12	13.75	13.50
17.00	19.75	20.50	21.50	22.25	15.00	14.50	14.12	13.75
17.50	20.50	21.25	22.25	23.25	15.37	14.87	14.50	14.00
18.00	21.00	22.00	23.00	24.00	15.75	15.25	14.74	14.37
18.50	21.75	22.75	23.75	25.00	16.12	15.62	15.12	14.75
19.00	22.50	23.50	24.75	26.00	16.50	16.00	15.50	15.00

Dioptre to millimetre conversion table $n = 1.336$

36.00–9.37	40.12–8.41	44.25–7.63	48.37–6.98	52.50–6.43
36.12–9.34	40.25–8.38	44.37–7.61	48.50–6.96	52.62–6.41
36.25–9.31	40.37–8.36	44.50–7.58	48.62–6.94	52.75–6.40
36.37–9.27	40.50–8.33	44.62–7.56	48.75–6.92	52.87–6.38
36.50–9.24	40.62–8.30	44.75–7.54	48.87–6.91	53.00–6.36
36.62–9.21	40.75–8.28	44.87–7.52	49.00–6.89	53.12–6.35
36.75–9.18	40.87–8.25	45.00–7.50	49.12–6.87	53.25–6.34
36.87–9.15	41.00–8.23	45.12–7.48	49.25–6.85	53.37–6.32
37.00–9.12	41.12–8.20	45.25–7.46	49.37–6.84	53.50–6.31
37.12–9.09	41.25–8.18	45.37–7.44	49.50–6.82	53.62–6.29
37.25–9.06	41.37–8.16	45.50–7.42	49.62–6.80	53.75–6.28
37.37–9.03	41.50–8.13	45.62–7.40	49.75–6.78	53.87–6.26
37.50–9.00	41.62–8.10	45.75–7.38	49.87–6.77	54.00–6.25
37.62–8.97	41.75–8.08	45.87–7.36	50.00–6.75	54.12–6.23
37.75–8.94	41.87–8.06	46.00–7.34	50.12–6.73	54.25–6.22
37.87–8.91	42.00–8.03	46.12–7.32	50.25–6.72	54.37–6.21
38.00–8.88	42.12–8.01	46.25–7.30	50.37–6.70	54.50–6.19
38.12–8.85	42.25–7.99	46.37–7.28	50.50–6.68	54.62–6.18
38.25–8.82	42.37–7.96	46.50–7.26	50.62–6.67	54.75–6.16
38.37–8.79	42.50–7.94	46.62–7.24	50.75–6.65	54.87–6.15
38.50–8.76	42.62–7.92	46.75–7.22	50.87–6.63	55.00–6.13
38.62–8.73	42.75–7.89	46.87–7.20	51.00–6.62	55.12–6.12
38.75–8.70	42.87–7.87	47.00–7.18	51.12–6.60	55.25–6.10
38.87–8.68	43.00–7.85	47.12–7.16	51.25–6.58	55.37–6.09
39.00–8.65	43.12–7.82	47.25–7.14	51.37–6.57	55.50–6.08
39.12–8.62	43.25–7.80	47.37–7.12	51.50–6.55	55.62–6.07
39.25–8.59	43.37–7.78	47.50–7.10	51.62–6.54	55.75–6.05
39.37–8.57	43.50–7.76	47.62–7.08	51.75–6.52	55.87–6.04
39.50–8.54	43.62–7.74	47.75–7.06	51.87–6.50	56.00–6.03
39.62–8.51	43.75–7.71	47.87–7.05	52.00–6.49	
39.75–8.49	43.87–7.69	48.00–7.03	52.12–6.47	
39.87–8.46	44.00–7.67	48.12–7.01	52.25–6.46	
40.00–8.43	44.12–7.65	48.25–6.99	52.37–6.44	

Index

QUASAR® 205
AND *Boston® XO*

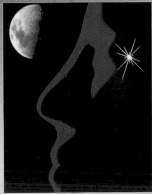
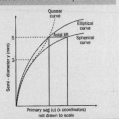
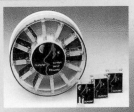

Subscribe to
Optician

And receive your own personal copy every week

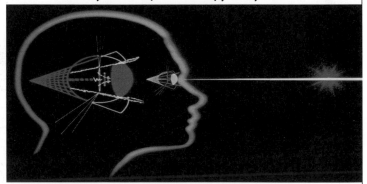

- exclusive news coverage
- latest job vacancies
- fashion trends
- approved continuing education
- clinical and technical features

- business management information AND a range of supplements throughout the year:
  - eyestyle
  - eyecontact
  - optical technician
  - recruitment
  - optical yearbook
  - wallplanner

For current subscription rates simply telephone 01444 475634 or fax 01444 445447 Quote code 124.

Or fill in the coupon below and return it to: Optician Subscriptions, FREEPOST RCC2619, HAYWARDS HEATH, RH16 3BR (please affix stamp if posted outside the UK)

Optician

☐ **Please send me the current subscription rates for Optician**

| Title | Initial | Surname |

Job title

Address ☐ home ☐ practice

Postcode   Telephone   Code 124

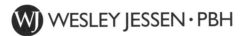

Instructions for the CD-ROM

System requirements

IBM PC or compatible, 486 DX or higher, running Windows 3.1 or Windows 95, with 16 MB RAM, 10 MB of hard disk free, 16 colour monitor with a screen resolution set to 800 × 600 or higher, and a CD-ROM drive.

To install and use the CD-ROM

In Windows Program Manager, choose Run from the File menu (the Start menu in Windows 95), type in d;\setup.exe (where d is the CD-ROM drive) and press Enter. Follow the on-screen instructions.

These programs have been designed with ease-of-use in mind so that you should find all the information you need to make them work on the screen. The procedures to which they relate are described in the book.

You will find that you can move between text entry boxes by using the Tab key. To move backwards, use Shift+Tab. Otherwise use the mouse to position the cursor in the correct box. Boxes which have up and down arrows beside them (the arrows are called Spin buttons) can be controlled either by clicking on the arrows with the mouse or by holding down the Ctrl key and pressing the up and down arrow keys. You may find that you need to type in a figure instead of using the spin buttons; for instance if you want to set the displayed value to zero in certain cases. Once all the necessary data have been entered, you can press Tab once more to highlight the Calculate button. If you then press the Enter key, the calculation will be performed.

If you receive an error message when you press Calculate, check the values that you have set to make sure that they fall within the allowable range. If you are unsure about any of the values, refer to the relevant chapter in the book.

From the main menu you can select:

- Examples
- Gallery
- Tools
- Comparative fluorescein
- Soft torics

Examples

To create a colour version of the black and white illustrations in the book, select the figures from the drop down list, e.g. Figure 9.4 Average periphery. Then click on Draw the selected examples. Having done that the values for the cornea/lens specification can be amended and redrawn either by clicking:

A   Draw spherical Rx
B   Draw Quasar
C   Draw Asphericon

Gallery

From the gallery menu a red cross next to the chapter number indicates that there are colour illustrations to view. Click on the cross to expand the menu and then click on the caption to view a thumbnail picture. Click on View this slide to view the full size picture and accompanying text.

Tools

The tools menu provides a number of useful calculation functions related to contact lens practice.

Comparative fluorescein

The comparative fluorescein enables side-by-side comparisons of the fluorescein patterns for spherical Rx, toric Rx, Quasar and Asphericon lens geometries. To use, select Option under Lens then click on Lens Rx and specify details of the lens geometry. Always click Apply to make sure that the specified geometry will be used. This is very important. In the Cornea specify appropriate values and then click on Draw to generate the simulation. In

Mode, the Continuous provides 'realistic' simulations and Discrete causes the simulations to generate five micron banding. This will show you a detailed analysis of the lens/cornea relationship.

Soft torics

This has two components: LARS axis adjustment and Mislocation.

LARS AXIS ADJUSTMENT

This is intended to specify the axis direction based on the observed mislocation of a diagnostic lens. To use the lens on the graphic display, either click and drag or use the spin control at the base of the picture. (Positive numbers indicate anticlockwise rotation and negative numbers indicate clockwise rotation.) Remember to specify the ocular Rx rather than the spectacle Rx; if necessary use the calculator provided in Tools to obtain the ocular Rx.

MISLOCATION

Refer to the step-by-step instructions in the book. Chapter 23 pages 255 and 256.

There is no technical support available for this product. If you experience any problems, please make sure that your system meets the requirements detailed above and that you have followed the installation procedure correctly. If problems persist, then in the first instance write to the publishers at:

Butterworth-Heinemann, Linacre House, Jordan Hill, Oxford OX2 8DP, UK.